Sheila

MANUAL OF SMALL ANIMAL ENDOCRINOLOGY

Edited by
Maureen Hutchison
BSc BVMS MRCVS

Published by the
British Small Animal
Veterinary Association,
Kingsley House, Church Lane,
Shurdington, Cheltenham,
Gloucestershire GL51 5TQ.

Printed by Grafos S.A.,
Barcelona, Spain.

The publishers cannot take any responsibility
for information provided on dosages and methods
of application of drugs mentioned in this publication.
Details of this kind must be verified by individual users
in the appropriate literature.

First published 1990
Reprinted 1993

ISBN 0 905214 13 7

CONTENTS

PART ONE

Chapter One

A. David J. Watson

Chapter Two

Keith L. Thoday

Chapter Three

John K. Dunn

Chapter Four

Michael E. Herrtage

Chapter Five

Elspeth M. Milne

Chapter Six

W. Edward Allen and Gary C. W. England

Chapter Seven

W. Edward Allen and Gary C. W. England

Chapter Eight

Tim J. Gruffydd-Jones

CONTENTS

4

ACKNOWLEDGEMENTS

This new addition to the BSAVA Manual range has posed an enormous challenge to both the editor and authors. To fulfil our brief of producing a concise, easy-reference publication which none the less contains the most up-to-date information on such a complex and ever-expanding subject as endocrinology was no easy task! It would not have been possible at all without the co-operation of those contributors who generously gave of their time in cutting or re-drafting their manuscripts in order to produce a uniform overall format.

I would also like to thank Colin Price and David Parkes, who read and commented on some of the manuscripts; Michael Herrtage for his advice and for the copy used on the front cover; Caroline Sheard, who prepared the index and Michael Gorton Design for the lay-out and graphics. Finally, the book would never have reached full-term without the unswerving support of Simon Orr, Chairman of BSAVA Publications Committee.

Whether we have achieved our aim is for you, the reader, to decide.

Maureen Hutchison

FOREWORD

This book is another addition to the BSAVA Manual series. Designed to be easily read and followed by the busy practitioner, convenient enough to be referred to during a consultation, the Manual of Small Animal Endocrinology is no exception. Like many other areas, endocrinology has advanced rapidly over the last decade. Methods of confirming or aiding diagnosis have improved and are now, for the most part, readily available — though not yet in the practice laboratory.

This is a book with a difference. It is divided into three parts. The first part is conventional enough. There is a chapter on each endocrine gland. The anatomy and physiology are briefly covered and then the methods of diagnosis and treatment of conditions affecting the particular gland are fully discussed. The way the Manual is written ensures that this information is as recent as possible.

It is in the second part that this Manual deviates from most standard publications. Here there are four chapters covering typical presenting conditions that are relatively common in general practice but require detailed diagnosis and treatment. It is probably this part that the practitioner is likely to find most beneficial as one is guided through the labyrinth of differential diagnosis distinguishing between endocrinological and other disorders.

The third, the smallest part of the book, tidies up a few loose ends. This, together with the table of normal serum hormone levels of the dog and cat, completes the Manual of Endocrinology. The authors have followed their brief well. The length and format enable the Manual to be easily read with more than sufficient information available for the diagnosis and treatment of endocrinopathies in general practice. It also contains sufficient references to direct those readers who want to explore the subject in greater depth.

W. A. BRADLEY, B.V.Sc., M.R.C.V.S.

President, 1989-90

CHAPTER 1

THE PITUITARY GLAND

A. D. J. Watson B.V.Sc., Ph.D., F.R.C.V.S., F.A.A.V.P.T., M.A.C.V.Sc.

ANATOMY AND HISTOLOGY

The pituitary gland or hypophysis is a small ovoid structure which lies in a distinct fossa (the sella turcica) within the sphenoid bone ventral to the hypothalamus. The gland comprises tissues of two separate origins. The adenohypophysis (commonly termed the anterior lobe, but mostly located ventrally in dogs and cats) begins as a dorsal evagination (Rathke's pouch) from the oral cavity. It migrates upwards to partly surround the neurohypophysis, or posterior lobe, which protrudes ventrally from the hypothalamus and remains connected to it by the pituitary stalk. Part of the adenohypophysis, the intermediate lobe, fuses with the neurohypophysis and remains separated from the rest of the adenohypophysis by the hypophyseal, or Rathke's, cleft (Figure 1).

The adenohypophysis contains various types of endocrine cells (corticotrophs, thyrotrophs, gonadotrophs, somatotrophs, lactotrophs, melanotrophs) that secrete the pituitary trophic hormones. These cells are arranged in cords separated by an abundant capillary network. The neurohypophysis lacks secreting cells but contains special microglial cells and nerve fibres extending from several hypothalamic nuclei.

The hypothalamus, located dorsal to the pituitary, contains various structures important for regulation of adenohypophyseal and neurohypophyseal function. In addition, certain hypophyseal regions are involved in regulation of basic homeostatic mechanisms, including body temperature, thirst, eating, emotional responses, wakefulness and sympathetic responses (Figure 1).

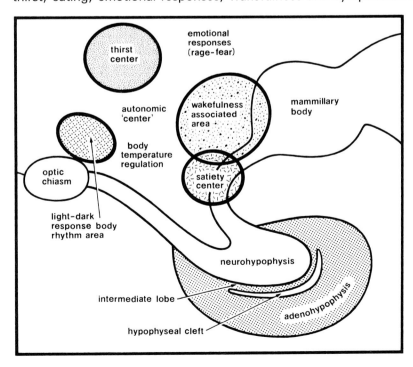

Figure 1

The canine pituitary gland and adjacent hypothalamic structures.
(Modified from Chastain and Ganjam 1986, with permission).

PITUITARY HORMONES

With increasing knowledge, it has become apparent that complex interactions exist between the various hormone arcs involving the adenohypophysis, and also between adenohypophyseal and neurohypophyseal mechanisms. None of these systems functions in isolation and all are influenced by other endocrine and non-endocrine factors. However, for the sake of simplicity, each hormone axis is considered here largely as a separate system. For more detailed information, the reader is referred to Williams (1981), Chastain and Ganjam (1986) and Feldman and Nelson (1987).

NEUROHYPOPHYSEAL HORMONES

Oxytocin and vasopressin are structurally related hormones produced by paraventricular and supraoptic nuclei in the hypothalamus. They are transported along axons in the pituitary stalk to the neurohypophysis and released from there into the general circulation (Figure 2).

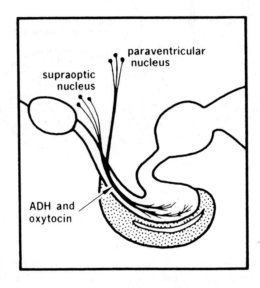

Figure 2
Hormone transport to the neurohypophysis.
ADH = vasopressin.
(From Chastain and Ganjam 1986, with permission).

Oxytocin

Suckling initiates release of oxytocin, which causes ejection of milk through contraction of myoepithelial cells within mammae. Oxytocin also promotes contraction of uterine smooth muscle.

Vasopressin (Antidiuretic Hormone, ADH)

Vasopressin secretion is controlled mainly by alterations in plasma osmolality, which are detected by osmoreceptors in the hypothalamus. Other controlling influences are changes in effective blood volume or blood pressure, detected by sensors in the cardiac atria and major vessels. Vasopressin modifies the permeability to water of cells in the distal convoluted tubules and collecting ducts of the kidneys. In the presence of vasopressin the cells are permeable and water can be resorbed. Without vasopressin activity, urine is dilute and voluminous.

ADENOHYPOPHYSEAL HORMONES

The activity of each endocrine cell type in the adenohypophysis is controlled by a corresponding releasing hormone from the hypothalamus. The releasing hormones are synthesized in neurones, transported in axons to the median eminence, then carried by capillaries to the adenohypophysis (Figure 3). Here they cause cells of the appropriate type to secrete preformed hormone into the systemic circulation.

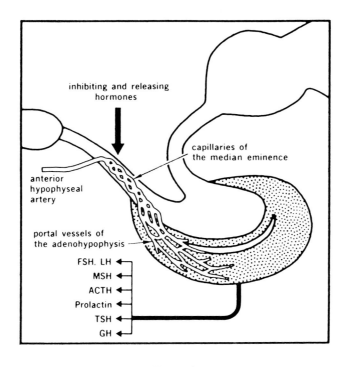

Figure 3
Transport of hypothalamic control hormones for the adenohypophysis.
FSH = follicle stimulating hormone, LH = luteinising hormone, MSH = melanocyte stimulating hormone,
ACTH = adrenocorticotrophic hormone, TSH = thyroid stimulating hormone, GH = growth hormone.
(From Chastain and Ganjam 1986, with permission).

In the adrenal, thyroid and gonadal systems, the pituitary hormone acts on the relevant target organ to stimulate production of another hormone; this in turn exerts an inhibitory feedback effect on synthesis of the specific hypothalamic releasing hormone. In contrast, growth hormone, prolactin and melanocyte stimulating hormone do not act through control of a target gland; inhibitory control of these hormones is achieved by production of a corresponding release-inhibiting hormone from the hypothalamus.

Adrenocorticotrophic Hormone (Corticotrophin, ACTH)

ACTH release from the pituitary is governed by corticotrophin releasing hormone (CRH) secreted by the hypothalamus.

ACTH stimulates glucocorticoid secretion by adrenocortical cells, the principal glucocorticoid in cats and dogs being cortisol (hydrocortisone). Cortisol secretion is subject to small and inconsistent fluctuations throughout the day in domestic pets, with highest concentrations in the early morning in dogs, and possibly in the evening in cats. High cortisol concentrations exert negative feedback at both hypothalamic (CRH) and pituitary (ACTH) level.

Thyroid Stimulating Hormone (Thyrotrophin, TSH)

The synthesis and release of thyroid hormones are controlled directly by TSH and indirectly by TRH. Normal values for these hormones are not known in dogs and cats. Secretion of thyroid hormones does not exhibit diurnal fluctuation in dogs and cats, but sporadic and unpredictable fluctuations occur in the basal level in dogs. Thyroid hormones exert a negative feedback mainly at pituitary level.

Follicle stimulating hormone (FSH) and luteinising hormone (LH)

A single gonadotrophin-releasing hormone (GnRH) controls release of both gonadotrophins (FSH and LH) from the adenohypophysis. The secretion of GnRH from the pituitary is affected by diurnal and seasonal factors which vary with the species. In females, FSH stimulates ovarian follicle growth (and thus oestrogen production), while LH stimulates ovulation and the formation and maintenance of the corpus luteum (and thus influences progesterone production). In males, FSH promotes spermatogenesis and LH stimulates testosterone secretion by interstitial cells of the testes. The sex steroids exert feedback inhibition on gonadotrophin secretion at both hypothalamic and pituitary levels. The complexities of hormonal regulation of reproduction are discussed in detail elsewhere in this manual (See Chapters 6, 7 and 8).

Growth hormone (Somatotrophin, GH)

GH secretion from the adenohypophysis is under dual control by GH-releasing hormone and GH-inhibiting hormone (somatostatin). Plasma GH concentrations normally show wide fluctuations, with brief surges of secretion occurring irregularly during a 24 hour period. GH has two opposing actions on many target tissues. There is an indirect growth-promoting or anabolic effect on bones and other tissues, which is mediated through somatomedin C produced mainly in the liver. There is also a direct insulin-antagonising, catabolic effect leading to lipolysis, hyperglycaemia and insulin resistance. Negative feedback control is effected by GH and somatomedin C on the hypothalamus and by somatomedin C on the pituitary. The importance of GH during growth is well understood but its physiological role in the adult remains unclear, even though GH secretion continues in later life.

Prolactin

Prolactin is similar in structure to GH and functions in the initiation and maintenance of lactation. Prolactin release is controlled by releasing hormone(s) and inhibitors (including dopamine) from the hypothalamus.

Melanocyte stimulating hormone (Melanotrophin, MSH)

Several forms of MSH are produced in the adenohypophysis, mainly the intermediate lobe. Factors controlling MSH release are not well described. MSH stimulates melanin synthesis by melanocytes.

PITUITARY-RELATED DISORDERS

Primary endocrine disorders with abnormal secretion of oxytocin, prolactin or melanocyte stimulating hormone are not recognised at present in small animals. A possible exception is pseudopregnancy, in which excess prolactin production might be implicated (see page 137).

PITUITARY TUMOURS

Signs

While various cell types can be involved in pituitary neoplasms, they produce clinical disease in three main ways.

1. A non-functional tumour can compromise adjacent pituitary and hypothalamic structures, causing insufficiency of one or more hormones and consequent signs.

2. An endocrinologically-active tumour may produce sufficient hormone (eg. ACTH) to cause a characteristic syndrome (eg. hyperadrenocorticism).

3. The tumour may compress or invade adjacent brain structures and produce predominantly neurological signs, such as central blindness (compression of optic chiasm or optic tracts), depression, somnolence, behavioural changes and disorders of thirst, appetite and temperature regulation.

Various combinations of central neurological signs and hormonal excesses or deficiencies, as described below, are possible (Figure 4).

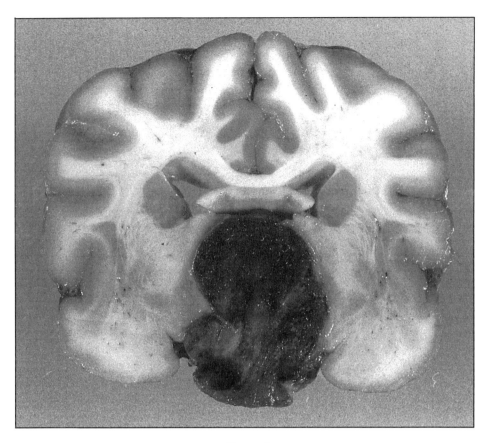

Figure 4

Cross section of brain of dog with neurological and endocrine abnormalities caused by an expanding pituitary tumour (chromophobe adenoma). The tumour secreted ACTH and produced pituitary dependent hyperadrenocorticism. Other hormonal deficits identified were hypothyroidism, deficiencies of follicle stimulating hormone and luteinising hormone, and impaired growth hormone secretion. The dog had shown behavioural change, mental depression and somnolence.

(From Allison et al 1983, with permission).

Diagnosis and Treatment

When pituitary neoplasia is suspected, hormonal function tests, selected on the basis of the signs shown, may aid diagnosis. Oedema of the optic disc and/or abnormal cerebrospinal fluid (increased pressure, cell count, protein content) are evident in some cases. Skull radiographs are usually unhelpful, as canine pituitary tumours tend to extend dorsally and rarely erode the sphenoid bone. Treatment is usually not feasible, although hypophysectomy or irradiation may be considered in specialist referral centres.

PANHYPOPITUITARISM

Panhypopituitarism denotes a deficiency of many of the adenohypophyseal hormones. Possible causes are congenital anomalies, neoplasms (pituitary adenoma or carcinoma, craniopharyngioma, metastases) and traumatic, inflammatory, vascular or degenerative lesions in the pituitary-hypothalamic region. Pituitary dwarfism in German shepherd dogs is often a form of panhypopituitarism.

Multiple endocrine abnormalities are usually present, but in various combinations. Clinical abnormalities vary accordingly. The sequence of insufficiency expected with increasingly extensive destruction of the adenohypophysis is GH, FSH-LH, TSH, ACTH. However, signs of GH deficiency may be inapparent in adults. If secondary hypogonadism, hypothyroidism or hypoadrenocorticism occur (due to lack of FSH-LH, TSH or ACTH respectively), signs are generally less severe than occur in primary dysfunction. Additional signs of vasopressin deficiency can be expected if the underlying lesion also damages the neurohypophyseal-hypothalamic area. Likewise, neurological signs may be present if adjacent brain structures are compromised.

13

CENTRAL OR NEUROGENIC DIABETES INSIPIDUS (CDI)

This syndrome results from an impairment of vasopressin production or release, which can be partial or complete. It is manifested by impaired renal water conservation, with consequent polyuria and compensatory polydipsia and is diagnosed more often in dogs than in cats. It occurs mostly as an acquired abnormality but is seen occasionally as a congenital defect in young animals. In most instances CDI is idiopathic and permanent. Other cases follow damage to the hypothalamus or neurohypophysis by head trauma, neoplasia, other space-occupying masses, infarcts and inflammatory lesions. The resulting central diabetes insipidus can be transient if the lesion resolves or the hypothalamus and proximal pituitary stalk are undamaged.

Signs and Findings

Affected individuals show excessive thirst and pass increased volumes of water-clear urine. The degree of polydipsia is variable depending on the extent of vasopressin lack and other factors, but typically exceeds 100 ml/kg/day. In extreme cases water-seeking behaviour may be bizarre, and regurgitation or vomiting can occur from gastric overload. Polyuria may cause some previously well house-trained animals to urinate indoors, especially at night, and exacerbate marginal or subclinical incontinence problems. Animals with idiopathic CDI show no other signs unless water intake is restricted, whereupon severe dehydration, coma and death may ensue. When caused by a tumour or other destructive lesion, additional hormonal defects or neurological signs may be present.

Diagnosis

The differentation of polyuria is discussed in more detail in Chapter 9. Central diabetes insipidus can be distinguished from possible alternative conditions by signs and abnormal results to laboratory tests.

Diabetes mellitus is suggested by the combination of polydipsia and polyuria with polyphagia, weight loss, hepatomegaly, glycosuria and hyperglycaemia.

Hyperadrenocorticism is likely if polydipsia and polyuria are accompanied by polyhagia, symmetrical alopecia, abdominal enlargement and hepatomegaly, especially if increased plasma alkaline phosphatase activity, eosinopenia and lymphocytopenia are present.

Renal failure should be considered if urine is inappropriately dilute (specific gravity < 1.030 in the dog, < 1.035 in the cat) in the presence of dehydration and/or azotaemia.

In bitches with pyometra, polyuria and polydipsia may be associated with depression, inappetence, vomiting, vulval discharge, uterine enlargement and leukocytosis. Pyometra occurs in metoestrus or in progestagen-treated individuals.

Patients with central diabetes insipidus typically have urine specific gravity below 1.007. However, similarly dilute urine may be found in renal diabetes insipidus, psychogenic polydipsia and normal animals.

Confirmation of diagnosis

1. Negative response to a Water Deprivation Test.
2. Positive response to vasopressin administration.

Several different protocols are available (see Chapter 9). Dogs with partial central diabetes insipidus and hyperadrenocorticism may show a subnormal increase in urine concentration when deprived of water; hyperadrenocorticism must then be excluded by other means. Diagnosis of central diabetes insipidus may be facilitated in the future by testing procedures which incorporate vasopressin assays (Biewenga *et al,* 1987), but these are not yet generally available.

Treatment

This is unlikely to be considered when central diabetes insipidus is a manifestation of a wider pituitary-hypothalamic dysfunction — as with an expanding tumour.

It is unecessary if the owner can tolerate the signs and access to water is reliable.

Synthetic vasopressin analogues can be used but are expensive. Ideally, treatment should be repeated only once mild polyuria and polydipsia recur, so that excessive water retention from over-dosing does not occur.

Desmopressin acetate (DDAVP, Ferring) is the most convenient form of therapy. It is administered as drops into the conjunctival sac: 2 to 4 drops twice daily is suggested initially. The dose should be adjusted according to individual response.

Vasopressin (Pitressin tannate in oil, Parke-Davis) may also be used, but is not readily obtainable in the United Kingdom. It is injected intra-muscularly at a dose rate of 1.25—5.00 units per animal, every 1 to 3 days as required. Adequate mixing and warming of the ampoule are important.

Chlorpropamide (Diabinese, Pfizer) may be used in partial central diabetes insipidus, as it sensitises the renal tubules to the action of residual vasopressin. Suggested doses are 10—40 mg/kg for dogs and 50 mg per cat. One or two weeks treatment may be needed before response occurs. The drug also stimulates insulin secretion, so regular feeding is advisable to prevent hypoglycaemia.

Thiazide diuretics can reduce paradoxically the urine volume by up to 50% in human central and nephrogenic diabetes insipidus, but results in animals have been variable. Hydrochlorthiazide (Direma, Elanco; Vetidrex, Ciba-Geigy) 2—4 mg/kg twice daily is suggested, together with a low sodium diet and potassium supplement. This is worth trying as it is a very much cheaper form of treatment than desmopressin.

EXCESSIVE VASOPRESSIN SECRETION

A syndrome of inappropriate excessive vasopressin secretion occurs in humans, as a rare primary idiopathic abnormality, or, more often, secondary to vascular, infectious or neoplastic disorders affecting lung or central nervous system, or following administration of some drugs.

Excessive water retention occurs, leading to hypo-osmolality of plasma and hyponatraemia. Hyponatraemia is due to the dilutional effects of retained water together with continuing urinary sodium losses. The natriuresis persists because aldosterone secretion is inhibited by hypervolaemia. Peripheral oedema is not a feature.

Mild cases can be managed by restricting water intake, but more severe cases may require drug therapy to inhibit the secretion or action of vasopressin.

The syndrome has been reported in a few dogs (Rijnberg et al, 1988). Two cases exhibited polyuria, polydipsia and episodes of neurological dysfunction (restlessness, unsteadiness, disorientation and screaming in one, ataxia and seizures in the other). In both cases the disorder was idiopathic. Another case was associated with a tumour in the thalamic-hypothalamic region (Houston et al, 1989).

ACROMEGALY

Acromegaly is a chronic disorder characterised by overgrowth of soft tissue and bone due to persistent growth hormone excess. The disease in man is usually caused by a pituitary tumour. A similar cause has been implicated in the few feline acromegalics identified (Feldman and Nelson, 1987). In bitches, acromegaly is induced in some individuals by progestagens (Eigenmann 1984, 1986). The site of growth hormone overproduction in acromegalic dogs is unknown but might involve pituitary, pancreas or other tissues. As growth hormone is diabetogenic in dogs and cats, mild glucose intolerance or overt diabetes mellitus may also occur.

Signs and Findings

Dogs with acromegaly are usually female, reflecting the role of progestational agents in the aetiology. A common finding is inspiratory stridor caused by excessive soft tissue formation in the tongue and around the mouth, pharynx and larynx. Panting, exercise intolerance and fatigue are likely. Other abnormalities are thickened skin with excessive folds (especially of head, neck and distal limbs), enlargement of the head, abdomen, limbs, paws and interdental spaces (Figures 5 and 6). Polyuria and polydipsia may occur if there is overt glucose intolerance. Findings in cats are similar (Figures 7 and 8) with the possibility of additional hormonal defects and neurological signs from a pituitary-hypothalamic mass.

Diagnosis

Canine cases may be recognised from the history and appearance. Feline cases may be more difficult. Acromegaly should be considered in both species if unusually high insulin dosage is required to control diabetes mellitus. Routine laboratory tests are non-contributory except for changes indicating glucose intolerance (ie. glycosuria, hyperglycaemia, abnormal glucose tolerance test results). Other non-specific abnormalities are mild hyperphosphataemia and increased plasma alkaline phosphatase and alanine aminotransferase (GPT) activity.

Diagnostic proof requires demonstration of persistent increases in plasma growth hormone or somatomedin C concentrations, but these assays are not currently available to practitioners in most countries.

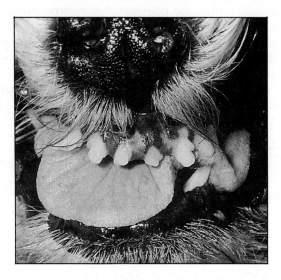

Figure 5
Mouth of acromegalic Dandie Dinmont, showing enlarged interdental spaces and tongue.
Acromegaly developed spontaneously in this dog, induced by persistent high plasma progesterone concentrations derived from functional ovarian tissue remaining after 'ovariectomy'.
(Courtesy of A. Rijnberk, Utrecht University).

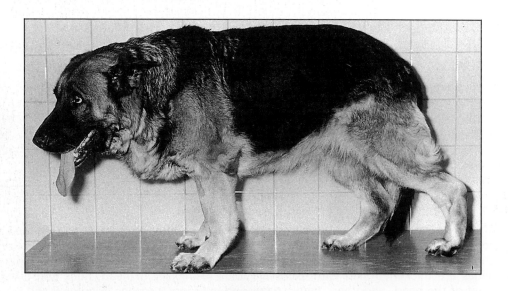

Figure 6
German shepherd bitch in which acromegaly occurred after repeated administration of progestagen for four years to prevent reproduction. Note heavy, thick appearance (compare with normal adult German shepherd in Figure 10), skinfolds around head and neck, large tongue and panting.
(Courtesy of A. Rijnberk, Utrecht University).

Treatment

Acromegaly induced by progestational agents in bitches is treatable by withdrawal of the drug or ovario-hysterectomy, depending on the cause. Growth hormone concentration falls rapidly after surgery and soft tissue changes regress in a few months. In drug-induced cases the process takes longer. If moderate hyperglycaemia (>10−12 mmol/l) persists, insulin administration should be considered to prevent complete β-cell exhaustion. However, care is needed because insulin requirement may decrease unpredictably as the effects of progestagen disappear. Some animals remain diabetic because of β cell exhaustion and persistent hypoinsulinaemia.

Information on the treatment of acromegalic cats is sparse. Medical treatments used in human cases (bromocriptine, somatostatin octapeptide) have not been effective in cats. The options of hypo-physectomy or pituitary irradiation might be considered in referral centres. Otherwise, prognosis is reasonable in the short term, with reported survivals of 8 to 30 months. Death or euthanasia is likely because of expansion of the pituitary tumour or development of congestive heart failure. In the meantime, high insulin doses may be needed and possibly treatment for heart failure.

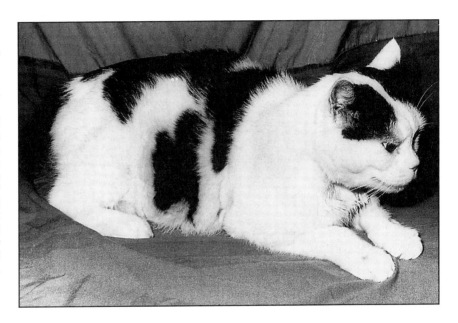

Figure 7
Acromegalic cat, aged 12 years. The cat had poorly controlled diabetes mellitus. Thick, coarse facial features, large body size and excessive skin folds were evident (compare with Figure 8). Acromegaly was confirmed by findings of persistently increased plasma somatomedin C concentrations and presence of a pituitary tumour on computed tomographic scanning.

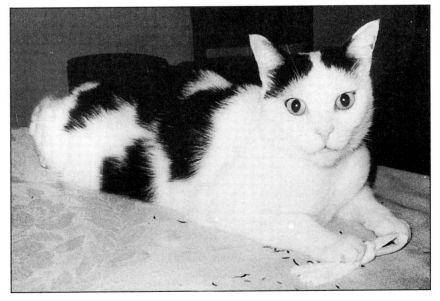

Figure 8
The same cat as in Figure 7 but 2.5 years earlier, showing normal conformation at that time.

PITUITARY DWARFISM

Dwarfism resulting from inadequate GH activity during the normal growth phase has been described often in dogs and occasionally in cats. A number of dog breeds have been affected but the prime example is the German shepherd dog (Allen *et al*, 1978) in which the disorder is inherited in autosomal recessive fashion. A cystic adenohypophysis was found in most of the affected German shepherds autopsied but pituitary structure was normal in a few. Although the clinical picture is dominated by the consequences of GH deficiency, other adenohypophyseal hormones may be diminished as well, causing various degrees of secondary hypothyroidism, hypoadrenocorticism and hypogonadism.

Signs and Findings

Abnormalities are evident usually from two or three months of age. Affected animals grow more slowly than their littermates and may need supplementary feeding from an early age to survive. Although of short stature, they retain near normal body proportions (Figure 9). They fail to develop a normal adult hair coat and soft puppy hairs are retained. Alopecia, hyperpigmentation and thinning of the skin ensue (Figure 10). Accompanying abnormalities include behavioural problems (aggression, fear biting), delayed dental eruption, short mandible, cardiac disorders, cryptorchidism, megaoesophagus and testicular atrophy or oestral abnormalities.

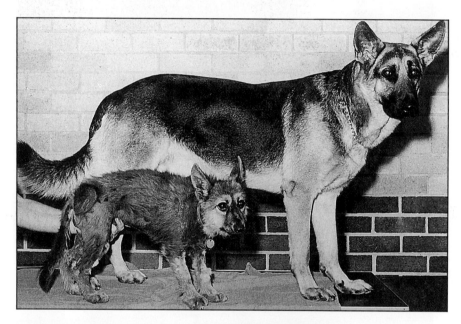

Figure 9
German shepherd dwarf
18 months old and normal
15 months old bitch for
comparison.
*(From Allan et al, 1978,
with permission).*

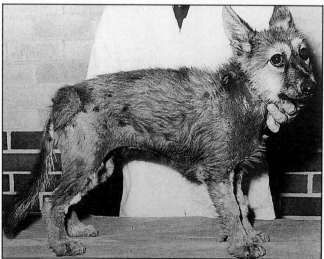

Figure 10
German shepherd dwarf shown in Figure 9.
Note alopecia and hyperpigmentation of neck
and flank, alopecia of thigh, and the persisting
puppy hair coat with a patch of primary guard
hair development over right hip.
(From Allan et al, 1978, with permission).

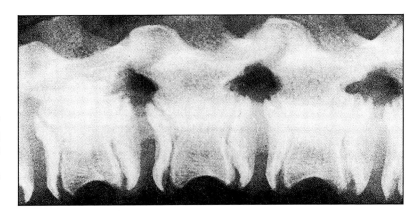

Figure 11
Spinal radiograph of dwarf
German shepherd showing
abnormal vertebral growth
plates.
*(From Allan et al, 1978, with
permission).*

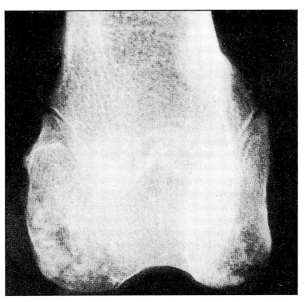

Figure 12
Post-mortem radiograph of distal femur of a
German shepherd with pituitary dwarfism,
showing disordered and incomplete calcification
(epiphyseal dysgenesis) suggesting concurrent
hypothyroidism.
(From Allan et al, 1978).

Skeletal radiographs may show delayed closure of growth plates in vertebrae and limbs (Figure 11). Epiphyses may have a 'moth-eaten', under-developed appearance which results from disordered and incomplete calcification (epiphyseal dysgenesis) and could suggest concurrent hypothyroidism (Figure 12).

Diagnosis

While the combination of proportional dwarfism and coat abnormalities is suggestive, other causes of poor growth may need to be excluded (Table 1).

Table 1
Some possible causes of small stature in dogs and cats*

Endocrine	Non-endocrine
Growth hormone deficiency	Poor diet
Hypothyroidism	Malassimilation
Hypoadrenocorticism	Portosystemic shunt
Hyperadrenocorticism	Glycogen storage disease
Diabetes mellitus	Cardiovascular defects
	Skeletal dysplasia
	Mucopolysaccharidosis

Modified from Feldman and Nelson, 1987

Growth hormone deficiency produces abnormalities and decreased elastin content of skin. A skin biopsy may be stained with Verhoef-van Gieson's stain to demonstrate elastin fibres.

Secondary thyroid or adrenal insufficiency may co-exist with growth hormone deficiency. To distinguish these conditions from primary deficits TSH and ACTH stimulation tests may be carried out.

Congenital hypothyroidism (cretinism) also causes stunting, but unlike growth hormone deficiency, body structures are disproportionate (i.e. short-broad skull, thick protruding tongue, short limbs and squarish trunk). As in growth hormone deficiency, the puppy coat is retained. However, in contrast, there is marked mental dullness and decreased activity. Goitre may or may not be present. These changes usually become apparent at three to eight weeks of age.

Definitive diagnosis in the live animal ideally requires demonstration of subnormal growth hormone levels by radioimmunoassay. The normal range for canine growth hormone (0-4 ng/ml) is at the limit of sensitivity of the assay. Therefore either clonidine or xylazine stimulation tests are carried out. Both these substances cause a short-lived rise in growth hormone levels in the normal dog.

Clonidine/xylazine stimulation test

10—30 µg/kg of clonidine or 100—300 µg/kg of xylazine are administered intravenously. After 15 minutes, a blood sample is taken for radioimmunoassay. Growth hormone levels in the normal dog will be in the order of 50-70 ng/ml at this time — returning to base-line within one hour. Rises are minimal in the pituitary dwarf.

Abnormally low somatomedin C concentrations are found concurrently. However, neither growth hormone nor somatomedin C assays are generally available in the United Kingdom. If a hospital or research laboratory was willing to carry them out, a number of control samples should be simultaneously processed to ensure the validity of the result.

Treatment

Bovine and porcine growth hormone may be administered (Scott and Walton, 1986) but at date of publication (1990) are very expensive and almost impossible to obtain in most countries. With treatment (see regime for growth hormone-responsive dermatosis on page 21), skin and hair usually improve within six-eight weeks, but growth may be limited because growth plates tend to close rapidly. In addition to GH, or as an alternative, replacement therapy with thyroid hormone, glucocorticoid or both should be considered, if these are deficient. Long term prognosis is reported to be poor, with most patients dying by three-eight years of age despite therapy.

GROWTH HORMONE RESPONSIVE DERMATOSIS

An endocrine pattern of alopecia which responds to growth hormone administration has been recognised in dogs. Although affected individuals have impaired ability to secrete growth hormone in response to the clonidine and xylazine stimulation tests, the cause of this defect and its relationship to the dermatosis is uncertain. The underlying abnormality could involve the pituitary, hypothalamus or other tissues. Few affected dogs have been examined post-mortem: the pituitary was normal in one of these cases and 'moderate atrophy' was found in another. The report of two affected Airedale terrier litter-mates suggests genetic factors may be involved in the aetiology.

Clinical findings

Pomeranians, chow chows, keeshonds and perhaps poodles are predisposed; males are affected more often than females. The onset is usually at one to three years of age, but may be later. There is symmetrical alopecia and hyperpigmentation of the trunk, neck, tail, caudal pinnae and proximal limbs (see Figure 13). Hair in these regions is easily epilated. The skin becomes thin, hypotonic and scaly in time. Affected animals are otherwise normal.

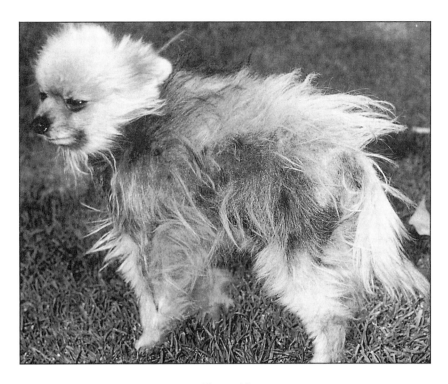

Figure 13

A three year old male Pomeranian with presumed GH-responsive dermatosis. Note alopecia affecting trunk and proximal limbs and hyperpigmentation. TSH response, ACTH response and dexamethasone suppression tests gave normal results. The testes were normal on palpation. Dermatohistopathology was compatible with GH deficiency, but GH production and response to GH therapy were not assessed in this case.

Diagnosis

The diagnosis is made by exclusion. The presence of clinical findings and laboratory abnormalities is used to rule out alternative causes of alopecia and hyperpigmentation (see Chapter 10). Growth hormone assays could provide confirmation if they were available but basal levels are not diagnostic and demonstration of a subnormal response to a clonidine or xylazine stimulation test would be required (Scott and Walton, 1986).

Responses to ACTH and TSH should be assessed in these patients as well because both hyperadrenocorticism and hypothyroidism impair growth hormone secretory capacity. Such detailed hormonal evaluation is impractical in most cases. Skin biopsy may be helpful. Decreased dermal elastin occurs in 40% of cases (Scott and Walton, 1986), although microscopic skin changes otherwise resemble those in many other endocrinopathies.

Treatment

At present growth hormone preparations are expensive and difficult to obtain. As untreated cases are otherwise well, the problem is an aesthetic one which informed owners may accept. However, trials have shown that affected dogs respond well to bovine and porcine growth hormone, but not to the ovine variety. A suggested regime is —

> 2.5 units for dogs weighing less than 14Kg
>
> 5.0 units for dogs weighing more than 14Kg

The unit dose is given sub-cutaneously at 2 day intervals for ten treatments.

Some treated dogs apparently recover completely and remain normal for long periods but others relapse on cessation of treatment. The prolonged remission after growth hormone treatment is puzzling as it contrasts with the need for continual replacement therapy in other hormonal deficiency states.

PITUITARY-DEPENDENT HYPERADRENOCORTICISM

The majority of hyperadrenocorticoid dogs have bilateral adrenal hyperplasia and in most of them an ACTH-secreting pituitary tumour can be identified. However, it is possible that in some cases of pituitary-dependent hyperadrenocorticism, the underlying abnormality may be excessive cortico-trophin releasing hormone (CRH) production by the hypothalamus, causing hyperplasia of pituitary corticotrophs and subsequent adenomatous change.

Human cases of pituitary-dependent hyperadrenocorticism are also seen, where the cause is ectopic production of ACTH, CRH or other substances with similar activity by a tumour involving neither the pituitary nor the hypothalamus. It is possible that there are similar diverse causes in the dog. However, generally the signs and findings resemble those produced by a hyperfunctional adrenal tumour.

In a few cases the pituitary-dependent form can be diagnosed confidently on clinical grounds alone, as when hyperadrenocorticoid signs occur in the absence of glucocorticoid therapy in a patient with signs of a space-occupying lesion in the pituitary-hypothalamic area. Otherwise, investigation and treatment of pituitary-dependent hyperadrenocorticism are as discussed in the chapter on the adrenal gland. Pituitary-dependent hyperadrenocorticism is rare in the cat. (For further details see page 95)

SECONDARY AND TERTIARY HYPOADRENOCORTICISM (See also page 101.)

Most clinical cases of hypoadrenocorticism are primary, caused by destruction of the adrenal glands and characterised by deficiencies of both glucocorticoid and mineralocorticoid activity.

In the secondary form, glucocorticoid deficiency results from a lack of ACTH but mineralocorticoid production is unimpaired. This can occur when prolonged glucocorticoid therapy ceases abruptly or destructive lesions involve the adenohypophysis.

If a lesion destroys the hypothalamus, secretion of corticotrophin releasing hormone may be impaired, causing ACTH deficiency. There is, therefore, a tertiary deficiency in glucocorticoid production. Mineralocorticoid secretion remains unimpaired.

Signs and findings

Clinical signs may be precipitated by stress and comprise weakness, depression, inappetence, vomiting, diarrhoea and collapse.

Patients with iatrogenic disease will usually have additional physical changes suggesting hyper-adrenocorticism e.g. polydipsia, polyuria, polyphagia, symmetrical alopecia, abdominal enlargement and hepatomegaly.

Those with pituitary or hypothalamic lesions have evidence of other hormone deficiencies (diabetes insipidus or hypothyroidism), hormone excesses (acromegaly) or neurological dysfunction (central blindness, depression, altered behaviour, disorders of thirst, appetite and temperature regulation). Blood leukocyte changes suggestive of glucocorticoid deficiency (lymphocytosis, eosinophilia) may be evident in some cases.

Diagnosis

In all three forms of hypoadrenocorticism tests show low or normal plasma cortisol concentrations with a subnormal response to the ACTH stimulation test. The secondary, iatrogenic form can be diagnosed from the history of systemic or topical glucocorticoid therapy and the primary form identified by concurrent plasma electrolyte abnormalities (low sodium, high potassium). Further differentiation of the three forms is rarely needed but the following protocol could be employed:

1.   Measurement of basal plasma ACTH concentrations (availability of this assay is limited at present) and/or evaluating the cortisol response to repeated ACTH administrations. This will distinguish the primary form from the other two. Primary hypoadrenocorticism is characterised by high basal ACTH concentration and no increase in cortisol after administration of ACTH. Secondary and tertiary forms have low basal ACTH concentrations and should respond to ACTH administration.

2.   Determination of hormonal responses to several doses of corticotrophin releasing hormone. This should differentiate spontaneous secondary and tertiary insufficiencies. No increase in ACTH or cortisol is expected in spontaneous secondary hypoadrenocorticism, but both should increase in the tertiary form.

Treatment

Iatrogenic cases should be given replacement therapy with prednisolone initially at 0.2 mg/kg each morning with gradual withdrawal over several months. Doses should be increased x 2—10 at times of stress. Similar treatment may help patients with pituitary-hypothalamic lesions, although it does not solve the underlying problem.

PITUITARY-DEPENDENT HYPERTHYROIDISM

In man, hyperthyroidsim is sometimes caused by excessive thyroid stimulation due to overproduction of thyroid stimulating hormone (TSH), thyrotrophin releasing hormone (TRH) or other thyroid stimulating factors. These processes have not been identified in dogs and cats, where primary thyroid abnormalities are usually implicated in naturally occurring hyperthyroidism. However, the role of TSH and TRH in cats with hyperthyroidism and bilateral thyroid adenomatous hyperplasia awaits evaluation.

SECONDARY AND TERTIARY HYPOTHYROIDISM (See also pages 48 and 49)

The majority of hypothyroid dogs (95%) have primary thyroid disease. Secondary hypothyroidism (TSH deficiency, caused by pituitary defect) and tertiary hypothyroidism (TRH deficiency, hypothalamic defect) are uncommon, but have both been observed as congenital or acquired abnormalities (Belshaw 1983). All forms of hypothyroidism are rare in the cat.

Signs

Signs may be limited to those described for primary hypothyroidism (see chapter on the Thyroid) or there may be additional endocrine or neurological manifestations of pituitary-hypothalamic dysfunction. The hypothyroid signs may be obscured by more obvious accompanying defects, as when congenital secondary hypothyroidism occurs in pituitary dwarfism.

Diagnosis and treatment

Diagnosis and treatment of hypothyroid disorders is described elsewhere (see 'Thyroid' chapter). Differentiation of the various forms of hypothyroidism is generally unnecessary, since replacement therapy with thyroid hormones is identical in all cases. However, thyroid stimulation tests are sometimes indicated to investigate possible pituitary-hypothalamic defects. If plasma thyroxine concentration increases in a hypothyroid patient after TSH administration, then secondary or tertiary hypothyroidism is present rather than a primary dysfunction. Some patients with secondary or tertiary hypothyroidism might respond only after TSH administration is repeated on several consecutive days, because thyroid atrophy is present. An alternative to repeated stimulation tests — which are expensive — is thyroid biopsy.

Assessment of thyroxine response to TRH administration could theoretically help to distinguish secondary and tertiary hypothyroidism. Some response might occur in tertiary deficiency but no response would be expected in the secondary form. However, repeated administration of TRH may be necessary to clarify the diagnosis in the presence of thyroid atrophy from previous understimulation.

SECONDARY AND TERTIARY HYPOGONADISM

Hypogonadism can occur secondarily when FSH and LH are lacking because of a pituitary deficit and as a tertiary phenomenon if gonadotrophin releasing hormone (GnRH) is deficient. Other pituitary-hypothalamic defects may occur concurrently. The result is testicular hypoplasia or atrophy in males or persistent anoestrus in females. Hormonal assays would indicate low plasma concentrations of FSH, LH and sex steroids in both forms and impaired response of these hormones to GnRH in secondary hypogonadism.

REFERENCES

ALLISON, R. M. M., WATSON, A. D. J. and CHURCH, D. B. (1983) Pituitary tumour causing neurological and endocrine disturbances in a dog. *J. small Anim. Pract.* **24**, 229.

ALLAN, G. S., HUXTABLE, C. R. R., HOWLETT, C. R., BAXTER, R. C., DUFF, B. and FARROW, B. R. H. (1978) Pituitary dwarfism in German shepherd dogs. *J. small Anim. Pract.* **19**, 711.

BIEWENGA, W. J., VAN DEN BROM, W. E. and MOL, J. A. (1987) Vasopressin in polyuric syndromes in the dog. *Front. Horm. Res.* **17**, 139.

BELSHAW, B. E. (1983) Thyroid Diseases. In: *Textbook of Veterinary Internal Medicine, Diseases of the Dog and Cat* (ed. S. J. Ettinger) 2nd edn, p.1592. W. B. Saunders, Philadelphia.

CHASTAIN, C. B. and GANJAM, V. K. (1986) *Clinical Endocrinology of Companion Animals.* Lea and Febiger, Philadelphia.

EIGENMANN, J. E. (1984) Acromegaly in the dog. *Vet. Clin. N. Am: Small Anim. Pract.* **14**, 827.

EIGENMANN, J. E. (1986) Disorders associated with growth hormone oversecretion: diabetes mellitus and acromegaly. In: *Current Veterinary Therapy IX, Small Animal Practice* (ed. R. W. Kirk) p 1006. W. B. Saunders, Philadelphia.

FELDMAN, E. C. and NELSON, R. W. (1987) *Canine and Feline Endocrinology and Reproduction.* W. B. Saunders, Philadelphia.

HOUSTON, D. M., ALLEN, D. A., KRUTH, S. A., POOK, H., SPINATO, M. T. and KEOGH, L. (1989). Syndrome of inappropriate antidiuretic hormone secretion in a dog. *Can. Vet. J.* **30**, 423.

RIJNBERK, A., BIEWENGA, W. J. and MOL, J. A. (1988) Inappropriate vasopressin secretion in two dogs. *Acta endocr. Copenh.* **117**, 59.

SCOTT, D. W. and WALTON, D. K. (1986) Hyposomatotropism in the mature dog: a discussion of 22 cases. *J. Am. Anim. Hosp. Ass.* **22**, 467.

WILLIAMS, R. H. (1981) *Textbook of Endocrinology* 6th edn. W. B. Saunders, Philadelphia.

CHAPTER 2

THE THYROID GLAND

Keith L. Thoday B.Vet.Med., Ph.D., D.V.D., M.R.C.V.S.

ANATOMY AND HISTOLOGY

Thyroidal gross and microscopic anatomy is similar in both dogs and cats. The gland, which lies within the cervical fascia between the sternothyroideus muscles and the trachea, consists of two lobes, only rarely connected by an isthmus. The anterior poles of the lobes are positioned just below the cricoid cartilage and extend downward over the first five to six (cat) or eight (dog) tracheal rings. A fibrous capsule surrounds each lobe. Dorsally, the lobes are in close proximity to the carotid sheath and the vagosympathetic trunk. The right recurrent laryngeal nerve is dorsal to medial to the right thyroid lobe.

The thyroid glands are not palpable in healthy dogs or cats. The normal thyroid : body weight ratio is 100 mg/kg in mature animals.

One external (cranial) and internal (caudal) parathyroid gland is normally associated with each thyroid lobe. The external parathyroids are usually located near the cranial pole of each lobe in fascia external to the thyroid capsule. The internal parathyroids are more variable in position but usually lie within the thyroid parenchyma at the caudal pole of each lobe.

The main arterial supply in both dogs and cats is the cranial thyroid artery, a branch of the common carotid artery. In the dog, this artery divides into dorsal and ventral branches which enter the gland and divide further into lobar branches. In the cat, the cranial thyroid artery enters the thyroid before branching to supply the lobe, plus both parathyroids. A caudal thyroid artery may be seen in some dogs but is not present in most cats. Venous drainage of both the thyroid and parathyroids is via the caudal thyroid vein which, together with the small cranial thyroid vein, drains into the internal jugular vein.

The principle nerve supply to the thyroid is derived from the cranial cervical ganglion and the cranial laryngeal nerve.

Accessory thyroid and parathyroid tissue is common in both dogs and cats in practically any position between the tongue and the heart.

The thyroid capsule gives off septa or trabeculae which are continuous with sparse interstitial connective tissue which divides the lobes into interconnected lobules. The gland is relatively homogenous, consisting of numerous follicles which are completely closed and surrounded by a network of delicate reticular fibres. They are lined with a single layer of cells with a secretory polarity directed towards the follicular lumen. In the resting state, the cells are low cuboidal or sometimes squamous but, when stimulated, the cells become cuboidal or columnar and the colloid is dissolved. Parafollicular cells (light or C cells) are considered to be the source of calcitonin.

PHYSIOLOGY

IODOTHYRONINES

Hormone synthesis, secretion and metabolism

The thyroid gland is unique among the endocrine glands in that an integral part of its hormones is a micronutrient, iodine, which is available in only limited amounts. The daily maintenance iodine requirement in a normal diet of an adult dog weighing 10 to 15 kg is 140 μg whereas for adult cats it is from 150 to 400 μg per cat. Most iodine in the diet is reduced to iodide in the gastrointestinal tract and absorption of iodide begins immediately (Belshaw et al., 1975).

Inorganic iodide enters the thyroid follicular cells and is transformed into the metabolically active thyroid hormones 3, 5, 3^1, 5^1 tetraiodothyronine (T4) and 3, 5, 3^1 triiodothyronine (T3). All body T4 is initially secreted by the thyroid. By contrast, T3 production in the euthyroid state is variably a result of thyroidal secretion and extra-thyroidal conversion of T4 to T3. Thyroid hormones are carried in blood bound to plasma proteins.

Only non-protein bound (free) hormone is metabolically active, the bound fraction acting as a reservoir in situations of rapid increase or decrease of hormone supply to tissues. In dogs, the free T4 (FT4) concentrations range from 0.103 to 0.303 per cent of the total plasma T4 (TT4) concentration (Furth et al., 1968, Refetoff et al., 1970) while in cats the corresponding figures are 0.083 to 0.105 per cent (Thoday, unpublished data). In dogs, the T4 plasma half-life has been variably reported as 10.3 hours (Furth et al., 1968) to 15.9 hours (Kallfelz and Erali, 1973) and the T3 plasma half-life 5—6 hours (Fox and Nachreiner, 1981).

T4 has been described by many workers as a prohormone with its activity being dependent on its mono-de-iodination to T3. While this conversion is responsible for approximately 85 per cent of its activity, T4, like T3 does have intrinsic thyromimetic actions, although T3 is three to five times more potent.

CONTROL OF THYROID FUNCTION

The hypothalamic-pituitary-thyroid-extrathyroidal axis

Detailed information about this axis in dogs and cats is unavailable although it is assumed, from indirect evidence, to be similar to that of man. Thus, peptidergic neurones in the thyrotropic area of the hypothalamus secrete the tripeptide amide thyrotropin releasing hormone (TRH) into the hypophyseal portal system. TRH acts on the thyrotrope cells of the anterior pituitary, influencing thyroid stimulating hormone (TSH) production in a tonic and permissive way.

The thyroid is under the direct control of TSH. Within minutes of TSH administration, there is enhancement of iodide binding to protein, iodothyronine synthesis, thyroglobulin secretion into the follicular lumen and ingestion of colloid via pseudopod formation. Increased trapping of iodide follows after several hours.

The lack of homologous TSH assays for dogs and cats (see later) has inhibited the detailed investigation of the hypothalamic-pituitary-thyroid-extrathyroidal axis of these species. However, studies on a homologous canine TSH assay together with those determining serum T4 concentrations after TSH administration in dogs and cats indicates a functional hypothalamic-pituitary-thyroid axis comparable to that of man.

Inhibition of thyroid hormone production is achieved via a negative feedback system whereby plasma FT4 and free T3 (FT3) act directly on the pituitary. Small doses of thyroid hormones suppress and large doses completely abolish the TRH-induced release of TSH (Belshaw, 1983). Extrathyroidal thyroid hormone metabolism may also act as a regulator of thyroid function by de-iodination of T4 to either T3 or the metabolically inactive rT3.

Other mechanisms affecting thyroid hormone concentrations

Iodine intake. Thyroglobulin stored within the thyroid follicles allows for continued hormone secretion during iodine deficiency. During such times, there may be preferential T3 secretion relative to T4. Because T3 is more potent that T4, this mechanism serves to maintain euthyroidism despite iodine deficiency.

A gradual increase in iodide intake, with a consequent increase in thyroidal iodide concentrations, results in increased stores of thyroid hormones. Beyond a certain level, excess iodide administration has an antithyroid effect as iodide binding to thyroglobulin is progressively inhibited. This has been termed the Wolff-Chaikoff effect which serves to prevent massive thyroid hormone release after an iodide overload.

Inherent rhythms. Circadian variations in thyroid hormone secretion do not occur in cats (Hoenig and Ferguson, 1983) or dogs (Kemppainen *et al.*, 1984). *Thus the time of day is not critical when sampling dogs and cats for thyroid hormone determinations.*

Effects of sex. For any given age, female and neutered female cats have higher serum TT4 concentrations than males and neutered males. Similar but not statistically significant differences occur with serum total T3 (TT3) concentrations. Neutering does not affect feline TT4 and TT3 concentrations (Thoday *et al.*, 1984).

Effects of age. Neonatal dogs (up to 100 days of age) have higher, and old dogs lower, TT4 concentrations than healthy adults (Book, 1977; Ray and Howanitz, 1984). TT4 concentrations of cats vary highly significantly with age, decreasing in a non-linear manner until approximately five years of age and then rising again. Serum TT3 concentrations also show a non-linear decrease with age but level out rather than increase at very high ages (Thoday *et al.*, 1984).

Effects of breed and heredity. TT4 and TT3 concentrations tend to be lower in large and giant breeds of dogs and in certain breeds such as the German shepherd dog, cocker spaniel, boxer, beagle, Labrador retriever, Alaskan malamute and Siberian husky (Blake and Lapinski, 1980; Muller *et al.*, 1983). Pedigree cats tend to have higher TT3 concentrations at any given age than domestic short and long-haired cats taken as one group (Thoday *et al.*, 1984). Related cats, unlike unrelated cats living in the same environment, have similar TT3 but not TT4 concentrations (Thoday *et al.*, 1984).

Effects of obesity. Overeating results in increased T3 production in man but such people are euthyroid. The plasma TT3 and TT4 concentrations of obese dogs are elevated (Gosselin *et al.*, 1980). Similar investigations have not been carried out in the cat.

Effects of disease and malnutrition. In man, a number of conditions (diabetes mellitus, hepatic and renal conditions, other chronic disease states, surgery, starvation, malnutrition) are associated with reduced extrathyroidal T4 to T3 conversion and, except in chronic renal failure, increased plasma rT3. This decrease in circulating T3 is probably a mechanism to conserve body protein during illness and has been termed the 'low T3' or 'euthyroid sick' syndrome. The plasma TT4 concentration may also be reduced in the euthyroid sick syndrome (usually in acute, severe conditions) and is termed specifically the 'low T4 state of medical illness'. The FT4 concentration remains the same and patients are euthyroid.

The euthyroid sick syndrome has been investigated in dogs. In a group of dogs with a variety of medical conditions in an intensive care unit, all had sub-normal TT4 concentrations (Ferguson, 1984). Depressed plasma TT4 and increased rT3 concentrations are commonly noted in dogs with liver and kidney disease, hyperadrenocorticism and diabetes mellitus (Larsson, 1987). Accompanying low TT3 concentrations, as occurs in man, are rare. No comparable studies have been carried out in cats.

Effect of drugs. A number of drugs have been shown to alter plasma thyroid hormone concentrations in man, either by changes in peripheral metabolism or in plasma or cellular binding.

In dogs, plasma T4 concentrations may be depressed by, for example, diphenylhydantoin, phenobarbitone, phenylbutazone, o,p'DDD, glucocorticoids and salicylates (Belshaw, 1983; Muller *et al.*, 1983; Ferguson, 1984). Plasma T3 concentration is lowered by prednisolone (Woltz *et al.*, 1983). Dogs maintained on these drugs do not develop signs of hypothyroidism, euthyroidism probably being maintained by adequate levels of FT4 and FT3. Such studies have not been carried out in cats.

The clinical importance of these observations is that such animals may falsely be diagnosed as hypothyroid by basal plasma T4 measurement, whereas the increase after TSH stimulation is almost parallel to that of healthy dogs. Studies to determine the exact mechanism by which drugs affect plasma T4 concentration in dogs have not been reported.

As a large number of other drugs may decrease (e.g. androgens, cholecystographic agents, diazepam, heparin, imidazoles, penicillin, primidone, phenothiazines, amiodarone) T4 and/or T3 or increase (e.g. 5-fluorouracil, halothane, narcotic antagonists, amiodarone, insulin, thiazides) T4 and /or T3 in man (Ferguson, 1984) and as such drugs have found veterinary uses, in the absence of species specific studies, it is probably safer to assume that the use of any drug *may* affect plasma T4 or T3 concentrations in dogs and cats and to use diagnostic techniques for thyroid disorders which circumvent possible areas of confusion.

CALCITONIN

Calcitonin, a polypeptide hormone produced by the thyroid parafollicular cells, decreases plasma calcium and phosphate concentrations.

The principle actions of calcitonin involve:

1. Reduction of bone resorption (which could release both calcium and phosphate) due to temporary blockage of both osteocytic and osteoclastic osteolysis.

2. Increased phosphate deposition in bone and soft tissue.

3. Reduced renal reabsorption of calcium and phosphate and, to a lesser extent, sodium, potassium, magnesium and chloride.

4. Decreased renal activation of vitamin D.

5. Increased small intestinal secretion of sodium, potassium, chloride and water.

Although parathyroid hormone is the main factor in the regulation of plasma calcium concentration, the combined control mechanism with calcitonin provides a highly sensitive, dual negative feedback mechanism. The action of calcitonin is probably directed at the prevention of post-prandial hypercalcaemia and to reduce maternal skeletal demineralisation during gestation.

CURRENTLY USED CLINICAL TESTS OF THYROID FUNCTION

MEASUREMENT OF CIRCULATING HORMONES UNDER BASAL CONDITIONS

Assay of total thyroxine and triiodothyronine

Principles. Measurement of the total (protein bound plus free) blood thyroid hormone concentrations is currently the simplest and most economical way of evaluating canine and feline thyroid gland function. Most laboratories use radioimmunoassay (RIA) which offers a unique combination of specificity, sensitivity, precision and practicality. Enzyme-linked immunosorbent assay (ELISA) offers a cheaper and potentially safer alternative but is currently less reliable diagnostically than RIA (Larsson and Lumsden, 1980). Whichever laboratory or technique is used, it is essential that the methods have been modified for the much lower TT4 and TT3 concentrations and the different plasma/serum matrices occurring in dogs and cats. For example, in the author's laboratory the reference range for TT4 in cats is 8.5—46.2 nmol/l, which is totally in the hypothyroid range of human sera run in a similar assay (reference range 70.0—150.0 nmol/l).

Either serum or heparinised plasma may be submitted for thyroid hormone determinations and give comparable results. T4 and T3 are extremely stable and temperature of storage, repeated freezing and thawing and haemolysis do not significantly affect TT4 and TT3 concentrations (Reimers *et al.,* 1982; Donne and Wildgoose, 1984). Transfer to the laboratory by post is not, therefore, a problem for the practitioner.

Diagnostic applications. Although there are occasional exceptions, basal TT3 measurements provide little additional diagnostic information over basal TT4 concentrations to the small animal practitioner. A low TT4 concentration supports a diagnosis of hypothyroidism in the presence of compatible historical and clinical features. However, both TT4 and TT3 concentrations are influenced by a large number of variables of non-thyroidal origin (see previous) and definitive diagnosis requires dynamic function testing using TSH.

A single basal TT3 and/or TT4 measurement will confirm the diagnosis of hyperthyroidism in most affected dogs and cats.

Assay of free thyroxine and triiodothyronine

Principles. Only the free thyroid hormones are metabolically active, the protein bound hormones simply acting as a reservoir to maintain the free concentrations between narrow limits. FT4 and FT3 are, therefore, potentially more valid estimates of thyroid function than TT4 and TT3. The standard technique for the determination of free thyroid hormones is by the technically demanding and difficult technique of equilibrium dialysis. However, recently, RIA kits have been produced commercially for the determination of FT4 and FT3 in man and these have received some veterinary attention.

Diagnostic applications. Basal FT4 concentrations are, as would be expected, significantly lower in hypothyroid than in euthyroid dogs (Ekersall and Williams, 1983; Feldman and Nelson, 1987) However, FT4 concentrations appear to be depressed in some non-thyroidal disease conditions in the same way as TT4 (Feldman and Nelson, 1987) and currently this diagnostic technique should not be used as the sole method of diagnosis of hypothyroidism in dogs.

FT4 concentrations are elevated in hyperthyroid cats (Thoday, unpublished observations).

Assay of thyroid stimulating hormone

Principles. In human medicine, the currently available highly specific and sensitive plasma TSH assays are used, sometimes together with plasma T4 (total or free) concentrations, as a first line approach to the investigation of both hypo and hyperthyroidism. In primary hypothyroidism, there are elevated plasma TSH and low plasma T4 concentrations while in secondary hypothyroidism, both plasma TSH and T4 are low. In hyperthyroidism, because of increased negative feedback effects of the raised concentrations of thyroid hormones on the pituitary, plasma TSH is undetectable. TSH is a species specific polypeptide which, although biologically active, is immunologically distinct between species. Although Nachreiner (1981) reported that an RIA kit for measuring human TSH gave reliable values in dogs, other workers have reported that there is a significant overlap in TSH concentrations between euthyroid and hypothyroid dogs (Larsson, 1981; Ferguson, 1984) using such methods.

Diagnostic applications. Although Quinlan and Michaelson (1981) have developed an homologous RIA for canine TSH, a laboratory service using it is not available in the U.K.

A reliable TSH assay would be of considerable value in the further delineation of canine and feline thyroid disorders and is urgently awaited.

Assay of plasma calcitonin

Principles. Plasma calcitonin, produced by the C cells of the thyroid, may be measured by RIA.

Diagnostic applications. In humans, thyroidal medullary carcinoma elevates the plasma calcitonin concentration. However, raised concentrations may also occur in pregnancy and lactation and as a result of acute pancreatitis, renal failure, gastrinoma and thyroiditis. Dynamic function tests using calcium or pentagastrin may be used to refine diagnosis.

Medullary carcinoma of the thyroid also occurs in dogs but detailed investigations into the hormonal status of such cases has not been reported.

MEASUREMENT OF CIRCULATING HORMONES — DYNAMIC FUNCTION TESTS

The TSH stimulation test

Principles. As previously discussed, TSH stimulates a number of steps in thyroid hormone synthesis. In the absence of specific assays for canine TSH, the measurement of TT4 concentrations before and after TSH administration provides the most convenient method for the definitive diagnosis of canine hypothyroidism (Oliver and Waldrop, 1983). However, TSH is expensive and difficult to obtain as there are currently no British suppliers. Because the majority of T3 is produced by mono-de-iodination of T4, serum TT3 determination after TSH stimulation is diagnostically unreliable. The test can also be used in cats although, because feline hypothyroidism is extremely rare, its main application is to the diagnosis of borderline hyperthyroidism.

Diagnostic application. In veterinary medicine, the TSH stimulation test has been most widely applied to the diagnosis of primary hypothyroidism in dogs (Belshaw, 1983). In such cases, there is no significant increase in plasma TT4 concentration after TSH administration. The changes in TT3 concentration in response to TSH are not consistent enough to be used in a clinical situation.

A suggested regimen for this test is shown in Table 1 and its method of interpretation is shown in Table 2. Some authors have suggested using 1 I.U. TSH per dog on grounds of cost. However, in one study (Thoday, unpublished data) two of five euthyroid dogs failed to double their basal TT4 after 4 hours when 1 I.U. TSH was used, whereas this occurred when subsequently they were tested with 5 I.U. TSH. The author therefore currently uses 5 I.U. TSH for the test. There are many other regimens, with some workers using 0.1 I.U. TSH per kg body weight.

The test will differentiate hypothyroxinaemia due to non-thyroidal illness or drug administration (responses similar to euthyroid animals) from primary hypothyroidism (Belshaw, 1983). It may also be used to differentiate secondary and tertiary hypothyroidism from the primary form of the disease (Chastain *et al.*, 1979). In secondary and tertiary hypothyroidism, one dose of TSH usually leads to TT4 increases similar to those seen in non-thyroidal illness or as a result of drug administration. A small percentage of cases may require repeated administration of TSH for three consecutive days before a significant increase is seen (Ferguson, 1984), as prolonged TSH deficiency may lead to thyroid atrophy, limiting the thyroid's ability to respond to exogenous TSH.

Table 1
Suggested regimen for TSH stimulation test in dogs.

1. Collect blood sample into heparinised or plain tube.
2. Administer 5 I.U. bovine TSH intravenously.
3. Collect second blood sample *four* hours later as 1.
4. Separate plasma or serum by centrifugation for transport to laboratory.
5. Request measurement of TT4.

Interpretation: Euthyroid dogs should at least double their basal TT4 *and* fall within or above the normal post-TSH TT4 range for that laboratory.

Table 2
Interpretation of TSH stimulation test in dogs — some examples.

When:	TT4 basal reference range	:	13 — 52 nmol/l
	Post-TSH TT4 reference range	:	26 to 104 nmol/l
1.	Euthyroid response:		
	(a) Basal TT4	—	23 nmol/l
	Post-TSH TT4	—	68 nmol/l
	(b) Basal TT4	—	10 nmol/l
	Post-TSH TT4	—	35 nmol/l
2.	Hypothyroid response:		
	(a) Basal TT4	—	7 nmol/l
	Post-TSH TT4	—	11 nmol/l
	(b) Basal TT4	—	7 nmol/l
	Post-TSH TT4	—	21 nmol/l
	(c) Basal TT4	—	17 nmol/l
	Post-TSH TT4	—	20 nmol/l

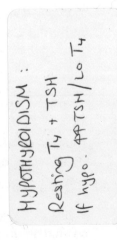

HYPOTHYROIDISM :
Resting T4 + TSH
If hypo. ↑↑TSH/Lo T4

In **cats,** the TSH stimulation test is used less commonly than in dogs because naturally occurring, acquired hypothyroidism has not been described. It may be used to confirm the diagnosis of cretinism. In addition, while a TSH stimulation test is not required for the diagnosis of hyperthyroidism in most affected cats, it has been suggested that it might be of value when resting thyroid hormone concentrations are borderline or only slightly increased (Peterson, 1982; Peterson et al., 1983).

The TSH stimulation test has been optimised and validated for use in cats (Thoday, 1986a) and this regimen and the method of interpretation is shown in Table 3. It has been suggested that the thyroid glands of hyperthyroid cats fail to respond to TSH because either they are secreting thyroid hormones independently of TSH control or that T4 and T3 are already being produced maximally (Peterson et al., 1983).

Table 3
Suggested regimen for, and interpretation of, the TSH stimulation test in cats

1. Collect blood sample into heparinised or plain tube.
2. Administer 0.5 I.U./kg, bovine TSH intravenously.
3. Collect second blood sample *six* hours later as 1.
4. Separate plasma or serum by centrifugation for transport to laboratory.
5. Request measurement of TT4.

Interpretation:
In the author's laboratory, in healthy cats, (normal range for TT4, 8.5—46.2 nmol/l), this regimen leads to a TT4 concentration of greater than 55 nmol/l six hours after TSH administration and to an increment in the serum TT4 of greater than 20 nmol/l. In hyperthyroid cats, there may be little or no TT4 response to TSH, but a normal response may also be obtained.

The TRH stimulation test

Principles. TRH, released by the hypothalamus, stimulates synthesis and release of TSH by the thyrothrophs of the anterior pituitary. TSH subsequently stimulates production of T4 and T3 by the thyroid.

In human medicine, measurements of plasma TSH before and after TRH administration have proved to be very valuable in the investigation of patients with suspected primary hyperthyroidism, where there is no significant rise due to suppression of the thyrotrophs. It may also be of value in differentiating between secondary (pituitary) and the rare tertiary (hypothalamic) forms of hypothyroidism. In pituitary hypothyroidism there is little or no TSH response, whereas in the hypothalamic form there may be delayed TSH response.

In small animals, where TSH assay is not available, elevations of TT4 after TRH administration indicate a functionally intact pituitary-thyroid axis.

Diagnostic applications. The TRH stimulation test has been recommended as a sensitive test of thyroid function in small animals. A failure of a significant increase in TT4 after TRH administration would indicate either primary or secondary hypothyroidism.

Lothrop et al.,(1984) recommended a test procedure of serum TT4 determination before and six hours after the intravenous administration of 0.1 mg/kg TRH to both dogs and cats. Using this method, 28 of 31 healthy dogs had an incremental increase of at least 1.5 times the basal TT4 concentration. However, Evinger et al., (1985), using an intravenous dose of 0.2 mg TRH/dog, found the largest increase of TT4 at four hours after TRH administration.

The value of this test in separating euthyroid and hypothyroid dogs in a clinical situation remains to be studied. In addition the effects of non-thyroidal illness and drug administration on the response to TRH have not yet been evaluated. No clinical evaluations of the TRH stimulation test in abnormal cats have been published.

RADIONUCLIDE STUDIES

Thyroidal radioiodine uptake (RIU)

Principles. Administered radioiodine is concentrated by the thyroid in the same way as dietary iodide. RIU, therefore, directly assesses the functional status of the thyroid. The peak uptake of radioiodine is inversely proportional to dietary iodine uptake. Generally, the higher the RIU, the more active is the thyroid (Peterson, 1984). Because ^{125}I has a longer half-life, ^{131}I or ^{123}I are usually used.

Diagnostic applications. In euthyroid dogs and cats, the peak radioiodine uptake is approximately 15% and 9% respectively (Belshaw, 1983; Peterson et al., 1983). RIU is increased in hyperthyroidism and in conditions of dietary iodine deficiency and decreased in hypothyroidism. *The test requires specialist facilities and is not available to most practitioners.*

Thyroid imaging. (Thyroid scanning, scintigraphy)

Principles. Scanning the thyroid with a gamma camera after administration of a suitable radionuclide serves to delineate areas with relatively high or low uptake. The radionuclides most commonly used are ^{131}I, ^{123}I and a radioisotope derived from molybdenum, technetium—99m as pertechnetate ($^{99m}T_cO_4$). Similar images are produced by each. Technetium is trapped and concentrated like iodide within follicular cells but unlike iodide, is neither incorporated in thyroglobulin nor stored in the thyroid. Its rapid uptake and short half-life (6.0 hours) give it considerable advantage for scintigraphy work.

Diagnostic applications. The thyroid scan has found its main use in *feline hyperthyroidism* to determine unilateral or bilateral lobe involvement and thus whether unilateral or bilateral thyroidectomy, with the latter's greater potential for post-operative sequelae, must be carried out. In unilateral lobe involvement, the production of TSH and therefore the function of the contra-lateral lobe is suppressed because of the high circulating concentrations of thyroid hormones, and a single area of radioactive uptake corresponding to the affected tissue is visualised on the scan (Figure 1). Where both lobes are involved in the disease, two areas of radioactive uptake are seen (Figure 2). The thyroid scan is also of value in determining abnormal thyroid lobe position or metastasis from malignant thyroid tumours.

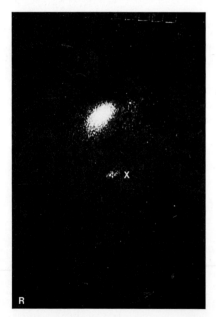

Figure 1

Thyroid scan of a hyperthyroid, 14-year-old, neutered male, domestic short-haired cat with unilateral (right sided) thyroid adenomatous hyperplasia. The uninvolved left thyroid lobe cannot be visualised. The small area of radioactivity is a marker. The image was produced by a five minute gamma camera scan using a pinhole collimator, 20 minutes after the intravenous administration of 45 MBq (1.2 mCi) technetium—99m.

Reproduced, with permission, from Thoday (1988).

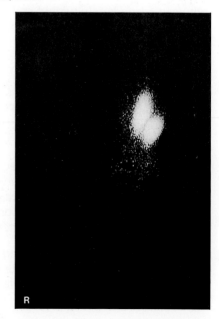

Figure 2

Thyroid scan of a hyperthyroid, 14-year-old, neutered female, domestic short-haired cat with bilateral adenomatous hyperplasia. The image was produced by a five minute gamma camera scan using a pinhole collimator, 20 minutes after the intravenous administration of 28 MBq (0.76 mCi) technetium—99m.

Reproduced, with permission, from Thoday (1988)

Plate 2:1 *(below)*
Non-functional papillary adenocarcinoma removed from a five-year-old,
entire female, Persian cat (TT4, 30 nmol/l; TT3, 0.60 nmol/l). The swelling had been
noticed by the owner in association with cervical discomfort. Excision was curative.

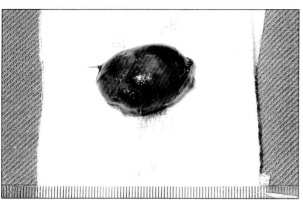

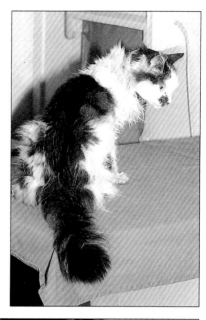

Plate 2:2 *(right)*
Hyperthyroid, 15-year-old, neutered male, domestic long-haired cat showing poor
bodily condition and typical anxious expression (TT4, 160 nmol/l; TT3, 2.17 nmol/l).

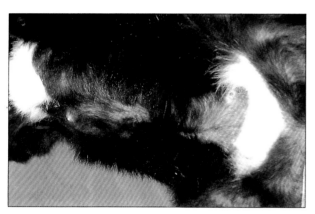

Plate 2:3   Hyperthyroid, 16-year-old, neutered female,
domestic short-haired cat showing diffuse thinning of hair
over the ventral thorax, abdomen and medial thighs
(TT4, 156.0 nmol/l; TT3, 2.30 nmol/l).

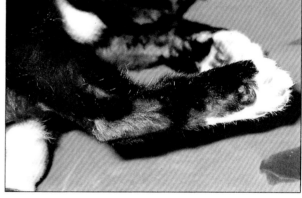

Plate 2:4
The cat in Plate 2:3 showing patchy alopecia
over the caudal hocks.
Plates 2:2, 2:3 and 2:4 reproduced by permission, Thoday (1988)

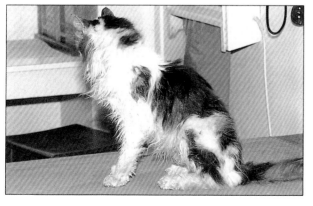

Plate 2:5
The cat in Plate 2:2. The coat condition is poor
with numerous mats.

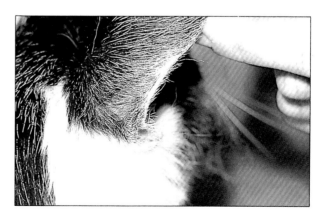

Plate 2:6   Hyperthyroid, 13-year-old, neutered male,
domestic short-haired cat showing hyperaemia of the right
pinna (TT4, 146.3 nmol/l; TT3, 1.91 nmol/l).

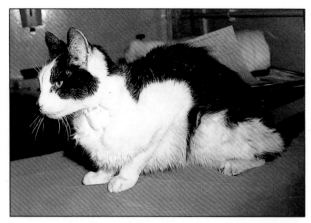 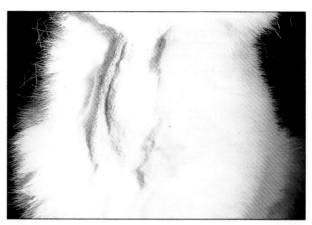

Plates 2:7a and 2:7b
The cat in Plate 2:6. There is severe weight loss and unilateral (left-sided) goitre.
Reproduced, with permission, from Thoday (1988).

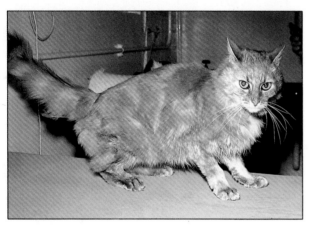 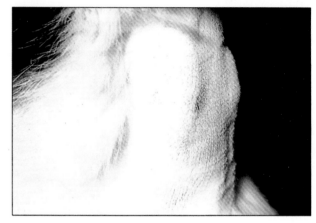

Plates 2:8a and 2:8b
Hyperthyroid, 11-year-old, neutered female, domestic long-haired cat with bilateral goitre
(TT4, 370.7 nmol/l; TT3, 4.2 nmol/l).

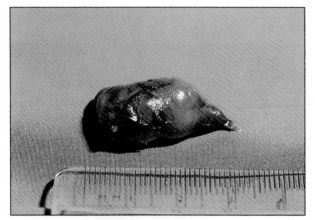 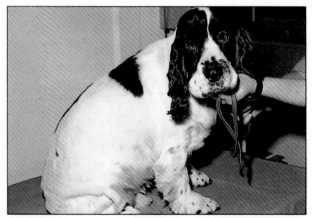

Plate 2:9
Hyperfunctional thyroid lobe removed by the
extracapsular technique.

Plate 2:10
Hypothyroid, seven-year-old, male cocker spaniel
showing obesity and tragic facial expression
(basal TT4 <5.0 nmol/l; post-TSH TT4, 7.2 nmol/l).

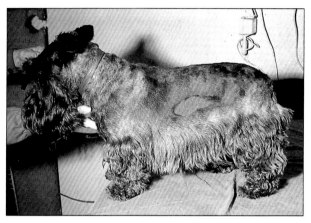

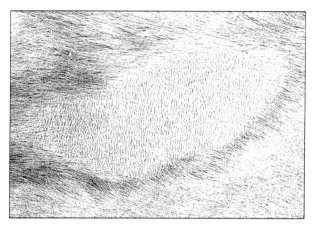

Plates 2:11a   Plate 2:11b

Hypothyroid, eight-year-old, female Scottish terrier with focal trunk alopecia and cutaneous hyperpigmentation.
The alopecia was bilaterally symmetrical (basal TT4, 10.3 nmol/l; post-TSH TT4, 18.7 nmol/l).

Plate 12:2
Hypothyroid, nine-year-old,
male miniature dachsund with diffuse
trunk alopecia and mild seborrhoea sicca.
The dog also had pinnal alopecia
which began at nine months of age,
was apparently unrelated to the hypothyroidism
and which, unlike the trunk alopecia,
did not respond to thyroid hormone treatment.

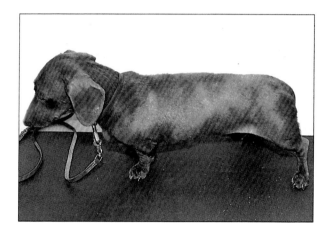

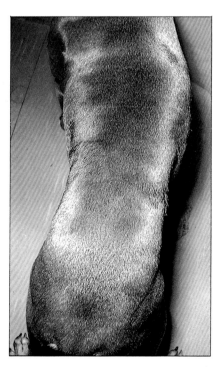

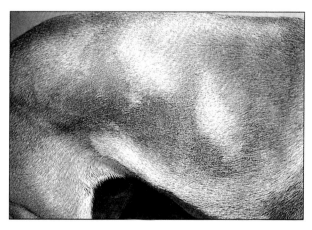

Plate 2:13a   Plate 2:13b

Hypothyroid, four-year-old, female boxer with bilaterally symmetrical, non-pruritic trunk alopecia and cutaneous
hyperpigmentation (basal TT4, 7.7 nmol/l; post-TSH TT4 10.6 nmol/l).

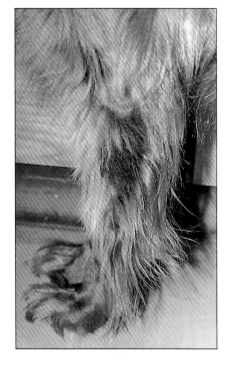

Plate 2:14
Hypothyroid, three-year-old, female Irish setter
with hypertrichosis ('carpet coat').
Much of the hair is paler than is normal
(basal TT4 < 5.0 nmol/l; post-TSH TT4 < 5.0 nmol/l).

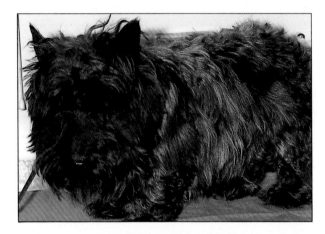

Plate 2:15a (above) and 2:15b (below)
Hypothyroid, five-year-old, male Scottish terrier. The dog shows
tragic facies. Alopecia was limited to the ventrum and was
associated with multi-focal hyperpigmentation and seborrhoea
oleosa (basal TT4, 17.4 nmol/l; post-TSH TT4 18.1 nmol/l).

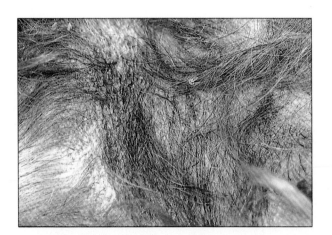

Plate 2:16
The dog in Plate 2:10 showing intertriginous, superficial
pyoderma. There was marked accompanying pruritus.

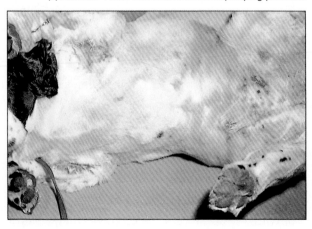

At the University of Edinburgh, the technique is carried out as shown in Table 4.

Thyroid scanning will also show reduced uptake of the radioisotope in canine hypothyroidism.

While immensely helpful, particularly in the evaluation of the hyperthyroid cat, this technique requires specialised equipment and may only be carried out at licensed centres. Several veterinary schools in the United Kingdom are equipped and licensed.

Table 4

Technique for thyroid imaging of hyperthyroid cats

1. Induce anaesthesia using ketamine hydrochloride.

2. Administer approximately 37 MBq (1 mCi) technetium—99m intravenously.

3. 20 minutes later, carry out a five minute gamma camera scan using a pinhole collimator.

THYROID BIOPSY

Principles. The histological examination of thyroid tissue is helpful in a number of situations. In dogs, it is essential in any form of goitre. It will also distinguish between euthyroidism, primary and secondary hypothyroidism. In suspected hyperthyroid cats, biopsy may be used to confirm that a mass is of thyroidal origin and to identify the specific histological abnormality.

Diagnostic applications

In dogs, thyroid biopsy may be carried out by a closed technique (fine needle aspirate, or by taking a core with a special needle such as a Vim Tru-Cut or Franklin-modified Vim-Silverman), or by an open technique by wedge biopsy, removal of the caudal quarter or by excision. Because the thyroid gland has a rich blood supply, great care must be exercised with respect to haemostasis. Biopsy will diagnose neoplasia and distinguish between the important causes of primary hypothyroidism (lymphocytic thyroiditis and idiopathic necrosis and atrophy). It will also distinguish between euthyroidism and primary and secondary hypothyroidism. The vacuoles present in the colloid of healthy thyroids are absent from those with secondary hypothyroidism.

In cats, closed biopsy is rarely indicated and the open technique is used to sample a lobe which is equivocally abnormal in size, colour or location at the time of unilateral thyroidectomy, thus indicating whether further surgery may be required. Because biopsy results may demonstrate absence of pathology, the procedure may reduce the incidence of post-operative hypoparathyroidism or prevent the lifelong administration of thyroid hormone replacement therapy (Black and Peterson, 1983). The biopsy should be taken from the caudal aspect of the gland which is the least vascular and which ensures preservation of the external parathyroid (Black and Peterson, 1983).

The sample can be removed with a wedge biopsy. Haemorrhage is controlled with digital pressure or with a deep, horizontal mattress suture. Another technique involves using a suture of polyglycolic acid or silk to amputate the caudal tip of the gland after ligation of the caudal vasculature.

CLINICAL CONDITIONS OF THE THYROID GLAND

THYROIDITIS

Thyroidal inflammatory disease may be acute or chronic. Acute thyroiditis is rare, usually infectious and associated with spread from localised extra-thyroidal disease.

Chronic thyroiditis appears to be of importance only in dogs. Lymphocytic thyroiditis, an autoimmune disorder, is probably the most important cause of canine hypothyroidism and is discussed subsequently. A familial, chronic, lymphocytic thyroiditis has also been described in research beagles but hypothyroidism does not usually result, presumably because enough functional gland remains.

THYROID NEOPLASIA

While neoplasms of the thyroid gland occur in both dogs and cats, there are marked variations in incidence and behaviour of such tumours between the species. In dogs, thyroid neoplasia is relatively rarely recognised clinically and most tumours are non-functional ('cold') and malignant. In cats, thyroid tumours are common and usually functional ('hot') and benign.

The term goitre is applied to an enlargement of the thyroid gland, irrespective of cause. In practice, goitre in both cats and dogs is usually associated with neoplasia.

CANINE THYROID NEOPLASIA

Neoplasms of the canine thyroid may result in euthyroidism, hypothyroidism or hyperthyroidism. In one series of cases, 54% of affected dogs were euthyroid, 40% were hypothyroid due to destruction of normal thyroid tissue by the tumour and 6% were hyperthyroid (Feldman and Nelson, 1987). Resultant hypo- and hyperthyroidism will be considered under the relevant sections.

Aetiology

Most investigators agree that of tumours detected clinically, more than 80% are malignant. Thus, all thyroid tumours in dogs should be considered malignant until proven otherwise.

Benign tumours. Most benign thyroid tumours (adenomas) in dogs are small, solid, focal, non or normally functioning masses which are not detected clinically (Feldman and Nelson, 1987).

Malignant tumours. Thyroid carcinomas may be of follicular or parafollicular (C cell) origin. The latter are uncommon. Tumours of follicular origin may be subclassified into a number of types but these classifications are somewhat subjective and of limited importance to the practitioner and thus will not be considered further.

Thyroid carcinomas are usually large and solid and local invasion and metastatic spread are common. The major lymphatic drainage is cranial from the thyroid, the retropharyngeal lymph nodes most commonly being involved, together with the lungs. Spread to almost any other tissue is possible. Thyroid neoplasia may occur in association with other endocrine neoplasia, the so-called multiple endocrine neoplasia (MEN) syndromes.

Breed, sex and age predispositions

Canine thyroid tumours are usually found in middle-aged to old animals. Beagles, boxers and golden retrievers are reported to be over-represented but there is no sex predisposition.

Historical and clinical features

In the absence of effects on thyroid function, affected dogs are usually presented because of a cervical mass. Other signs that have been reported include coughing, respiratory distress, polyuria, polydipsia, depression, weight loss, anorexia, vomiting or regurgitation, dysphagia, dysphonia and pain (Feldman and Nelson, 1987).

Physical examination reveals the presence of a firm, asymmetrical, variably (often non) mobile swelling. The submandibular lymph nodes may also be enlarged.

Investigative procedures

Non-specific tests

Radiology. Thoracic radiographs may reveal pulmonary metastatic spread.

Haematological and biochemical changes. Where tumours do not affect function, these are unremarkable.

Specific tests

Circulating thyroid hormone concentrations. Determination of TT4 and TT3 concentrations is mandatory in all cases of suspected thyroid neoplasia.

Radionuclide studies. In animals where normal function is maintained, such scans add little to the overall diagnostic investigation.

Biopsy. Because of the highly vascular nature of the canine thyroid tumour, fine needle (21 to 23 gauge) aspiration is the biopsy technique of choice. Even so, the sample may often be contaminated with blood making cytological diagnosis difficult. In such situations, it may be necessary to resort to open biopsy.

Treatment

Thyroid tumours which do not affect function may be treated in four ways: by surgery, chemotherapy, cobalt irradiation or by a combination technique. Cobalt irradiation will not be available to practitioners and, although in combination with partial surgical resection, may be the technique of choice for invasive thyroid malignancies, will not be considered further. Whatever technique is chosen, the prognosis remains guarded because of the potential of malignant thyroid tumours to recur locally or metastasise.

Surgery. Thyroid adenomas or small, non-invasive carcinomas may be relatively simply removed by unilateral thyroidectomy (ideally) or thyroparathyroidectomy after ligation of the local vasculature. Large masses may require bilateral thyroidectomy but in such cases an attempt should always be made to preserve both external parathyroid glands. Invasion of local structures may prevent complete excision but partial excision may reduce some of the signs previously discussed. The retropharyngeal lymph nodes should be examined and removed if metastasis is suspected.

Post-operative complications. After unilateral canine thyroidectomy, no special post-operative care is required. With bilateral thyroidectomy, monitoring for temporary or permanent hypoparathyroidism (hypocalcaemia) is required. The procedures and treatment regimens are the same for dogs and cats and are discussed in detail under post-operative complications of feline thyroidectomy. (page 45).

Long-term management. After bilateral thyroidectomy, T4 supplementation (Eltroxin, Glaxo) at a dose of 10-20 μg/kg twice daily is required. T4 therapy has also been recommended in thyroid carcinomas with or without associated surgery to reduce TSH secretion and thyroid stimulation.

Chemotherapy. This mode of therapy should be considered when total surgical removal of the tumour is not possible or metastasis is suspected or confirmed.

Doxorubicin (Adriamycin, Farmitalia C.E.) at a dose of 30 mg/m^2 body surface area administered intravenously every three weeks is the currently preferred treatment regimen. Treatment should be continued for six cycles or until the tumour has totally regressed or side-effects develop. Acute reactions to doxorubicin include anaphylaxis, gastrointestinal dysfunction, hypotension and cardiac arrhythmias (Susaneck, 1983) and should be treated using an antihistamine (H^1 receptor antagonist) such as chlorpheniramine maleate (Piriton injection, Allen and Hanburys). Dogs that have shown previous adverse reactions to doxorubicin should be pretreated with such an antihistamine. Chronic side-effects include weight loss, anorexia, bone marrow hypoplasia, alopecia, testicular atrophy and, most importantly, cardiomyopathy.

Combination therapy using vincristine (Oncovin, Lilly) at a dose of 0.5 mg/m^2 intravenously once weekly and cyclophosphamide (Endoxana, WBP) at a dose of 100-150 mg/m^2 intravenously every three weeks, together with doxorubicin may be attempted when doxorubicin therapy alone is ineffective.

FELINE THYROID NEOPLASIA

Neoplasms of the feline thyroid are usually functional (i.e. cause hyperthyroidism) or occasionally do not affect function (i.e. affected animals are euthyroid). There are no documented cases of feline thyroid neoplasia resulting in hypothyroidism.

Aetiology

Benign tumours. There is considerable uncertainty about the classification of benign feline thyroid tumours and Lucke (1968) was doubtful whether a true distinction should be made between what she termed nodular (adenomatous) goitre and single or multiple adenomas, except on the basis of size. Benign tumours are usually, but not invariably, associated with excessive hormone production.

Malignant tumours. Thyroid carcinoma, the primary cause of hyperthyroidism in the dog, rarely causes hyperthyroidism in the cat. When carcinomas occur, they usually co-exist with adenomatous changes. Plate 2.1 shows a non-functional papillary adenocarcinoma excised from a five year old, entire female, Persian cat.

Breed, sex and age predispositions. These are as for feline hyperthyroidism (see subsequently).

Historical and clinical features. In the absence of thyrotoxicosis (considered subsequently), benign thyroid tumours may be an incidental finding at post-mortem examination or, as with cases of non-functional thyroid carcinoma, animals may be presented by the owners because of a palpable cervical swelling. Other signs in one case of non-functional thyroid carcinoma seen by the author included local cervical discomfort and inappropriate urination and defaecation which resolved after successful surgical removal of the tumour.

Investigative procedures

Non-specific tests

> **Haematological and biochemical changes.** Where tumours are non-functional, these are unremarkable.

Specific tests

> **Circulating thyroid hormone concentrations.** Determination of TT4 and TT3 concentrations is mandatory in all cases of suspected thyroid neoplasia.

> **Biopsy.** Fine needle aspirate biopsy may be carried out to confirm the origin and nature of the thyroid tumour.

Treatment

Non-functional thyroid tumours in cats are usually treated by surgery. No special pre-operative treatment is required. The surgical technique and post-operative management is as described in detail under feline hyperthyroidism.

MEDULLARY CARCINOMA OF THE THYROID

Medullary carcinoma (parafollicular carcinoma, C cell tumour) arises from the parafollicular cells of the thyroid. In humans, they have a capacity for multiple hormone secretion (calcitonin, serotonin, adrenocorticotrophic hormone (ACTH) and prostaglandin E_2 and $F_2\alpha$ and medullary carcinoma may be associated with other APUD cell tumours. Medullary carcinoma of the thyroid has also been recognised in dogs (Leav *et al.*, 1976).

Although the acute effect of administered calcitonin is to decrease plasma calcium concentrations, humans and dogs with medullary carcinoma are usually eucalcaemic. Diarrhoea, possibly due to the production of serotonin or prostaglandins by the neoplasm, is the most marked symptom of canine medullary carcinoma.

A diagnosis of medullary carcinoma should always prompt a search for tumours of other embryologically related cells (e.g. phaeochromocytoma).

Treatment of canine medullary carcinoma is surgical removal.

ACCESSORY/ECTOPIC THYROID TUMOURS

Accessory thyroid carcinoma has been recorded in dogs in thyroid tissue in the pericardial sac and immediately anterior to the heart (Thake et al., 1971; Leav et al., 1976) and at the base of the tongue (Feldman and Nelson, 1987).

Noxon, et al., (1983) described hyperthyroidism associated with multinodular adenomatous goitre of one thyroid and an adenoma in possibly ectopic thyroid tissue in the jugular furrow of a cat. Surgical removal of the adenoma alone was curative.

HYPERTHYROIDISM

Hyperthyroidism (thyrotoxicosis) is a multisystemic disorder resulting from excessive circulating concentrations of T3 and/or T4. Although only first confirmed in 1979, feline hyperthyroidism is now considered to be one of the most common disorders of older cats. The literature on the condition has recently been reviewed in detail by Thoday (1988). Canine hyperthyroidism is a rare condition.

FELINE HYPERTHYROIDISM

Aetiology

Benign thyroid tumours, usually classified as thyroid adenomas (adenomatous hyperplasia) because of the difficulties in distinguishing between the two pathological changes, cause between 98 and 99% of cases. Functional thyroid carcinoma is causal in 1—2% of cases (Peterson et al., 1983).

The factors initiating feline hyperthyroidism are unknown. Thyroid antibodies (significantly correlated to bilateral goitre) and antinuclear antibody (ANA) have been described in affected animals.

Breed, sex and age predispositions

Hyperthyroidism is a disease of middle-aged to old cats, with no case yet being recorded in an animal below six years of age. There are no breed or sex predispositions.

Historical and clinical features

The signs of feline hyperthyroidism vary from mild to severe with most individuals showing dysfunction of a number of organ systems. Table 5 lists the important historical features of the disease reported in three published, independent series of the condition.

Physical appearance. Most hyperthyroid cats show mild to severe weight loss. Muscular weakness, tremor, heat intolerance and intermittent fever may also be seen. Central nervous system abnormalities such as hyperactivity, nervousness, an anxious facial expression (Plate 2:2) and aggressiveness are common.

Cutaneous signs of dry coat, greasy seborrhoea, patchy alopecia (Plates 2:3, 2:4) and matting (Plate 2:5) associated with failure to groom and increased nail growth, are frequent findings.

Gastrointestinal features. Polyphagia is one of the most frequently seen symptoms of the condition, alternating, in approximately 20% of cases, with short periods of inappetance. Other common gastrointestinal symptoms include vomiting (related or unrelated to feeding), increased frequency of defaecation, diarrhoea, increased faecal volume, steatorrhoea and excessive flatus.

Polyuria/polydipsia. Approximately 75% of cats show polyuria/polydipsia.

Cardiovascular features. A large number of cardiovascular abnormalities may be seen in hyperthyroid cats. Hyperaemia of the skin of the ears (Plate 2:6) and of the mucous membranes, suggestive of hypertension, may be observed. The area of cardiac auscultation may be increased. Tachycardia (rate up to 360 beats per minute), with or without premature beats, a strong femoral pulse, prominent precordial impulse, gallop rhythms and arrhythmias and apical left and/or right-sided systolic murmurs are all common. Cardiomegaly usually due to hypertrophic or rarely congestive cardiomyopathy may occur. Some cats are presented in congestive cardiac failure with pulmonary oedema and pleural effusion.

Table 5
Historical and clinical findings in three independent series of cases of feline hyperthyroidism

Clinical findings	Percentage of cases affected		
	Peterson *et al* (1983) (131 cases)	Hoenig *et al* (1982) (24 cases)	Holzworth *et al* (1980) (10 cases)
Weight loss	98	83	100
Polyphagia	81	79	70
Hyperactivity	76	38	70
Tachycardia	66	79	70
Polyuria/polydipsia	60	71	40 – 50
Vomiting	55	33	40
Cardiac murmur	53	NS	50
Diarrhoea	33	54	50
Increased faecal volume	31	NS	50
Anorexia	26	NS	NS
Polypnoea (panting)	25	33	NS
Heat intolerance	25	8	NS
Intermittent fever	25	8	70
Muscle weakness	25	NS	NS
Muscle tremor	18	NS	NS
Congestive cardiac failure	12	NS	NS
Increased nail growth	12	NS	NS
Dyspnoea	11	NS	NS
Skin changes	7	58	30
Ventral neck flexion	3	NS	NS
Hyperaemia of mucous membranes and skin	NS	NS	30
Voice change	NS	8	NS
Palpable thyroid lobe(s)	90	88	100

NS = not specified

Reproduced, with permission, from Thoday (1988).

Respiratory features. Respiratory abnormalities, in particular tachypnoea and dyspnoea, occasionally accompanied by sneezing, occur in approximately 33% of cases.

Apathetic hyperthyroidism. Approximately 8-10% of affected cats present with depression rather than hyperactivity and inappetance rather than polyphagia, often in association with severe cardiac abnormalities. Clinicians should be aware of this form of the disease which is comparable with so-called apathetic (masked) hyperthyroidism of man.

Goitre. Palpable thyroid enlargement is present in approximately 96% of affected cats (Thoday, 1986a). Goitre may be unilateral or bilateral. Plates 2:7a and 2:7b and 2:8a and 2:8b illustrate unilateral and bilateral goitre respectively in hyperthyroid cats. As the thyroid gland of healthy cats is not palpable, the detection of a neck mass must make the clinician highly suspicious of hyperthyroidism, although it must be remembered that not all thyroid masses are hyperfunctional. The detection of feline goitre may, on occasions, be difficult even for those with experience in the field. Affected glands are freely mobile and commonly migrate ventrally. They may also become retro-tracheal or intra-thoracic. Each side of the neck should be palpated with the ends of the fingers *with great care* along the jugular furrow, supporting the contra-lateral side with the thumb of the same or the other hand. Anterior migration of suspected intra-thoracic lobes for diagnostic purposes may be made possible by heavily sedating or anaesthetising animals and holding them vertically with the head pointing downwards.

Investigative procedures

As hyperthyroidism is a multisystemic disorder, a large number of procedures have been used in its investigation. They may be divided into those tests which specifically incriminate abnormal thyroid function and non-specific tests which may still be helpful to the practitioner because they may be performed 'in-house' and lend support to the performance of specific diagnostic procedures which are usually more expensive and require external laboratory support.

Non-specific tests

Radiology. Thoracic radiographs reveal cardiomegaly in up to 50% of cases (reviewed by Thoday, 1988). A lateral radiograph is most helpful in detecting this change (Van den Broek and Darke, 1987). An example is shown in Figure 3a. Evidence of pulmonary oedema and/or pleural effusion may be seen if there is associated heart failure.

Electrocardiography. Numerous electrocardiographic disturbances have been reported in hyperthyroid cats. The most frequent changes are sinus tachycardia (rate greater than 240 beats per minute) and an increase in R wave amplitude (greater than 0.9 mV) in lead II, suggestive of left ventricular enlargement. Other important changes include prolonged QRS duration, short Q-T interval, atrial and ventricular premature complexes, left anterior fascicular block, right bundle-branch block, first and second degree atrioventricular block, atrial or ventricular tachycardia and ventricular pre-excitation.

Echocardiography. Bond *et al.,* (1983) reported echocardiographic abnormalities in 29 of 30 affected cats. The most important changes were left ventricular hypertrophy, aortic root and left atrial enlargement and increased parameters of contractibility. Facilities for ultrasonography are likely to become available to an increasing number of practitioners.

Haematological changes. While haematological changes (raised packed cell volume (PCV), erythrocytosis, occasionally mild anaemia) may be found in hyperthyroid cats, the changes are of little diagnostic value.

Biochemical changes. There are alterations in many biochemical parameters in hyperthyroidism, the most common being mild to moderate elevations in one or more of the following: serum alkaline phosphatase (AP), alanine aminotransferase (ALT) and aspartate aminotransferase (AST). Peterson *et al.,* (1983) reported that 127 of 131 cases of feline hyperthyroidism had elevations of at least one of AP, ALT, AST or lactate dehydrogenase (LDH). On biopsy, the liver shows only mild, non-specific changes.

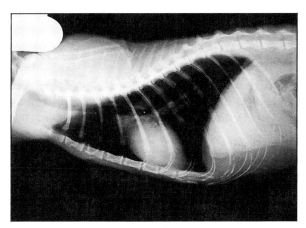 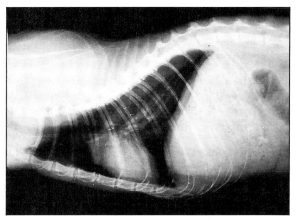

Figure 3a.
Lateral thoracic radiograph of a hyperthyroid, 12-year-old, neutered male, domestic short-haired cat showing cardiac enlargement. The cranial and caudal cardiac borders are rounded (TT4, 296.7 nmol/l; TT3, 5.57 nmol/l). The dimensions used to determine heart size were the apicobasilar length and the craniocaudal width.

Figure 3b.
Lateral thoracic radiograph of the same cat in Figure 3a, 11 weeks after successful surgical treatment showing reduction in cardiac size (TT4, 24.8 nmol/l; TT3, 0.55 nmol/l).

The serum cholesterol concentration is in the normal range. Mild to moderate hyperphosphataemia occurs in approximately 20% of hyperthyroid cats.

Faeces examination. Mild to marked steatorrhoea is common in hyperthyroid cats. Peterson *et al.,* (1981) reported 48-hour faecal fat contents of 5.5—35.3 g fat (normal was less than 3.5 g).

Specific tests

Circulating thyroid hormone concentrations. TT4 and TT3 concentrations are elevated above the normal range in most hyperthyroid cats. Occasionally, TT3 concentrations are at the high end of the reference range, which may reflect either early, mild disease or animals with severe, concurrent non-thyroidal illnesses.

FT4 is, not suprisingly, also elevated in affected cats.

TSH stimulation test. Where the TT3 and/or TT4 concentrations are elevated, this test adds nothing to the diagnosis of the disease. A failure to respond to TSH (see page 29) in animals with high-normal TT4 and suspected hyperthyroidism, supports the diagnosis. A normal response, however, does not exclude the condition (Thoday, 1986a).

Radionuclide studies

Thyroidal radioiodine uptake. The mean thyroidal RIU of 32 hyperthyroid cats, 24 hours after the intravenous administration of ^{131}I was 39.1% (mean normal value was 9.2%) (Peterson *et al.,* 1983). Because many factors, including high dietary iodine, renal disease and numerous drugs may decrease thyroidal RIU, such measurements are a relatively insensitive, and from a practitioner's viewpoint, an unnecessarily complicated test for hyperthyroidism. Thyroidal RIU is, therefore, most useful in determining the ^{131}I dose for treatment of hyperthyroidism.

Thyroid imaging. In feline hyperthyroidism, thyroid imaging, usually using technetium—99m as pertechnetate, is a very useful procedure to determine unilateral or bilateral lobe involvement; alterations in position of the lobes; the site of hyperfunctional accessory/ectopic thyroid tissue and the presence of regional or distant metastasis from a functional thyroid carcinoma. Where thyroid imaging facilities are not available, the clinician can only make the decision on whether to remove one or both thyroid lobes on their gross appearance at the time of surgery.

Pertechnetate is concentrated primarily in three tissues: the thyroid, the salivary glands and the gastric mucosa. In addition, the heart may be visualised, but this is merely because of its contained blood. Healthy cats show a consistent thyroid/salivary ratio of pertechnetate uptake of approximately one (Beck *et al.,* 1985), whereas in hyperthyroid animals, the ratio is much higher (and the salivary glands are therefore less easily seen) because of the increased thyroidal uptake.

Treatment.

Feline hyperthyroidism may be treated in three ways: by surgery, with radioactive iodine (^{131}I) or by long-term use of an antithyroid drug. Because radioiodine therapy requires specialist facilities and long-term medical therapy has problems with continued owner compliance, surgical thyroidectomy is the treatment of choice for most thyrotoxic cats.

Surgery. Feline thyroidectomy is a relatively simple procedure. However, because hyperthyroidism is a multisystemic disease, affected cats have increased anaesthetic and surgical risks which can be minimised by suitable pre-operative treatment.

Pre-operative treatment. The two most widely used drugs have been propylthiouracil (PTU) and methimazole (MMI). PTU is now considered to be too toxic for use in cats. MMI is not available in the UK but carbimazole (CBZ) (Neo-Mercazole, Nicholas), which is metabolised to methimazole in plasma and is the preferred drug in humans in this country, is effective and safe in cats and is the pre-operative treatment of choice. At a dosage of 5 mg three times daily, most hyperthyroid cats become euthyroid in one to three weeks.

Propranolol (Inderal, ICI), a β1 and β2—adrenergic receptor antagonist, prevents many of the cardiovascular and neuromuscular effects of excess thyroid hormones and controls the tachycardia and hyperexcitability associated with feline hyperthyroidism, at a dosage of 2.5—5.0 mg three times daily. It may be used together with CBZ in severe cases of hyperthyroidism and tapered and stopped as the CBZ-induced euthyroidism develops.

In man, pre-operative potassium iodide reduces thyroid size and vascularity. Similar beneficial effects occur in cats, a dosage of 10 mg three times daily for 10 days prior to surgery being satisfactory (Thoday, 1986a). It should be administered in dilute solution (10 mg/ml) to reduce the possibility of gastric irritation and vomiting (Thoday, 1985).

Anaesthesia. A regimen should be used which minimises the risk of death from cardiac arrhythmia. Premedication with acetylpromazine, induction with ketamine hydrochloride (Vetalar, Parke, Davis) and maintenance with nitrous oxide or halothane alone or in combination is satisfactory.

Anticholinergic agents such as atropine should not be used as they may cause sinus tachycardia and enhance anaesthetic-induced cardiac arrhythmias. Glycopyrolate (Robinul, Robins) is the anticholinergic of choice if required.

Surgical technique. The cat is positioned in dorsal recumbency with the forelimbs pulled caudally and the neck slightly extended. After incising the skin from the larynx to the manubrium, the sternohyoideus and sternothyroideus muscles are separated by blunt dissection to reveal the thyroid lobes.

Where thyroid imaging facilities are not available, the clinician can only decide on whether to carry out a unilateral or bilateral thyroidectomy on the gross appearance of the lobes. In cases of unilateral pathology, the unaffected lobe should appear atrophic to normal. However, in one study, approximately 15% of cats with subsequently proven bilateral lobe involvement had one lobe which could have been mistaken grossly as being normal at the time of surgery (Peterson and Turrel, 1986) and unilateral thyroidectomy in such cases results in eventual recurrence of the disease.

Thyroidectomy may be either extracapsular or intracapsular.

Extracapsular technique. The cranial and caudal thyroid vessels are ligated and transected. Dissection of the loose cervical fascia surrounding the gland allows its removal (Plate 2:9) (Black and Peterson, 1983). The internal parathyroid is embedded in the substance of the thyroid and cannot be preserved. Disadvantages of this technique include possible sacrifice of the external parathyroid or temporary/permanent damage to this gland's blood supply with the risk of post-operative hypocalcaemia either immediately or on further thyroidectomy if the contralateral lobe subsequently becomes involved in the disease process.

Intracapsular thyroidectomy circumvents these problems (Birchard *et al.,* 1984; Peterson *et al.,* 1984). Here, the caudal thyroid vein is ligated and transected. A nick incision is then made in an avascular area of the ventral, caudal thyroid capsule and extended with scissors until the entire capsule is opened. The thyroid parenchyma is then bluntly dissected using sterile cotton-buds leaving the thyroid capsule, the external parathyroid and its blood supply, intact. If thyroid tissue fragments during separation from the capsule, all pieces must be removed. If there is bilateral lobe involvement, the procedure is repeated for the other lobe. One disadvantage of this technique is the frequent, profuse haemorrhage during blunt dissection. More importantly, spillage of cystic fluid together with viable thyroid cells or leaving tiny remnants of thyroid tissue on the capsule may result in eventual recurrence of the hyperthyroidism.

Whatever the technique used, after examining the surgical field for haemostasis, the incision is closed routinely. After bilateral thyroidectomy, plasma calcium concentration should be monitored daily for five days or until it has stabilised in the reference range.

Post-operative complications. Reported early post-operative complications include hypoparathyroidism, Horner's syndrome and voice changes.

Hypoparathyroidism, resulting from injury, devascularisation or inadvertent surgical removal of the external parathyroids, results in hypocalcaemia which may be seen as heightened neuromuscular irritability with muscle tremors, tetany and generalised convulsions. As only one parathyroid gland is required to maintain normocalcaemia, hypoparathyroidism only occurs after bilateral thyroidectomy. A marginal fall in plasma calcium concentration is common in cats after thyroparathyroid surgery. In the author's laboratory (plasma calcium reference range 2.1—2.9 mmol/l) clinical signs of hypoclacaemia do not usually occur if the plasma calcium concentration remains above 1.2 mmol/l and no treatment is usually given to these cases. In most cats with iatrogenic hypoparathyroidism, clinical signs develop within one to three days of surgery.

Treatment of hypoparathyroidism involves the use of calcium with or without vitamin D. A number of regimens have been recommended (reviewed by Thoday, 1988). The currently used regimen at the Royal (Dick) School of Veterinary Studies is shown in Table 6 (see also page 70).

In most cases, iatrogenic hypocalcaemia in cats resolves spontaneously days, weeks or months after surgery. In such cases, the hypocalcaemia probably results from reversible parathyroid damage or ischaemia, or accessory parathyroid tissue may become functional (Peterson, 1984).

Table 6
Currently used regimen at the Royal (Dick) School of Veterinary Studies, University of Edinburgh
for the management of iatrogenic hypocalcaemia in cats

(A)   ACUTE PHASE

  1.   Initially, administer 10—15 mg/kg elemental calcium intravenously over 10—20 minutes, simultaneously auscultating the heart. Stop if bradycardia develops. This is equivalent to:

       1.0—1.5 ml/kg 10% calcium gluconate (Calcium Gluconate injection B.P.)

       or

       1.0—1.5 ml/kg 10% calcium glubionate (Calcium Sandoz Ampoules 10%, Sandoz).

  2.   Once signs are controlled, administer by slow, continuous, intravenous infusion:
       —2.5 ml/kg 10% calcium gluconate/glubionate in 150 ml isotonic saline over eight hours. Repeat if required.

(B)   MAINTENANCE

  Begin oral therapy as soon as it can be tolerated. Administer:

  1.   50—75 mg/kg/day elemental calcium orally as
       —500 —750 mg/kg/day calcium gluconate (Calcium Gluconate Tablets B.P.) (600mg) in three or four *divided* doses.

       or

       —400 —600 mg/kg/day calcium lactate (Calcium Lactate Tablets B.P.) (300 mg, 600 mg less readily available) in three or four *divided* doses.

  2.   0.03 mg/kg dihydrotachysterol (Tachyrol, Duphar [tablets], once daily. AT 10, Sterling Research [solution]), once daily.

  Once the plasma calcium concentration is stable, decrease the dihydrotachysterol by 0.01 mg/kg every alternate day. Subsequently, assess calcium and dihydrotachysterol requirement according to plasma calcium concentration.

Horner's syndrome. resulting from injury to the cervical sympathetic trunk, may occur as a sequel to feline thyroidectomy.

Voice changes. The recurrent laryngeal nerves lying close to the thyroid lobes, are less than 1 mm in diameter, and may be damaged during thyroidectomy in cats. Resultant signs include temporary or permanent voice changes, cough and harsh respiratory sounds.

Long-term management. Following thyroidectomy for hyperthyroidism, elevated plasma TT3 and TT4 concentrations become normal or subnormal within 24 and 48 hours respectively. After hemithyroidectomy for unilateral lobe involvement, TT4 and TT3 concentrations become subnormal because of atrophy of the contralateral lobe but return to the normal range within eight weeks. Most cats which have undergone bilateral thyroidectomy do not require any thyroid hormone supplementation, plasma concentrations returning to normal within three to six months. During this time, exogenous thyroid hormones are not required as they delay a return to T4 and T3 self-sufficiency because of their negative feedback effects on TSH production.

Permanent hypothyroidism should be confirmed by the demonstration of subnormal plasma TT4 and TT3 concentrations and failure to show normal increase in these hormones after TSH stimulation. In such cases, suitable replacement therapy is 10 μg/kg thyroxine sodium (Eltroxin, Glaxo) twice daily.

After successful surgery, the symptoms, signs and laboratory abnormalities of hyperthyroidism resolve (Figure 3b). In a small number of cases, there may be some residual changes of cardiomyopathy. Because hyperthyroidism may recur in cases of initially unilateral or bilateral thyroid lobe involvement, it is recommended that all hyperthyroid cats treated surgically should have their serum TT4 and TT3 concentrations monitored at six to twelve month intervals to ensure early diagnosis of any relapse.

Radioactive iodine. In human medicine, radioactive iodine (^{131}I) provides a simple, effective and safe treatment for hyperthyroidism. After concentration within the gland, radioactive iodine selectively irradiates and destroys functional thyroid tissue. However, dosages have to be carefully calculated as hypothyroidism results from overdosage and persistent or recurrent hyperthyroidism results from inadequate therapy. [131]I has been used successfully to treat feline hyperthyroidism (reviewed by Thoday, 1988). However, as this technique is unlikely to be available to the practitioner, it will not be further considered here.

Long-term anti-thyroid drug therapy. This therapeutic approach has been suggested for the management of feline hyperthyroidism where unrelated medical conditions increase the surgical risk, owners refuse surgical treatment and radioiodine therapy is unavailable (Peterson, 1981, 1982).

As discussed previously with respect to pre-operative treatment, propylthiouracil (PTU), methimazole (MMI) and carbimazole (CBZ) reduce the plasma TT4 and TT3 concentrations in most hyperthyroid cats to the reference range within one to three weeks. All suffer a number of disadvantages.

These drugs do not remove the underlying thyroid pathology and, if they are discontinued or given irregularly by the owner, the thyroid hormone concentrations increase again. It may also be difficult to maintain the euthyroid state without regular changes in the dosages of the drug.

Minor adverse reactions to PTU in cats are common and include lethargy, vomiting, inappetence, facial swelling and pruritus. More serious side-effects include hepatopathy, immune-mediated haemolytic anaemia, thrombocytopenia and a positive serum ANA titre. For these reasons, *the use of PTU for control of feline hyperthyroidism is no longer recommended* (Peterson and Turrel, 1986).

Both MMI and its parent compound CBZ appear to be better tolerated and safer than PTU in cats. Since MMI is not available in the UK, *CBZ is the drug of choice for the long-term medical management of feline hyperthyroidism.* The drug is used initially as described under pre-operative treatment (see page 44. Although the author has yet to see side-effects other than transient vomiting and depression with CBZ, haematological abnormalities (transient to severe leucopenia, eosinophilia, lymphocytosis, severe thrombocytopenia) have been recorded with MMI in cats and complete blood and thrombocyte counts should therefore be performed at two week intervals, especially between the second and twelfth weeks of therapy when these effects usually occurred (Peterson and Turrel, 1986). Granulocytopenia and thrombocytopenia are reasons for discontinuing the drug.

The long-term maintenance dosage of CBZ is 5 mg two or three times daily. To maintain TT4 and TT3 concentrations in the reference range and to monitor for serious adverse reactions, complete blood and thrombocyte counts and serum thyroid hormone concentrations should be carried out at three monthly intervals and CBZ dosages adjusted accordingly.

CANINE HYPERTHYROIDISM

Aetiology

The only reported cause of canine hyperthyroidism is functional thyroid neoplasia (see page 38).

Historical and clinical features

The historical and clinical features of canine hyperthyroidism are very similar to the feline condition and the reader is referred to this section for a full review. However, in dogs, the cervical mass is more prominent and may be the reason for presentation to the veterinary surgeon.

Investigative procedures

Non specific tests
As in the feline condition, these tests are helpful in supporting the diagnosis (see page 39).

Specific tests

Circulating thyroid hormone concentrations. Elevated TT3 and/or TT4 concentrations confirm the diagnosis of hyperthyroidism. Where significant elevations of both TT4 *and* TT3 are found, thyroid carcinoma should be assumed to be present.

Thyroid biopsy. Cytological examination of needle aspirates may confirm the nature of the mass.

Radionuclide studies. Where facilities exist, thyroid imaging with technetium is useful to confirm the presence of a mass, to delineate it and to identify any metastases. An RIU test will confirm that the mass traps iodide which is important therapeutically as such tumours may be treated with radioiodine.

Treatment

Functional canine thyroid tumours may be treated by surgery with or without chemotherapy, by irradiation with radioiodine, by cobalt irradiation or by chemotherapy alone. The principles of each of these modes of therapy have been discussed previously (see page 39). Where metastasis has already occurred, radioiodine therapy has the advantage of being effective against both primary and secondary tumours. Drugs that simply reduce TT4 and TT3 concentrations (e.g. PTU, MMI, CBZ) should not be used alone because they are not cytotoxic to the causal thyroid carcinoma. However, such drugs, potassium iodide and propranolol may all be used for pre-operative treatment of canine hyperthyroidism. Initial doses of PTU and propranolol for dogs are 3.3 mg/kg and 1-5 mg/kg respectively, three times daily.

HYPOTHYROIDISM

Hypothyroidism is a multisystemic disorder associated with a deficiency of thyroid hormone activity. Canine hypothyroidism is the commonest endocrine disorder in dogs. In cats, only congenital hypothyroidism, which is extremely rare, has been confirmed.

CANINE HYPOTHYROIDISM

Aetiology

Hypothyroidism may be classified as congenital or acquired, primary, secondary or tertiary, naturally-occurring or iatrogenic. Congenital hypothyroidism (resulting from thyroidal agenesis or inadequate maternal intake of iodine during gestation) is termed cretinism. The prefixes primary, secondary and tertiary describe the site of the lesion and refer to the thyroid, pituitary and hypothalamus respectively.

Table 7 lists possible causes of canine hypothyroidism. However, approximately 90% of cases are due to naturally-occurring, acquired, primary diseases (lymphocytic thyroiditis and idiopathic necrosis and atrophy).

Primary hypothyroidism. *Lymphocytic thyroiditis,* an autoimmune disorder involving both humoral and cell-mediated components, is probably the most important cause of canine hypothyroidism. The resulting thyroidal destruction is progressive, with signs of hypothyroidism developing when more that 75% of the gland has been destroyed. It has been suggested that *idiopathic necrosis and atrophy* may be the end result of lymphocytic thyroiditis although the possibility that it is an unrelated degenerative disorder has also been proposed. Neither condition is goitrous. *Non-functional neoplasia* (see page 38) and *thyroidal aplasia/hypoplasia* are rare primary causes of hypothyroidism.

Secondary hypothyroidism. TSH deficiency results in inadequate thyroidal stimulation and reduced thyroid hormone production. This may be *congenital* (usually accompanied by growth hormone deficiency) resulting in pituitary dwarfism, or *acquired* as a result of pituitary neoplasia. These cases may show neurological abnormalities or signs of other endocrine system involvement (e.g. diabetes insipidus and hyper or hypo-adrenocorticolism. Less than 5% of clinical cases of canine hypothyroidism are due to secondary causes.

All other causes of hypothyroidism in dogs are extremely rare.

Table 7
Possible causes of canine hypothyroidism

```
(A)   NATURALLY-OCCURRING
      1.    Primary (Reduced T4/T3 production)
            (a)   Congenital
                  (i)    Thyroid aplasia or hypoplasia
            (b)   Acquired
                  (i)    Lymphocytic thyroiditis
                  (ii)   Idiopathic necrosis and atrophy
                  (iii)  Neoplasia

      2.    Secondary (Reduced TSH production)
            (a)   Congenital
                  (i)    Hypopituitarism (pituitary dwarfism)
            (b)   Acquired
                  (i)    Pituitary neoplasia
                  (ii)   Other pituitary lesions (e.g. trauma)

      3.    Tertiary (Reduced TRH production)
            (a)   Congenital
            (b)   Acquired

      4.    Defective thyroid hormone production
            (a)   Congenital
                  (i)    Dyshormonogenesis
            (b)   Acquired
                  (i)    Iodine deficiency

      5.    Other defects
            (i)    T4 or T3 antibodies
            (ii)   Abnormalities of intestinal T4 absorption?      'Poor converters'
            (iii)  Abnormal plasma protein binding?
            (iv)   Abnormalities of T4 -> T3 conversion?

(B)   IATROGENIC
      1.    Primary (Reduced T4/T3 production)
            (i)    Thyroid ablation (surgery, radioiodine)
            (ii)   Antithyroid drugs (e.g. PTU, MMI, CBZ)

      2.    Secondary (Reduced TSH production)
            (i)    Pituitary ablation
            (ii)   Pituitary irradiation
```

Tertiary hypothyroidism. TRH deficiency should result in TSH deficiency and reduced thyroid hormone production. This tertiary (hypothalamic) hypothyroidism has been rarely but definitively described in man and suspected in a small number of dogs.

Defective thyroid hormone production. Iodine deficiency is likely to be extremely rare in the UK because commercial pet food contains more than adequate amounts of this micronutrient.

Breed, sex and age predispositions

Reported breed predispositions to hypothyroidism vary according to the country of origin of the report and are not necessarily applicable to the UK. Males and females are equally affected. The age at onset is most commonly between six and ten years but may be younger, particularly in large or giant breeds.

Historical and clinical features

The signs of canine hypothyroidism vary from mild to severe and involve one or a large number of organ systems in any combination and thus the condition has been well-described as "the great impersonator". Table 8 lists the important historical and clinical features of the condition. It is essential for the practitioner to remember that an animal may exhibit any one sign in isolation or any combination of the signs listed.

General features. Affected animals may show lack of endurance progressing to lethargy with or without mental depression. Because these changes are insidious, owners are frequently unaware they have occurred or, in an older animal, merely attribute them to ageing, until successful treatment results in resolution. Classically, hypothyroid dogs are obese (Plate 2:10) but more commonly are of normal weight or may even be thin. Most affected dogs have a normal (although often low end of the range) rectal temperature. Subnormal temperatures are uncommon.

Table 8
Important historical and clinical features of canine hypothyroidism

A. GENERAL FEATURES
   Lack of endurance
   Lethargy
   Mental depression
   Weight gain, loss, no change
   Normal, low-normal, reduced
      body temperature

B. GASTROINTESTINAL FEATURES
   Abnormalities uncommon
   Appetite usually normal
   Occasionally, may show:
      Vomiting
      Diarrhoea
      Constipation

C. CARDIOVASCULAR FEATURES
   Low normal heart rate to bradycardia
   Weak apex beat
   Cardiac arrhythmias

D. REPRODUCTIVE FEATURES
   Decreased libido
   Irregular oestrous cycles/anoestrus
   Infertility (male and female)
   Testicular atrophy
   Gynecomastia
   Galactorrhoea

E. OCULAR FEATURES
   Blepharoptosis
   Corneal lipidosis
   Keratoconjunctivitis sicca
   Corneal ulceration
   Uveitis
   Retinopathy

F. NEUROMUSCULAR FEATURES
   Myopathy
   Myalgia
   Neuropathy
   Excessive wear of dorsal nails
   Laryngeal paralysis

G. CUTANEOUS FEATURES
   Lack of primary pruritus
   Alopecia (patchy, bilaterally symmetrical)
   Coat dull, dry, easily epilated,
      fails to regrow after clipping
   Hypertrichosis
   Skin thick, (myxoedema), cool,
      hyperpigmented, tragic facies
   Comedones
   Seborrhoea
   Hyperkeratotic plaques (particularly pinnae)
   Pyoderma (with or without secondary pruritus)
   Easy bruising
   Poor wound healing

Gastrointestinal features. Most affected dogs have no gastrointestinal abnormalities. The appetite is usually normal. Rarely, diarrhoea, constipation or vomiting may be noted.

Cardiovascular features. Most affected dogs have a normal heart rate although it may be towards the low end of the range. Rarely bradycardia may be noted. There may be a weak apex beat and various cardiac arrythmias may be noted.

Reproductive features. Hypothyroid bitches commonly fail to exhibit oestrous cycles. There may be decreased libido and infertility in both sexes, testicular atrophy and, rarely, gynecomastia and galactorrhoea.

Ocular features. These are rare in hypothyroid dogs, with the most common abnormality being blepharoptosis. Corneal lipidosis (arcus lipoides) is occasionally seen.

Neuromuscular features. Signs attributable to neuromuscular dysfunction include muscle wasting (particularly temporals and masseters), stiffness and weakness. Excessive wear of the dorsal part of the nails is a subtle but not uncommon sign. Facial palsy and laryngeal paralysis have also been associated with hypothyroidism. Treatment of the thyroid dysfunction appears to reverse these abnormalities provided it is given in the early stages.

Cutaneous features. The cutaneous signs of hypothyroidism are legion. Classically, there is bilaterally symmetrical, non-pruritic alopecia which spares the distal limbs (Plates 2:11, 2:12, 2:13). The remaining haircoat is easily epilated and fails to regrow, or regrows only slowly after clipping. There are varying degrees of hyperpigmentation and thickened, non-pitting skin (myxoedema). However, there are so many variations from this picture in hypothyroid dogs — including no skin changes, that the clinician must be perpetually on his guard to eliminate this diagnosis in dermatological cases. Alopecia, with or without pigmentation, may be focal, multifocal or asymmetric. It commonly affects the tail ('rat-tail'), the dorsal muzzle and, in giant breeds, the distal limbs. In some breeds, classically the boxer and the Irish setter, hair may fail to be shed resulting in hypertrichosis ('carpet-coat'). This hair may be paler than normal (Plate 2:14).

Skin over the dorsum is often thickened and that over the eyes may droop giving a tragic facial expression (facies) (Plates 2:10 and 2:15a). Seborrhoea is common and may be dry, greasy (Plate 2:15b) or associated with inflammation. Comedones are common, particularly over the dorsum and hyperkeratotic plaques may occur around the borders of the pinnae.

Superficial (folliculitis) (Plate 2:16) or deep (furunculosis) focal, multifocal or generalised pyoderma occurs frequently. It is, therefore, *essential to screen the thyroid function of all dogs presented with recurrent skin infections at any site whether or not they have other evidence of hypothyroidism.* In the presence of seborrhoea or pyoderma, hypothyroidism may be accompanied by pruritus.

Poor wound healing and easy bruising have also been reported.

Investigative procedures

Hypothyroidism, like hyperthyroidism, is a multisystemic disorder. Thus, a number of non-specific tests may support the clinical diagnosis.

Non-specific tests

Radiology. Radiographic examination of the skeleton of congenitally hypothyroid dogs may reveal epiphyseal dysplasia of the long bones, delayed epiphyseal closure of the carpal and tarsal bones with valgus deformities and vertebral abnormalities (Feldman & Nelson, 1987).

Electrocardiography. ECG abnormalities may include sinus bradycardia, low voltages in all leads, flattening or inversion of the T wave and arrhythmias.

Haematological changes. A physiological, hypoplastic (normocytic, normochromic) anaemia (an adaption to reduced oxygen usage) with decreased packed cell volume (<36 l/l), red blood cell count and haemoglobin concentration, is seen in approximately 25% of hypothyroid dogs.

Secondary nutritional anaemias, as seen in some hypothyroid humans, are very rare in dogs. Lepttocytes (red blood cells with large cellular envelopes or membranes reflecting increased membrane cholesterol loading), may also be seen (Feldman & Feldman, 1977). Elevations of the erythrocyte sedimentation rate (ESR) are also common.

Biochemical changes. There are alterations in a number of biochemical parameters in hypothyroidism, but these are variable and inconsistent. Increases in plasma lipid concentrations are the classical changes. Hypercholesterolaemia, although not pathognomonic for hypothyroidism, occurs in 33% (Muller *et al.,* 1983) to 75% (Feldman & Nelson, 1987) of cases. Plasma cholesterol concentrations are influenced by feeding and should be taken after a minimum of 12 hours' starvation. Hypertriglyceridaemia and changes in lipoprotein electrophoresis may also occur.

Serum creatinine phosphokinase (CPK) is commonly elevated whether or not myopathy is detectable clinically. Mild to marked elevations of AP, ALT, AST,and LDH may also occur.

Urine changes. Urine analysis is usually normal in hypothyroid dogs. Proteinuria has been occasionally recorded as a result of immune-complex glomerulonephritis in lymphocytic thyroiditis.

Skin biopsy. In canine hypothyroidism, this may reveal many non-diagnostic changes consistent with endocrinopathy (orthokeratotic hyperkeratosis, epidermal atrophy, epidermal melanosis, follicular keratosis, follicular dilatation, follicular atrophy, a predominance of telogen hair follicles and sebaceous gland atrophy). Histological findings very suggestive of hypothyroidism include vacuolated and/or hypertrophied arrector pilae muscles, thickened dermis and increased dermal mucin (Scott, 1982).

Specific tests

Circulating thyroid hormone concentrations. As previously discussed, a low circulating TT4 or FT4 concentration will support but not confirm a diagnosis of hypothyroidism in the presence of compatible historical features. Definitive diagnosis relies on the results of TSH stimulation testing. Where the TT4 is extremely low, the diagnosis may reasonably be presumed. For example, the author has never seen a normal TT4 response to TSH stimulation in a dog with a TT4 of 7 nmol/l or less (normal TT4 range with this technique is 13—52 nmol/l).

There is little additional diagnostic value in practice to be obtained from measurement of TT3 or FT3 concentrations.

Combination of FT4 and cholesterol concentrations. Recently a novel combination has been said to increase the diagnostic accuracy of non-dynamic function testing. Using the equation:

$$k = 0.7 \times FT4 \text{ concentration (nmol/l)} - \text{cholesterol concentration (mmol/l)},$$

a k-value < -4 gave a definitive diagnosis of hypothyroidism whereas a k-value of $> +1$ indicated thyroid normality or failure to respond to thyroid supplementation (Larsson, 1988).

The TSH stimulation test. Currently, despite the present difficulties in the UK in obtaining the drug, the determination of circulating TT4 concentrations before and after TSH administration remains the most convenient method for the definitive diagnosis of canine hypothyroidism. While some practitioners dismiss its use because of the involved expense, this is minimal compared to that of long-term, unnecessary thyroid hormone supplementation (which is also ill-advised). The regimen for this test and its interpretation are described on page 29.

Recently, the diagnostic accuracy of the test has been been refined by combining the TT4 and the increase in TT4 concentrations after TSH administration (Larsson, 1988).

Using the equation:

$$k = 0.5 \times \text{basal TT4 concn (nmol/l)} + \text{increase in TT4 concn after TSH (nmol/l)},$$

all dogs with a k – value of < 15 were hypothyroid while dogs with k > 30 were not hypothyroid or were unresponsive to treatment.

When a TSH stimulation test is required in an animal that is already receiving thyroid hormone supplementation, the drug should be discontinued for a minimum of four weeks prior to the test to allow any induced thyroidal suppression to recover.

The TRH stimulation test. The principles and clinical application of this test have been discussed on page 31. The test is theoretically of greater diagnostic value than the TSH stimulation test because it will indicate both primary and secondary hypothyroidism. However, as TRH does not directly stimulate the thyroid, the test also has a greater potential margin of error and the value of the test in separating euthyroid and hypothyroid dogs has yet to be critically evaluated.

Radionuclide studies. These techniques have been considered previously. They are unlikely to be carried out under practice conditions.

Thyroid biopsy. Thyroid biopsy will distinguish between euthyroidism, primary hypothyroidism and secondary hypothyroidism. In addition, it will distinguish between lymphocytic thyroiditis and idiopathic necrosis and atrophy. The technique and its interpretation are discussed on page 37.

Treatment

Hypothyroidism may be treated in three ways: using dessicated thyroid, L-thyroxine (T4) or L-triiodothyronine (liothyronine sodium, T3).

The drug of choice for the treatment of canine hypothyroidism is thyroxine sodium, T4, (Eltroxin, Glaxo) at a dosage of 10 μg/kg twice daily. Rarely, a dog will require 20 μg/kg twice daily but the lower dosage should always be used initially. Attitudinal responses may occur within two to three weeks but treatment should be continued for 12 weeks before effectiveness is assessed. In some severe cases, normalisation of the skin and hair may take as long as six months.

It is difficult to unintentionally overdose dogs with thyroid hormones. Possible signs of overdosage are those of thyrotoxicosis e.g. restlessness, panting, diarrhoea, polyuria/polydipsia and tachycardia but they are extremely rare. Even where there is pre-existing cardiac disease, there are usually few problems with T4 treatment but in such cases an increasing dosage regimen should be used beginning on 2.5 μg/kg twice daily, increasing by 2.5 μg/kg twice daily every week until the full therapeutic dosage is reached.

Liothyronine sodium (T3, Tertroxin, Pitman-Moore) is effective in the treatment of canine hypothyroidism but is less physiological (any residual endogenous T4 production is inhibited by negative feedback) and is shorter-acting. Although cases have been reported, the author has yet to see a dog with hypothyroidism respond to T3 after failure of T4. Such therapeutic failure in a correctly diagnosed animal usually indicates inadequate T4 dosage which should be increased. Where required, the T3 dosage regimen is 4.4 μg/kg three times daily. If response is satisfactory, a dose of 6.6 μg/kg twice daily may be tried to improve long-term owner compliance.

Desiccated thyroid (dry thyroid, thyroid extract) is a naturally-occurring product, with batch to batch variations in potency and shelf-life. It has no advantages over T4 and its use should be avoided.

At the dosages given above, the treatment of canine hypothyroidism with T4 is usually straightforward and monitoring by physical examination alone suffices in most cases. Where response is inadequate or side-effects are noted, TT4 and TT3 concentrations should be assessed. If twice daily therapy with T4 is being administered, this should be carried out twice — at four-eight hours after dosing (peak time of action) and 12 hours after dosing (i.e. immediately before the next dose is due). Both should be in the euthyroid range. With T3 supplementation, on three times daily therapy, samples should be taken at two to three hours and eight hours after dosing for TT3 only (TT4 will be undetectable).

Treatment of secondary and tertiary hypothyroidism is essentially the same as the primary disease but additional hormonal therapy (e.g glucocorticoids) may be required. Hypothyroidism resulting from T4 or T3 antibodies has been reported to respond to increased dosages of hormone with or without glucocorticoid therapy.

In congenital hypothyroidism many of the signs of cretinism resolve but lameness and arthritis may develop subsequently to abnormal development of joints and bones.

FELINE HYPOTHYROIDISM

Cretinism has been described in the cat but is extremely rare. Arnold *et al.,* (1984) reported a case of primary goitrous hypothyroidism and dwarfism (which they attributed to dyshormonogenesis) in a 14 week-old kitten.

Although there are numerous anecdotal reports of the acquired condition, none has been confirmed by TT4 and TT3 measurements before and after TSH stimulation leaving a case of definitively diagnosed, naturally-occurring, acquired feline hypothyroidism yet to be described.

Iatrogenic feline hypothyroidism occasionally results from the surgical or medical treatment of thyrotoxicosis. The management of the iatrogenic condition is discussed on page 46.

FELINE SYMMETRIC ALOPOECIA

Feline symmetric alopoecia (previously termed feline endocrine alopoecia) is a condition of multiple aetiology, which, when a specific cause cannot be established, may respond to a number of hormonal regimens. Prior to diagnosis, it is essential to eliminate diseases of known aetiology which result in a similar clinical appearance. At least some cats with idiopathic feline symmetric alopoecia (IFSA) may have low functional thyroid reserve (Thoday, 1986a and b).

Eighty per cent of cats with IFSA show acceptable to excellent regrowth of hair on T3 (Tertroxin, Pitman-Moore) therapy, at an initial dose of 20 μg/cat twice daily, increasing by 10 μg twice daily every third day to a maximum of 50 μg twice daily. In many cases the response may be maintained using 30 μg T3 twice daily but intermittent higher dosages as above may be given at the first sign of recurrence of hair loss.

REFERENCES AND FURTHER READING

ARNOLD, V., OPITZ, M., GROSSER, I., BADER, R. and EIGENMANN, J. E. (1984). Goitrous hypothyroidism and dwarfism in a kitten. *J. Am. Anim. Hosp. Ass.* **20**, 753.

BECK, K. A., HORNOFF, W. J. and FELDMAN, E. C. (1985). The normal feline thyroid. Technetium pertechnetate imaging and determination of thyroid to salivary gland radioactivity ratios in 10 normal cats. *Vet. Radiol.* **26**, 35.

BEIERWALTES, W. H. and NISHIYAMA, R. H. (1968). Dog thyroiditis: occurrence and similarity to Hashimoto's struma. *Endocrinology,* **83**, 501.

BELSHAW, B. E. (1983). Thyroid diseases. In *Textbook of Veterinary Internal Medicine: Diseases of the Dog and Cat,* (ed. S.J. Ettinger), 2nd edn., p. 1592. W.B. Saunders, Philadelphia.

BELSHAW, B. E., BARANDES, M., BECKER, D. V. and BERMAN, M. (1974). A model of iodine kinetics in the dog. *Endocrinology,* **95**, 1078.

BELSHAW, B. E., COOPER, T. E. and BECKER, D. V. (1975). The iodine requirement and influences of iodine intake on iodine metabolism and thyroid function in the adult beagle. *Endocrinology,* **96**, 1280.

BIRCHARD, S. J., PETERSON, M. E. and JACOBSON, A. (1984). Surgical treatment of feline hyperthyroidism: Results of 85 cases. *J. Am. Anim. Hosp. Ass.* **20**, 705.

BLACK, A. P. and PETERSON, M. E. (1983). Thyroid biopsy and thyroidectomy. In: *Current Techniques in Small Animal Surgery,* (ed. M.J. Bojrab), 2nd edn., p. 388. Lea & Febiger, Philadelphia.

BLAKE, S. and LAPINSKI, A. (1980). Hypothyroidism in different breeds. *Canine Pract.* **7**, 48.

BOND, B. R., FOX, P. R. and PETERSON, M. E. (1983). Echocardiographic evaluation of 30 cats with hyperthyroidism. *Procs. Am. Coll. Vet. Int. Med. 39.*

BOOK, S. A. (1977). Age related changes in serum thyroxine and ^{125}I-triiodothyronine resin sponge uptake in the young dog. *Lab. Anim. Sci.* **27**, 646.

CHASTAIN, C. B., McNEEL, S. V., GRAHAM, C. L. and PEZZANITE, S. C. (1983). Congenital hypothyroidism in a dog due to an iodide organification defect. *Am. J. vet. Res.* **44**,1257.

CHASTAIN, C. B., RIEDESEL, D. H. and GRAHAM, C. L. (1979). Secondary hypothyroidism in a dog. *Canine Pract.* **6**,(5), 59.

DONNE, C. S. and WILDGOOSE, W. H. (1984). Magnetic antibody immunoassay thyroid function tests in general practice. *Vet. Rec.* **115**, 79.

ECKERSALL, P. D. and WILLIAMS, M. E. (1983). Thyroid function tests in dogs using radioimmunoassay kits. *J. small Anim. Pract.* **24**, 525.

EVINGER, J. V., NELSON, R. W. and BOTTOMS, G. D. (1985). Thyrotropin-releasing hormone stimulation testing in healthy dogs. *Am. J. vet. Res.* **46**, 1323.

FELDMAN, B. F. and FELDMAN E. C. (1977). Routine laboratory diagnosis in endocrine disease. *Vet. Clins. N. Am.: Small Anim. Pract.* **7**, 443.

FELDMAN, E. C. and NELSON, R. W. (1987). *Canine and Feline Endocrinology and Reproduction,* p. 55. W. B. Saunders, Philadelphia.

FERGUSON, D. C. (1984). Thyroid function tests in the dog. Recent concepts. *Vet. Clins. N. Am.: Small Anim. Pract.* **14**, 783.

FOX, L. E. and NACHREINER, R. F. (1981). The pharmokinetics of T3 and T4 in the dog. *Procs. 62nd Conference of Res. Workers in Anim. Dis.,* 13.

FURTH, E. D., BECKER, D. V., NUNEZ, E. A. and REID, C. F. (1968). Thyroxine metabolism in the dog. *Endocrinology,* **82**, 976.

GOSSELIN, S. J., CAPEN, C. C., MARTIN, S. L. and TARGOWSKI, S. P. (1980). Biochemical and immunological investigations on hypothyroidism in dogs. *Can. J. Comp. Med.* **44**, 158.

HOENIG, M. and FERGUSON, D. C. (1983). Assessment of thyroid functional reserve in the cat by the thyrotropin-stimulation test. *Am. J. vet. Res.* **44**, 1229.

HOENIG, M., GOLDSCHMIDT, M. H., FERGUSON, D. C., KOCH, K. and EYMONTT, M. J. (1982). Toxic nodular goitre in the cat. *J. small Anim. Pract.* **23**, 1.

HOLZWORTH, J., THERAN,P., CARPENTER, J. L., HARPSTER, N. K. and TODOROFF, R. J. (1980). Hyperthyroidism in the cat: Ten cases. *J. Am. vet. med. Ass.* **176**, 345.

KALLFELZ, F. A. and ERALI, R. P. (1973). Thyroid function tests in domesticated animals: Free thyroxine index. *Am. J. vet. Res.* **34**, 1449.

KAPLAN, M. M. (1981). Interactions between drugs and thyroid hormones. *Thyroid Today,* **4**, 1.

KEMPPAINEN, R. J., MANSFIELD, P. D. and SARTIN, J. L. (1984). Endocrine responses of normal cats to TSH and synthetic ACTH administration. *J. Am. Anim. Hosp. Ass.* **20**, 737.

KENNEDY, R. L. and THODAY, K. L. (1984). Autoantibodies in feline hyperthyroidism. *Vet. Rec.* **114**, 575.

KENNEDY, R. L. and THODAY, K. L. (1988). Autoantibodies in feline hyperthyroidism. *Res. vet. Sci.,* **45**,300.

KENNEDY, R. L. and THODAY, K. L. (1989). Lack of thyroid stimulatory activity in the serum of hyperthyroid cats. *Autoimmunity,* **3**, 317.

LARSSON, M. (1981). Evaluation of a human TSH radioimmunoassay as a diagnostic test for canine primary hypothyroidism. *Acta. vet. Scand.* **22**, 589.

LARSSON, M. (1987). Diagnostic methods in canine hypothyroidism and influence of nonthyroidal illness on thyroid hormones and thyroxine-binding proteins. Ph.D. Thesis, University of Uppsala.

LARSSON, M. (1988). Determination of free thyroxine and cholesterol as a new screening test for canine hypothyroidism. *J. Am. Anim. Hosp. Ass.* **24**, 209.

LARSSON, M. and LUMSDEN, J. H. (1980). Evaluation of an enzyme-linked immunosorbent assay (ELISA) for determination of plasma thyroxine in dogs. *Zbl. Vet. Med. A.* **27**, 9.

LEAV, I., SCHILLER, A. L., RIJNBERK, A., LEGG, M. A. and KINDEREN, P.J. der (1976). Adenomas and carcinomas of the canine and feline thyroid. *Am. J. Path.* **83**, 61.

LOTHROP, C. D., TAMAS, P. M. and FADOK, V. A. (1984). Canine and feline thyroid function assessment with the thyrotropin-releasing hormone response test. *Am. J. vet. Res.* **45**, 2310.

LUCKE, V. M. (1964). An histological study of thyroid abnormalities in the domestic cat. *J. small Anim. Pract.* **5**, 351.

MAWDESLEY-THOMAS, L. E. and JOLLY, D. W. (1967). Autoimmune disease in the beagle. *Vet. Rec.* **80**,553.

MULLER, G. H., KIRK, R. W. and SCOTT, D. W. (1983). *Small Animal Dermatology,* 3rd ed. p 492, W. B. Saunders, Philadelphia.

NACHREINER, R. F. (1981). Laboratory diagnosis of endocrine diseases, *Procs. Am. Anim. Hosp. Ass.* **48**, 181.

NESBITT, G. H. (1983). *Canine and Feline Dermatology : a systematic approach.* p 91. Lea & Febiger, Philadelphia.

NOXON, J. O., THORNBURG, L. P., DILLENDER, M. J. and JONES, B. D. (1983). An adenoma in ectopic thyroid tissue causing hyperthyroidism in a cat. *J. Am. Anim. Hosp. Ass.* **19**, 369.

OLIVER, J. W. and WALDROP, V. (1983). Sampling protocol for thyrotropin stimulation test in the dog. *J. Am. vet. med. Ass.* **182**, 486.

PETERSON, M. E. (1981). Propylthiouracil in the treatment of feline hyperthyroidism. *J. Am. vet. med. Ass.* **179**, 485.

PETERSON, M. E. (1982). Diagnosis and treatment of feline hyperthyroidism. *Procs. 6th Kal Kan Symposium,* 63.

PETERSON, M. E. (1984). Feline hyperthyroidism. *Vet. Clins. N. Am: Small Anim. Pract.* **14**, 809.

PETERSON, M. E., BECKER, D. V., HURLEY, J. R. and FERGUSON, D. C. (1981). Spontaneous feline hyperthyroidism. *Prog. and Abstr. 62nd Ann.Meeting Endocrine Soc.* 203.

PETERSON, M. E., BIRCHARD, S. J. and MEHLHAFF, C. J. (1984). Anaesthethic and surgical management of endocrine disorders. *Vet. Clins. N. Am: Small Anim. Pract.* **14**, 914.

PETERSON, M. E., KINTZER, P. P., CAVANAGH, P. G., FOX, P. R., FERGUSON, D. C., JOHNSON, G. F. and BECKER, D. V. (1983). Feline hyperthyroidism: Pretreatment clinical and laboratory evaluation of 131 cases. *J. Am. vet. med. Ass.* **183**, 103.

PETERSON, M. E., LIVINGSTON, P. and BROWN, R. S. (1987). Lack of circulating thyroid stimulating immunoglobulins in cats with hyperthyroidism. *Vet. Immunol. Immunopathol.* **16**, 277.

PETERSON, M. E. and TURREL, J. M. (1986). Feline hyperthyroidism. In: *Current Veterinary Therapy IX: Small Animal Practice.* (ed. R. W. Kirk) p 1026. W. B. Saunders, Philadelphia.

QUINLAN, W. J. and MICHAELSON, S. (1981). Homologous radioimmunoassay for canine thyrotropin: Response of normal and x-irradiated dogs to propylthiouracil. *Endocrinology.* **108**, 937.

RAY, R. A. and HOWANITZ, P. (1984). RIA in thyroid function testing. *Diagnostic Med.* May, 55.

REFETOFF, S., ROBIN, N. I. and FANG, V. S. (1970). Parameters of thyroid function in serum of 16 selected vertebrate species: A study of PBI, serum T4, free T4 and the pattern of T4 and T3 binding to serum proteins. *Endocrinology,* **86**, 793.

REIMERS, T. J., McCANN, J. P., COWAN, R. G. and CONCANNON, P. W. (1982). Effects of storage, haemolysis, and freezing and thawing on concentrations of thyroxine, cortisol and insulin in blood samples. *Procs. Soc. Exper. Biol. Med.* **170**, 509.

SCHAER, M. (1981). The thyroid gland. In: *Pathophysiology in Small Animal Surgery* (ed. M.J. Bojrab), p 314. Lea & Febiger, Philadelphia.

SCOTT, D. W. (1982). Histopathologic findings in endocrine skin disorders of the dog. *J. Am. Anim. Hosp. Ass.* **18**, 173.

SUSANECK, S. J. (1983). Doxorubicin therapy in the dog. *J. Am. vet. med. Ass.* **182**, 70.

THAKE, D. C., HEVILLE, N. F. and SHARP, R. K. (1971). Ectopic thyroid adenomas at the base of the heart of the dog. *Vet. Pathol.* **8**, 421.

THODAY, K.L. (1985). The skin. In: *Feline Medicine and Therapeutics* (eds. E.A. Chandler, C.J. Gaskell and A.D.R. Hilbery), p 33. Blackwell Scientific Publications, Oxford.

THODAY, K. L. (1986a). Clinical, biochemical and immunological studies of feline thyroid function. Ph.D Thesis, University of Edinburgh.

THODAY, K. L. (1986b). The differential diagnosis of symmetric alopecia in the cat. In: *Current Veterinary Therapy IX: Small Animal Practice.* (ed. R. W. Kirk), p 545. W. B. Saunders, Philadelphia.

THODAY, K. L. (1988). Feline hyperthyroidism — A review of the literature. In: *Advances in Small Animal Practice 1* (ed. E.A. Chandler), p 120. Blackwell Scientific Publications, Oxford.

THODAY, K. L., SETH, J. and ELTON, R. A. (1984). Radioimmunoassay of serum total thyroxine and triiodothyronine in healthy cats: assay methodology and effects of age, sex, breed, heredity and environment. *J. small Anim. Pract.* **25**, 457.

VAN DEN BROEK, A. V. D. and DARKE, P. G. G. (1987). Cardiac measurements on thoracic radiographs of cats. *J. small Anim. Pract.* **22**, 473.

VOITH, V. L. (1970). *Accessory thyroids of the dog.* M.S. Thesis, The Ohio State University.

WINIWARTER, H. de (1935). Recherches sur les derives branchiaux (chat). Archives de Biologie, **46**, 369.

WOLTZ, H. H., THOMPSON, F. N., KEMPPAINEN, R. J., MUNNELL, J. F. and LORENZ, M. D. (1983). Effects of prednisone on thyroid gland morphology and plasma thyroxine and triiodothyronine concentrations in the dog. *Am. J. vet. Res.* **44**, 2000.

CHAPTER 3

THE PARATHYROID GLANDS

John K. Dunn B.V.M.&S., M.A., M.Vet.Sc., M.R.C.V.S.

ANATOMY AND HISTOLOGY

In the dog there are two pairs of parathyroid glands. The external glands are oval, purplish structures 2-5 mm in length and 0.5-1.0 mm in width, which are embedded in loose connective tissue cranial and dorsolateral to the anterior pole of the thyroid glands. The internal glands are smaller, flatter and embedded within the fibrous capsule of the thyroid glands. During development the external parathyroids are closely associated with the thymus. Consequently accessory parathyroid tissue may be present in the neck or cranial mediastinum.

Histopathologically the parathyroid glands are composed of two cell types; (a) chief cells and (b) oxyphil cells. Chief cells are concerned with the synthesis and secretion of parathyroid hormone (PTH). Oxyphil cells are biologically inactive and their numbers increase with age. Prolonged hypocalcaemia results in an increased number of 'water-clear' cells, the function of which is uncertain.

PARATHYROID HORMONE (PTH)

At any one time most chief cells are in a resting phase although each is constantly secreting a minimum level of PTH.

Low blood calcium (Ca), and to a lesser extent low magnesium (Mg) levels, stimulate PTH secretion. Although only small amounts of preformed hormone are stored, the parathyroid gland is capable of rapidly altering the rate of hormone secretion in response to minor fluctuations in blood calcium. A negative feedback system operates to maintain calcium levels within a narrow physiological range (approximately 2.2−2.7 mmol/l). Hyperphosphataemia indirectly stimulates PTH secretion by lowering blood calcium.

ACTIONS OF PARATHYROID HORMONE

Calcium ions play an important role in muscle contraction, nerve impulse conduction and the release of neurotransmitters. Calcium ions stabilise nerve cell membranes by decreasing their permeability to sodium.

The interaction of PTH with calcitonin secreted by C (parafollicular) cells of the thyroid gland, and the active renal metabolite of vitamin D, 1,25 dihydroxycholecalciferol (1, 25 $(OH)_2$ D_3), is responsible for calcium homeostasis. PTH target cells, are present in bone, kidney and gastrointestinal tract, although the action of PTH on the latter is indirect and mediated by 1,25 dihydroxycholecalciferol (Table 1.)

Action on bone

PTH mobilises calcium, and to a lesser extent phosphate, from bone to the extracellular fluid (ECF). The immediate effects of PTH on bone involve the osteocyte-osteoblast 'pump' which moves calcium from bone to ECF. The long term effects of prolonged PTH secretion include increased bone resorption (increased osteoclastic activity) and, paradoxically, an increase in bone formation due to an increase in the number of osteoblasts. Resorptive effects usually exceed the anabolic effects leading to a net negative skeletal balance. As mineral is removed from bone it is replaced by immature fibrous connective tissue. This fibrous osteodystrophy tends to be generalised although the changes are often accentuated in the cancellous bones of the skull.

Action on the kidney

The actions of PTH on renal tubular function can be summarised as follows:

1. PTH decreases phosphate reabsorption by the proximal convoluted tubule i.e. promotes urinary excretion of phosphate (and other ions)

2. promotes reabsorption of calcium in the distal convoluted tubule and decreases urinary excretion of magnesium, ammonia and H^+ ions

3. accelerates the conversion of vitamin D_3 to 1, 25 dihydroxycholecalciferol in the kidney thus indirectly increasing the intestinal absorption of calcium and phosphate.

These effects tend to increase serum calcium. However, it is the effects of PTH on the distal renal tubule and the 'acute' phase of bone resorption which are responsible for rapid minor adjustments in blood calcium (Table 1).

Table 1. Actions of parathyroid hormone.

1. Kidney	a)	Increases urinary excretion of phosphate, potassium, bicarbonate, sodium, amino acids, cyclic adenosine monophosphate.
	b)	Increases tubular reabsorption of calcium, magnesium, ammonia, H^+ ions.
2. Bone	a)	Immediate effect: Stimulates osteocytic/osteoclastic resorption of bone.
	b)	Longterm effect: Stimulates osteoblastic activity.
3. Intestine		Indirectly increases intestinal uptake of calcium and phosphate by increasing the renal production of 1, 25 dihydroxycholecalciferol.

Interpretation of serum calcium levels

A total serum calcium measurement includes albumin-bound calcium (50%), free ionised calcium (40%) and non-ionised calcium salts (10%). The value must be interpreted in association with the serum albumin concentration and acid-base status of the patient. Only the ionised fraction is physiologically active. Although hypoalbuminaemia lowers the total serum calcium concentration, the concentration of free ionised calcium usually remains unaltered. Alkalosis, by increasing the proportion of albumin-bound calcium, may effectively decrease the concentration of ionised calcium. A formula for correcting total serum calcium based on the serum concentration of albumin is:

Adjusted Ca (mg/dl) = measured Ca (mg/dl) — albumin (g/dl) + 3.5 (Finco, 1983).

DISORDERS OF PARATHYROID FUNCTION

PRIMARY HYPERPARATHYROIDISM

Primary hyperparathyroidism is a relatively rare disorder of older dogs (greater than 8 to 10 years of age), resulting from excessive secretion of PTH by neoplastic or hyperplastic chief cells. In dogs the most common cause is a functional adenoma of the chief cells affecting one gland only. Occasionally, ectopic accessory parathyroid tissue, displaced into the anterior mediastinum during embryological development of the thymus, may also become neoplastic. Similar lesions in cats are rare.

Parathyroid hyperplasia has been reported as a primary disease entity and generally involves more than one parathyroid gland (Feldman and Nelson, 1987a). More commonly, however, parathyroid hyperplasia is a feature of secondary renal or nutritional hyperparathyroidism (see pages 64 and 66). Non-affected chief cells atrophy since the normal negative feedback system in response to hypercalcaemia remains intact.

Clinical signs

The clinical signs of primary hyperparathyroidism are insidious in onset and relate to the known functions of PTH and the effects of hypercalcaemia on renal function. Systemic signs will be apparent in animals which have been severely hypercalcaemic for a prolonged period and are due to the direct effects of calcium on renal tubular function. Hence, some of the clinical signs may be those associated with renal failure and the uraemic syndrome (Table 2).

Table 2
Clinical signs of chronic renal failure and the uraemic syndrome.

1.	Depression
2.	Polydipsia
3.	Polyuria
4.	Vomiting
5.	Diarrhoea (often melaena due to platelet dysfunction)
6.	Oral ulceration
7.	Anaemia (non-regenerative)
8.	Dehydration
9.	Halitosis (uraemic breath)

Affected animals are frequently polydipsic and polyuric since chronic hypercalcaemia affects the normal concentrating ability of the renal tubules by altering their responsiveness to antidiuretic hormone (nephrogenic diabetes insipidus). Decreased excitability of gastrointestinal smooth muscle may result in vomiting and constipation. Other more non-specific signs include listlessness, depression, inappetence, muscle wasting, weakness, shivering and muscle twitching. The physiological effects of prolonged excessive secretion of PTH on bone may result in lameness, pathological fractures, facial bony swellings (hyperostosis) or, in advanced cases, 'rubber-jaw'.

On physical examination enlarged parathyroid glands are usually not palpable. In dogs the most common cause of hypercalcaemia is the hypercalcaemia of malignancy (less accurately termed pseudohyperparathyroidism) which is discussed more fully in the chapter on Paraneoplastic Syndromes. A thorough physical examination should, therefore, include a rectal examination and palpation of the mammary glands and all peripheral lymph nodes to rule out apocrine gland adenocarcinoma of the anal sac, mammary adenocarcinoma and lymphosarcoma as neoplastic causes of hypercalcaemia.

Laboratory findings

Routine haematology is frequently uninformative and abnormalities are either non-specific or relate to hypercalcaemia-induced renal failure. Biochemical abnormalities consist of persistent hypercalcaemia with a low or low normal serum phosphate concentration. Some animals are marginally hyperchloraemic due to increased proximal tubular reabsorption of chloride (Feldman and Nelson, 1987a). Prolonged hypercalcaemia results in renal damage (nephrocalcinosis) with increases in blood urea nitrogen (BUN), creatinine and phosphate. Serum alkaline phosphatase may be elevated in cases with advanced bone disease.

Electrocardiography

ECG alterations in response to severe hypercalcaemia include (1) bradycardia and (2) prolongation of the P-R interval with shortening of the Q-T interval.

Radiographic findings

These are non-specific for primary hyperparathyroidism. Skeletal demineralisation may be manifested as a generalised decrease in bone density. Earliest changes consist of radiolucency of the sockets of the teeth (lamina dura dentes), the vertebral bodies and dorsal spinous processes of the vertebrae. Subperiosteal cortical resorption of bone and bone cysts (osteitis fibrosa cystica) may be visualised in the long bones (especially the phalanges). Soft tissue mineralisation affecting stomach, lungs, heart and periarticular regions has been reported, but is more commonly a feature of secondary renal hyperparathyroidism. Urinary calculi, composed of calcium oxalate or calcium phosphate, are usually readily indentifiable. Nephrocalcinosis may appear as a diffuse, mild radiopacity of the kidneys (Carillo *et al.*, 1979; Berger and Feldman, 1987).

Parathyroid hormone assay

Assays to measure serum immunoreactive PTH are not widely available, are expensive and have yet to be critically evaluated in small animals. Most assays measure the dominant, more persistent C-terminal fragment since the biologically active N-terminal fragment has a very short half-life in the circulation. Furthermore, results from different laboratories using antibovine PTH sera, are difficult to interpret since reference preparations of PTH are not available.

Diagnosis

A diagnosis of primary hyperparathyroidism, in the absence of PTH assays, is based on excluding other causes of hypercalcaemia. Marginally high calcium levels (>3 mmol/l) should be interpreted cautiously and always repeated. Consideration should be given to the serum albumin concentration, the animal's acid-base status and age. Young dogs (i.e. less than 3 to 6 months of age) tend to have high normal serum concentrations of calcium and phosphate. Lipaemia may artificially elevate calcium levels.

Screening radiographs of the thorax, abdomen, skull and long bones should be taken.

A lymph node and/or bone marrow aspirate should be performed to rule out lymphosarcoma.

Response to glucocorticoids. The response to prednisolone (2mg/kg per os twice a day for two days) may help differentiate between primary hyperparathyroidism and hypercalcaemia associated with lymphosarcoma. A rapid fall in serum calcium within 48 hours is more consistent with a diagnosis of lymphosarcoma than primary hyperparathyroidism.

Differential diagnosis

The differential diagnosis of primary hyperparathyroidism includes other causes of hypercalcaemia in the dog (Tables 3 and 4).

Table 3
Differential diagnosis of hypercalcaemia.

1. Hyperparathyroidism
2. Hypercalcaemia of malignancy (see 'Paraneoplastic Syndromes')
3. Renal failure
4. Hypoadrenocorticism
5. Metastatic bone tumours with osteolysis
6. Hypervitaminosis D
7. Lipaemia

Table 4
Differential diagnosis of hypercalcaemia:
biochemical abnormalities

	Serum Ca	Serum PO₄	BUN	Alkaline Phosphatase
Primary hyperparathyroidism	↑	↓	± ↑	± ↑
Hypercalcaemia of malignancy	↑	↓	± ↑	± ↑
Renal disease	occasionally ↑ but usually low or normal	↑	↑	Normal
Hypervitaminosis D	↑	↑	Normal	Normal
Metastatic bone tumours (with osteolysis)	↑ (mild)	Normal or slightly elevated	Normal	± ↑

Hypercalcaemia of malignancy, the most common cause of hypercalcaemia in the dog, is discussed at length in the chapter on 'Paraneoplastic Syndromes'. The onset of clinical signs tends to be more rapid; consequently bone demineralisation is usually not evident. The term pseudohyperparathyroidism is reserved for a syndrome of hypercalcaemia associated with malignant tumours of non-parathyroid origin, without bony metastases, that secrete a parathyroid hormone-like peptide.

Hypercalcaemia associated with hypervitaminosis D can arise as a complication of prolonged vitamin D administration in hypoparathyroid dogs and cats. The hypercalcaemia is accompanied by concurrent hyperphosphataemia since vitamin D increases intestinal uptake of calcium and phosphate.

The hypercalcaemia of Addison's disease is usually mild and reversible with appropriate treatment for hypoadrenocorticism (Peterson and Feinman, 1982). Serum calcium concentrations in animals with chronic renal failure are generally low or low normal and associated with a variable degree of hyperphosphataemia. A small percentage of these dogs (often young dogs with congenital renal disease) develop hypercalcaemia (Finco and Rowland, 1978).

Exploratory surgery

Exploratory surgery of the neck is justified only if no other cause for the hypercalcaemia can be ascertained. All four parathyroids should be evaluated before deciding which, if any, of the glands should be removed. External parathyroid adenomas are usually confined to a single gland and should be removed without damaging the surrounding tissue. Internal parathyroid adenomas should be removed along with the thyroid gland on the same side. Enlargement of more than one gland is more indicative of parathyroid hyperplasia and warrants special consideration; the smallest or normal glands(s) should be left intact to maintain calcium homeostasis. Transient hypocalcaemia may develop within 5 days following removal of a parathyroid adenoma due to atrophy of the unaffected glands (Berger and Feldman, 1987). Treatment of hypocalcaemia is covered under treatment of hypoparathyroidism.

Medical treatment for severe hypercalcaemia

Severe hypercalcaemia requires urgent and aggressive medical therapy. The aims of therapy are to:

1. Correct the fluid deficit with intravenous 0.9% saline

2. Diurese with 0.9% saline (given intravenously at 2—3 times the maintenance rate to promote renal excretion of calcium) and frusemide (5mg/kg given initially as an intravenous bolus). Potassium supplementation may be necessary to prevent hypokalaemia. In view of the large volumes of fluid administered it is essential that renal function be checked beforehand and that urine output be monitored via an indwelling urinary catheter. Thiazide diuretics are contraindicated since they decrease calcium excretion by the kidney.

3. Glucocorticoids (see above) should be administered only after initial investigations are complete and a cause for the hypercalcaemia cannot be established.

4. Phosphate infusions or oral phosphate preparations have been advocated to lower calcium levels but are best avoided since they may potentiate metastatic calcification.

5. Mithramycin (Mithracin, Pfizer) is a cytotoxic drug which is also a potent inhibitor of bone resorption. In the dog, a single intravenous bolus injection of 25μg/kg may correct hypercalcaemia of malignancy within 48 hours (MacEwen and Siegel, 1977). Toxic side effects include renal and hepatic damage.

Prognosis for long term survival in dogs with a concurrent impairment of renal function is extremely poor.

RENAL SECONDARY HYPERPARATHYROIDISM

Renal secondary hyperparathyroidism is characterised by the excessive, but not autonomous secretion of PTH by hyperplastic chief cells. Progressive renal disease leads to a significant reduction in glomerular filtration rate and decreased renal excretion of phosphate, resulting in hyperphosphataemia. By virtue of the reciprocal relationship which exists between phosphate and calcium (mass/law equation), serum calcium concentrations decrease resulting in increased secretion of PTH. A concurrent deficiency of the active renal metabolite 1, 25 dihydroxycholecalciferol leads to decreased absorption of calcium from the gastrointestinal tract. Table 5 lists some acquired and congenital disorders which may progress to chronic renal failure (CRF) and secondary hyperparathyroidism. Increased prolonged secretion of PTH results in osteoclastic bone resorption and severe fibrous osteodystrophy. This is especially prominent in the cancellous bones of the skull of young animals (less than 5 years of age) with chronic renal failure resulting from congenital renal abnormalities. A higher incidence of congenital or inherited renal disease ('renal dysplasia') has been reported in cocker spaniels, Lhasa apsos, shih tzus and Norwegian elkhounds (Bovee, 1984; Steward and MacDougall, 1984).

Clinical signs of chronic renal failure are typical of the uraemic syndrome (see Table 2). In advanced cases teeth become loose in their sockets and the bones of the mandible become pliable ('rubber jaw').

Laboratory findings

Serum calcium is generally normal or even low although a small percentage of animals are hypercalcaemic (Finco and Rowland, 1978). Other biochemical findings include increased blood urea nitrogen (BUN), increased serum creatinine, increased serum phosphate and occasionally increased alkaline phosphatase in cases with overt bone disease. A normocytic, normochromic, non-responsive anaemia is usually evident on routine haematology. Urine specific gravity is similar to that of glomerular filtrate and plasma i.e. 1.008—1.012 (isosthenuria).

Table 5
Acquired and congenital disorders which may progress to chronic renal failure

Acquired renal disease	Congenital renal disease
Chronic interstitial nephritis	Renal cortical hypoplasia
Glomerulonephritis	Polycystic kidneys
Nephrosclerosis	Bilateral hydronephrosis
Renal amyloidosis	

Radiographic findings

Radiographically there is resorption of alveolar bone around the tooth roots with loss of the lamina dura. Cystic or radiolucent areas are visible in the bones of the skull resulting in a 'motheaten' appearance (Figures 1 and 2). Long bones are less severely affected although pathological fractures occur occasionally. Soft tissue metastatic calcification may be evident in the rugal folds of the gastric mucosa, subcutis, periarticular tissues, pleura, endocardium, myocardium, lung and arterial walls (Figures 3 and 4).

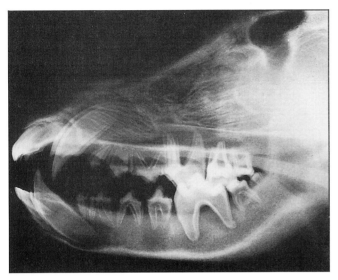

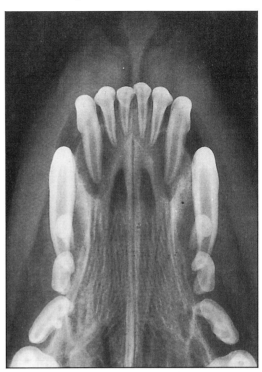

Figure 1 *(above)*. Lateral skull radiograph of a six month old male Dalmation with congenital renal hypoplasia and associated renal secondary hyperparathyroidism. There is diffuse loss of density of all the skull bones particularly around the tooth roots. As a result the teeth and soft tissues appear more prominent than usual.

Figure 2 *(right above)*. Intra-oral film of the maxillae and nasal chambers of a nine month old female Dalmation with chronic renal failure and renal secondary hyperparathyroidism. There is marked loss of alveolar bone resulting in the appearance of 'floating teeth'.

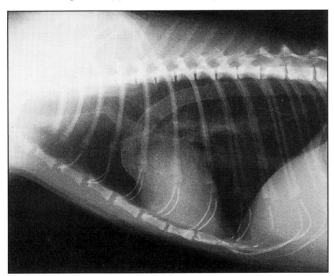

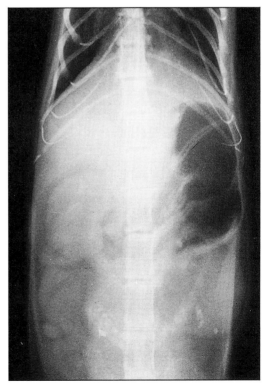

Figure 3 *(above)*. A lateral thoracic radiograph of a nine year old male domestic short-haired cat with chronic renal failure and renal secondary hyperparathyroidism. Note the mineralisation of the aorta, pulmonary arteries and anterior thoracic vessels.

Figure 4 *(right)*. Ventrodorsal view of the cranial abdomen of the cat in figure 3 showing calcification of the rugal folds of the stomach. Both kidneys are irregular in outline.

Treatment of chronic renal failure involves:

1. Correction of fluid deficits and diuresis with balanced electrolyte solutions or normal saline.

2. Cimetidine (Tagamet, Smith, Kline and French) is a histamine (H_2) receptor antagonist which blocks the synthesis of PTH in uraemic dogs (Jacob *et al,* 1981). Cimetidine may also minimise or prevent the gastric ulceration which occurs in uraemic animals. The dose for dogs is 5mg/kg per os BID.

3. Calcium and vitamin D administration has been advocated as a method of lowering serum phosphate levels if used in conjunction with a low phosphate diet (e.g. prescription diet K/D, Hills Pet Products). However, extreme caution is advised in view of their potential for inducing metastatic calcification.

4. Intestinal phosphate binders e.g. aluminium hydroxide or aluminium carbonate administered orally thirty minutes before a meal. The dose of phosphate binder should be adjusted until the serum phosphate concentration is normal (0.6—1.3 mmol/l). The average initial dose of aluminium hydroxide for a dog is 300—500mg per os three times daily (Polzin and Osborne, 1983). Side effects include constipation.

5. Peritoneal dialysis.

NUTRITIONAL SECONDARY HYPERPARATHYROIDISM

Nutritional secondary hyperparathyroidism is a disease of young growing dogs and cats fed on meat or meat and cereal diets which are either deficient in calcium or contain low or normal amounts of calcium but excessive levels of phosphorus. Diets consisting solely of liver or beef heart may have Ca: P ratio in excess of 1:40. Often there is a history of excessive supplementation with cod liver oil to provide a source of vitamin D.

Clinical signs

Young giant breeds of dogs and Siamese and Burmese cats are most commonly affected. Clinical signs, which may become apparent between 8 and 20 weeks of age, consist of fever and lameness associated with bone pain and/or pathological fractures. Affected animals show hind limb weakness and are reluctant to move or take very short, sharp steps. Young kittens tend to have a lordotic curve to their spine. Abnormalities in posture are common e.g. splaying of the toes and 'dropping' of the metacarpal and metatarsal bones so that the animal assumes a plantigrade stance. The carpal joints may be swollen with the limbs deviating laterally distal to the carpi. Pathological fractures of vertebral bodies may result in paraplegia.

Laboratory findings

Renal function is usually normal: consequently both calcium and phosphate levels are often normal because of compensatory renal control mechanisms. Alkaline phosphatase is normally elevated in all growing animals less than 6—9 months of age and is not necessarily indicative of bone disease.

Radiographic findings

The findings are somewhat similar to those of renal secondary hyperparathyroidism with a generalised loss of bone density and thinning of cortical bone (Figure 5). Flaring of the metaphyseal regions occurs and a band of increased radiodensity may be visible in the metaphysis adjacent to the growth plate in the region of the primary spongiosa. Pathological fractures are more common compared to renal secondary hyperparathyroidism, and are frequently of the folding or compression type (Figure 6). The growth plates are usually of normal width.

Treatment

Treatment is concerned with dietary management. The animal should be fed a balanced, commercially prepared diet containing calcium and phosphorus in a ratio of 1.2—2.0 : 1. Calcium and phosphorus requirements for growing puppies are 550mg/kg calcium and 450 mg/kg of phosphorus per day. Kittens require 200—400mg of calcium per day. Adult requirements are approximately half those of the young animal (Chastain and Ganjam, 1986).

Restricted exercise and strict confinement are essential for at least three weeks. Many animals show a dramatic clinical improvement within the first week but full skeletal recovery may take 2 to 3 months. The value of additional calcium supplementation or phosphate binders during the recovery phase is questionable and, if used, steps should be taken to ensure the supplement contains calcium and phosphorus in a 2:1 ratio. Non-steroidal anti-inflammatory drugs may be necessary for a few days during the acute phase of the disease. Corticosteroids are contraindicated since they may decrease blood calcium levels.

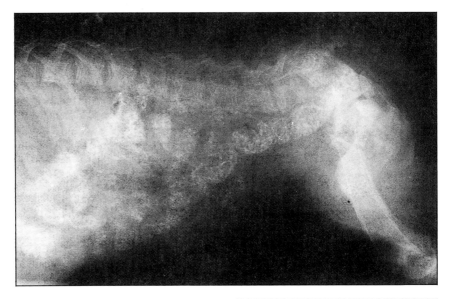

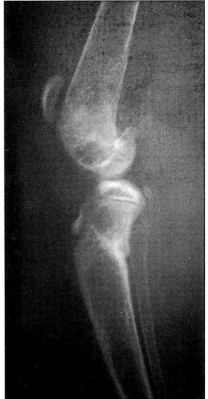

Figure 5 *(above)*
A lateral abdominal radiograph of an eight week old male Afghan pup with nutritional secondary hyperparathyroidism showing a generalised decrease in bone density and cortical thinning. There is a folding fracture with angulation in one femoral shaft. The mineral densities in the intestine are due to ingested bone meal.

Figure 6 *(right)*
Lateral radiograph of the stifle of a six month old male Chinchilla cat with nutritional secondary hyperparathyroidism. There is a resolving folding fracture in the proximal tibia shown by an oblique, ill-defined sclerotic line. 'Stress' lines are also visible in the distal femur.

HYPOPARATHYROIDISM

Primary or idiopathic hypoparathyroidism is a relatively rare metabolic disorder which can affect mature dogs of all breeds. A higher incidence in females has been reported (Sherding *et al*, 1980; Peterson, 1986). The most common cause of hypoparathyroidism is the iatrogenic form following removal of the parathyroid glands during thyroid surgery in hyperthyroid cats.

The disease is characterised by a transient or permanent deficiency of parathyroid hormone secretion resulting in inadequate mobilisation of calcium from bone, decreased calcium reabsorption from the renal tubule and decreased absorption of calcium from the gastrointestinal tract. Hence, hypocalcaemia develops. Concurrently, the increased renal tubular reabsorption of phosphate leads to hyper-phosphataemia. Primary hypoparathyroidism usually requires lifelong therapy to maintain normocalcaemia. Histological examination of parathyroid tissue removed from dogs with suspected or confirmed hypoparathyroidism has consistently shown lymphocytic and plasmacytic infiltration with fibrous tissue deposition compatible with immune-mediated destruction of the gland (Sherding *et al*, 1980).

Clinical signs

CNS and neuromuscular signs

Hypocalcaemia results in hyperexcitability of the peripheral and central nervous system. Clinical signs include focal muscle twitching or generalised tremors which progress to tetanic spasm and seizure activity (hypocalcaemic tetany). The seizures are often precipitated by noise, sudden movement or excitement and are of a tonic-clonic nature. Spasm of the facial muscles may be associated with facial rubbing. Affected animals are often febrile (due to increased muscle activity), walk with a stiff, hunched gait or are visibly ataxic.

Cataracts

Cataracts have been reported as a sequel to prolonged hypocalcaemia. These consist of small punctate or linear white opacities in the anterior and posterior cortical subcapsular regions. They do not affect vision and, in man, successful treatment halts cataract progression (Kornegay *et al,* 1980).

Miscellaneous signs

Vague, non-specific signs of hypoparathyroidism include anorexia, lethargy, listlessness, generalised weakness, vomiting, diarrhoea and weight loss. Behavioural changes such as restlessness, aggressiveness and disorientation may be noted by the observant owner. Prolonged panting and hyperventilation during a tetanic episode may produce a respiratory alkalosis which, by increasing the percentage of albumin-bound calcium, decreases the percentage of free-ionised calcium and exacerbates the clinical signs of hypocalcaemia.

Laboratory findings

Persistent hypocalcaemia accompanied by hyperphosphataemia in a dog with normal renal function is very suggestive of primary hypoparathyroidism. A low blood calcium level should be repeated and interpreted in association with the serum albumin concentration.

Electrocardiography

The main effect of hypocalcaemia on the ECG is prolongation of the $Q-T$ interval. T waves may become deeper and wider. The effect on heart rate is minimal; a mild tachycardia may be evident.

Diagnosis

Radiographic examination is generally uninformative and a diagnosis of primary hypoparathyroidism is based on the history, clinical signs, laboratory findings and the exclusion of other causes of hypocalcaemia. Parathyroid hormone assays are not routinely available. Parathyroid gland biopsies have been recommended but are difficult to perform.

Differential Diagnosis

Of the conditions listed in Table 6, only primary (or iatrogenic) hypoparathyroidism and eclampsia are likely to present with clinical signs of hypocalcaemia. Eclampsia occurs only during late pregnancy or during lactation. Disorders resulting in hypoalbuminaemia usually do not present with clinical signs of hypocalcaemia since ionised calcium levels remain normal. Only hypoparathyroidism and renal disease may present with hypocalcaemia and hyperphosphataemia. With acute and chronic urethral obstruction or acute ethylene glycol toxicity the hypocalcaemia is accompanied by increases in serum phosphate, BUN, creatinine and potassium. Hyperkalaemia potentiates the effects of hypocalcaemia and affected animals may occasionally seizure.

Table 6
Differential diagnosis of hypocalcaemia

Hypoparathyroidism (iatrogenic or acquired)

Eclampsia

Vitamin D deficiency (rare)

Acute renal failure (urethral obstruction or ethylene glycol toxicity)

Hypoalbuminaemia (protein losing enteropathy, malabsorption syndromes,
    liver disease, nephrotic syndrome)

Medullary C-cell carcinomas of the thyroid gland (excessive secretion of
    calcitonin)

Nutritional secondary hyperparathyroidism

Acute pancreatitis

Phosphate-containing enemas

Blood sample collected in EDTA

Repeated whole blood transfusions containing citrate as anticoagulant

Hypoparathyroidism in cats

Iatrogenic hypoparathyroidism may occur following bilateral thyroidectomy and clinical signs of hypocalcaemia usually occur post-operatively within 72 hours if no parathyroid tissue is preserved. Transient hypocalcaemia occasionally occurs following unilateral removal of the thyroid/parathyroid complex.

Clinical signs in the cat include lethargy, generalised weakness, anorexia, vomiting, prolapse of the third eyelid with rapid progression to muscle tremors and tetanic seizures. Serum calcium concentrations should be checked daily for 4 to 7 days post-operatively.

Treatment

Treatment of primary or acquired hypoparathyroidism involves the administration of calcium and vitamin D or vitamin D analogues. The aim is to maintain serum calcium within the low normal reference range (Table 7).

Treatment of hypocalcaemic tetany

10% calcium gluconate should be given intravenously at a dose of 5—15mg (0.5—1.5 ml) per kg BW over 10—30 minutes. ECG monitoring is advisable and the infusion is stopped if bradycardia develops. For short term maintenance 10% calcium gluconate may be added to intravenous fluids (not solutions containing bicarbonate) and given at a rate of 20mg (2ml)/kg over 6—8 hours. Alternatively, the dose of calcium gluconate used initially to control clinical signs may be diluted with an equal volume of normal saline and administered subcutaneously every 6—8 hours. Calcium chloride should **not** be given subcutaneously. Oral calcium and vitamin D therapy should be initiated immediately since it takes 24—48 hours before any affect is achieved (see below).

Table 7
Treatment of hypocalcaemia

1. **Hypocalcaemic tetany**

   Administer 5—15 mg (0.5—1.5 mls) /kg of 10% calcium gluconate intravenously over 10—30 mins. Can be added to intravenous fluids or given subcutaneously.

2. **Longterm maintenance**

   a) **Oral calcium**

Dog	Cat
50—100mg of elemental calcium /kg bodyweight daily divided into three equal doses	0.5—3 g per day in 3 equal doses
25mg/kg/day for maintenance	

   b) **Vitamin D$_2$ (ergocalciferol)**

Dog	Cat
4000—6000 units/kg/day	10,000 units daily
1000—2000 units/kg/day for maintenance	

   or

   c) **Dihydrotachysterol**

Dog	Cat
0.03mg/kg/day 2—3 days	0.03mg/kg once daily 3 days then 0.02 mg/kg once daily 4 days then
0.01mg/kg/day maintenance	0.01mg/kg maintenance reducing to weekly maintenance dose

   or

   d) **Calcitriol**

   Suggested dose in dogs
   0.06 micrograms/kg/day

   (Peterson, 1982; Feldman and Nelson, 1987b).

Long term management is best achieved with

A. **Oral calcium salts,** bearing in mind that different calcium preparations contain different amounts of elemental calcium. (Calcium gluconate tablets contain 9%, calcium lactate 13% and calcium carbonate 40% elemental calcium). The dose for the dog is 50—100mg/kg per day given in three divided doses reducing to 25 mg/kg day for maintenance. For cats the dose is 0.5—3g per day, again in three divided doses.

B. **Vitamin D_2** (ergocalciferol) is inexpensive but large doses are required to overcome the relative deficiency of 1, 25 dihydroxycholecalciferol that exists in hypoparathyroid animals. Vitamin D_2 is stored in fat and has a slow onset of action (approximately 3 weeks). Furthermore, vitamin D_2-induced hypercalcaemia is slow to reverse.

C. **Dihydrotachysterol (Tachyrol, Duphar)**

Dihydrotachysterol (DHT) is more potent than vitamin D_2. For the dog, the dose is 0.03 mg/kg per day for 2 to 3 days reducing to 0.01 mg/kg/day for maintenance. The dose of calcium can usually be tapered after 1—2 weeks of DHT before being discontinued. The dose of DHT for the cat is 0.03 mg/kg daily for 3 days then 0.02 mg/kg for 4 days then 0.01 mg/kg daily for maintenance. In many cases it is possible to reduce this dose further to a weekly maintenance dose. The advantages of DHT are that, although more expensive, it has a more rapid onset of action (1—7 days) and the hypercalcaemic effects, if they occur, are more rapidly reversed (4—14 days).

D. **Calcitriol (Rocaltrol, Roche)**

This is an analogue of 1, 25 dihydroxycholecalciferol and therefore no activation is required. Onset of action is extremely rapid.

Complications of vitamin D therapy

Prolonged vitamin D therapy can result in hypercalcaemia and nephrocalcinosis (secondary to prolonged calciuria). Regular monitoring of serum calcium levels is essential. Initially, this should be performed on a daily basis followed by weekly monitoring when clinical signs have abated. Once blood calcium and phosphate levels have stabilised, monthly checks shold be undertaken. All therapy should be discontinued immediately if an animal becomes hypercalcaemic. Ovariohysterectomy is recommended since oestrogens may alter the response to vitamin D.

REFERENCES

BERGER, B. and FELDMAN, E. C. (1987). Primary hyperparathyroidism in dogs: 21 cases (1976 – 1986). *J. Am. vet. med. Ass.,* **191,** 350.

BOVEE, K. C. (1984). Genetic and metabolic diseases of the kidney. In: *Canine Nephrology,* 339, Harwell Publishing Co.

CARRILLO, J. M., BURK, R. L. and BODE, C. L. (1979) Primary hyperparathyroidism in a dog. *J. Am. vet. med. Ass.,* **174,** 67.

CHASTAIN, C. B. and GANJAM, V. K. (1986). Hyperparathyroidism. In: *Clinical Endocrinology of Companion Animals,* 192, Lea and Febiger, Philadelphia.

FELDMAN, E. C. and NELSON, R. W. (1987a). The parathyroid gland — primary hyperparathyroidism. In: *Canine and Feline Endocrinology and Reproduction,* 328, W. B. Saunders Co. Philadelphia.

FELDMAN, E. C. and NELSON, R. W. (1987b). Hypocalcaemia — Hypoparathyroidism. In: *Canine and Feline Endocrinology and Reproduction,* p 357. W. B. Saunders Co, Philadelphia.

FINCO, D. R. and ROWLAND, G. N. (1978). Hypercalcaemia secondary to chronic renal failure in the dog: A report of four cases. *J. Am. vet. med. Ass.,* **173,** 990.

FINCO, D. R. (1983). Interpretations of serum calcium concentrations in the dog. *Comp. of Continuing Education,* **5,** 778.

JACOB, A. I., CANTERBURY, J. M., GAVELLAS, G., LAMBERT, P. W. and BOURGOIGNIE, J. J. (1981). Reversal of secondary hyperparathyroidism by cimetidine in chronically uraemic dogs. *J. Clin. Invest.* **67,** 1753.

KORNEGAY, J. N., GREENE, C. E., MARTIN, C., GORGACZ, E. J. and MELCON, D. K. (1980). Idiopathic hypocalcaemia in four dogs. *J. Am. Animal. Hosp. Ass.,* **16,** 723.

MACEWEN, E. G. and SIEGEL, S. D. (1977). Hypercalcaemia: A paraneoplastic disease. *Vet. Clins. of N. Am.* **7,** 187.

MACINTYRE, I. (1986). The hormonal regulation of extracellular calcium *Br. Med. Bull.* **42,** 343.

PETERSON, M. E. and FEINMAN, J. M. (1982). Hypercalcaemia associated with hyperadrenocorticism in sixteen dogs. *J. Am. vet. med. Ass.,* **181,** 802.

PETERSON, M. E. (1982). Treatment of feline and canine hypoparathyroidism. *J. Am. vet. med. Ass.,* **181,** 1434.

PETERSON, M. E. (1986). Hypoparathyroidism. In: *Current Veterinary Therapy IX, Small Anim. Pract.,* (ed. R.W. Kirk) p 39, W. B. Saunders Co. Philadelphia.

POLZIN, D. J. and OSBORNE, C. A. (1983). Conservative medical management of canine chronic polyuric renal failure. In: *Current Veterinary Therapy VIII: Small Anim. Pract.* (ed. R. W. Kirk) p 997, W. B. Saunders Co, Philadelphia.

SHERDING, R. G., MEUTEN, D. J., CHEW, D. J., KNAACK, K. E. and HAUPT, K. H. (1980). Primary hypoparathyroidism in the dog. *J. Am. vet. med. Ass.,* **176,** 439.

STEWARD, A. P. and MACDOUGALL, D. F. (1984). Familial nephropathy in the cocker spaniel. *J. small Anim. Pract.,* **25,** 15.

FURTHER READING

HAZEWINKEL, H. A. W. (1989). Nutrition in relation to skeletal growth deformities. *J. small Anim. Pract.,* **30,** 625.

CHAPTER FOUR

THE ADRENAL GLANDS

Michael E. Herrtage M.A., B.V.Sc., D.V.R., D.V.D., M.R.C.V.S.

Each adrenal gland is composed of a cortex and a medulla, which are embryologically and functionally separate endocrine glands. The cortex is essential for life, but the medulla is not. The most common disorders affect the adrenal cortex causing either hyperadrenocorticism (Cushing's disease) or hypoadrenocorticism (Addison's disease). Conditions affecting the adrenal medulla are rare, the most common being a tumour (phaeochromocytoma).

ANATOMY

The adrenal glands are located craniomedially to the kidneys in retroperitoneal fat. The right adrenal gland lies between the medial surface of the cranial pole of the right kidney and the lateral aspect of the caudal vena cava at the level of the 13th thoracic vertebra. The right phrenicoabdominal vein crosses the ventral surface of the gland before joining the caudal vena cava. The left adrenal gland is found craniomedially to the border of the left kidney at the level of the second lumbar vertebra. Medially it is bounded by the descending aorta just caudal to the cranial mesenteric artery and cranial to the left renal artery and vein.

The adrenal glands of the normal dog together weigh about 1 g. On cross-section, the adrenal cortex appears pale yellow whereas the medulla is dark brown. The cortex completely surrounds the medulla and consists of three distinct zones. The outer **zona glomerulosa** (arcuata) comprises about 25 per cent of the cortex, the middle **zona fasciculata** comprises approximately 60 per cent and the inner **zona reticularis** accounts for the remaining 15 per cent of the cortex. The zona reticularis is adjacent to the medulla, which comprises 10 to 20 per cent of the total volume of the adrenal gland.

PHYSIOLOGY OF THE ADRENAL CORTEX

The adrenal cortex produces about 30 different hormones, many of which have little or no clinical significance. The hormones can be divided into three groups based on their predominant actions: **mineralocorticoids,** which are important in electrolyte and water homeostasis, **glucocorticoids,** which promote gluconeogenesis, and small amounts of **sex hormones,** particularly male hormones that have weak androgenic activity.

Aldosterone is the most important mineralocorticoid and is produced by the zona glomerulosa. The principal glucocorticoid, cortisol, and the sex hormones are produced in the zona fasciculata and zona reticularis. Glucocorticoid and mineralocorticoid release are controlled by different mechanisms.

REGULATION OF GLUCOCORTICOID RELEASE

Glucocorticoid release is controlled almost entirely by adrenocorticotrophic hormone (ACTH) secreted by the anterior pituitary, which in turn, is regulated by corticotrophin releasing hormone (CRH) from the hypothalamus (Figure 1). CRH is secreted by the neurons in the anterior portion of the paraventricular nuclei within the hypothalamus and is transported to the anterior pituitary by the portal circulation, where it stimulates ACTH release. There is probably an internal or 'short loop' negative feedback control by ACTH on CRH. ACTH secreted into the systemic circulation causes cortisol release with levels rising almost immediately. Cortisol has direct negative feedback effects on (i) the hypothalamus to decrease formation of CRH and (ii) the anterior pituitary gland to decrease the formation of ACTH. These feedback mechanisms help regulate the plasma concentration of cortisol.

Secretion of CRH and ACTH is normally episodic and pulsatile and this results in fluctuating cortisol levels. Diurnal variation is superimposed on this type of release. It is usually stated that in the dog CRH, ACTH and thus cortisol levels are highest in the early hours of the morning and that in the cat, they are greatest in the evening. However, a true circadian rhythm of cortisol levels has been difficult to confirm in the dog and cat (Kemppainen and Sartin, 1984; Peterson et al., 1988). The episodic release of CRH and ACTH is perpetuated by the reciprocal effect of cortisol acting through negative feedback control. This reciprocal arrangement does not hold during periods of stress when both ACTH and cortisol are maintained at high levels, because the effects of stress tend to override the normal negative feedback control.

In summary, ACTH and CRH secretion are influenced by diurnal variation and stress as well as by negative feedback control.

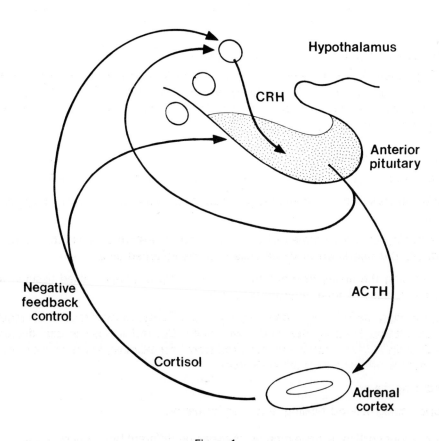

Figure 1
Regulation of glucocorticoid release.
The hypothalamic-pituitary-adrenal axis.

FUNCTIONS OF GLUCOCORTICOIDS

Cortisol has more diverse effects on the body than any other hormone. Its main effect is on carbohydrate, protein and fat metabolism to promote gluconeogenesis. Gluconeogenesis is the production of glucose at the expense of muscle and adipose tissue.

Effect on carbohydrate metabolism

Cortisol stimulates gluconeogenesis in the liver by inducing the formation of hepatic gluconeogenic enzymes. One of the effects of increased gluconeogenesis is a marked increase in glycogen stores within the hepatocytes. Cortisol also causes a moderate decrease in the rate of glucose utilisation by cells everywhere in the body. Both the increased rate of gluconeogenesis and the moderate reduction in the rate of glucose utilisation cause the blood glucose concentration to rise. The increase in blood glucose causes secondary hyperinsulinism that counters glucocorticoid activity. The net result in the normal animal is a balance between these opposing factors.

Effect on protein metabolism

Cortisol reduces protein stores in essentially all body cells except those of the liver. This reduction is caused by decreased protein synthesis and increased catabolism. The catabolic actions of glucocorticoids on muscle result in muscle wasting and weakness. Cortisol depresses amino acid transport into muscle cells and probably into other extrahepatic cells. This effect combined with increased catabolism leads to a rise in blood amino acid levels. The increased plasma concentration of amino acids, plus the fact that cortisol enhances transport of amino acids into the hepatic cells could also account for enhanced utilisation of amino acids by the liver to cause such effects as: (i) increased conversion of amino acids to glucose (gluconeogenesis), (ii) increased protein synthesis in the liver, (iii) increased formation of plasma proteins by the liver, (iv) increased deamination of amino acids by the liver.

Effects on fat metabolism

Cortisol increases lipolysis which results in the release of free fatty acids and glycerol from adipose tissue. Insulin counters this effect by inhibiting lipolysis and stimulating lipogenesis. Ketogenesis occurs if insulin's effects are exceeded. Adipose tissue tends to be redistributed to the abdomen and back of the neck in dogs with excess levels of glucocorticoids.

Anti-inflammatory effects

Glucocorticoids modify the inflammatory process and the immune response by:

1. Stabilising lysosomal membranes to reduce the release of proteolytic enzymes by damaged cells.

2. Decreasing capillary permeability, which prevents loss of plasma into the tissues and also reduces the migration of white cells into the inflamed area.

3. Depressing the ability of white blood cells to digest phagocytised tissues, thus blocking further release of inflammatory materials.

4. Suppressing the immune system, especially the T cells. Glucocorticoids decrease the number of circulating lymphocytes and eosinophils. Cortisol in excess can decrease antibody production but anamnestic antibody production, for example, booster vaccination, is relatively resistant compared to initial responses.

5. Reducing fever.

6. Suppressing wound healing and scar formation.

These effects of glucocorticoids have marked changes on different body systems and organ functions and are summarised in Table 1. A fuller explanation of the pathophysiology concerning excess glucocorticoid activity will be given in the discussion of hyperadrenocorticism.

REGULATION OF MINERALOCORTICOID RELEASE

Aldosterone release is influenced primarily by the renin-angiotensin system and by plasma potassium levels (Figure 2).

Renin is secreted into the blood by the cells of the juxtaglomerular apparatus, which consists of specialised cells in the wall of the afferent arteriole immediately proximal to the glomerulus and the specialised epithelial cells of the distal convoluted tubule adjacent to that arteriole, the macula densa. Renin release may be stimulated by stretch receptors in the juxtaglomerular apparatus in response to hypotension or reduced renal blood flow or by sodium and chloride receptors in the macula densa. Renin is also released by sympathetic nerve stimulation and is inhibited by angiotensin II, antidiuretic hormone, hypertension and increased reabsorption of sodium by the renal tubules.

Renin is an enzyme which splits circulating angiotensinogen, produced by the liver, into angiotensin I. Angiotensin I is converted to angiotensin II by a converting enzyme found almost entirely in the pulmonary capillary endothelium.

Angiotensin II is a powerful vasoconstrictor and stimulates aldosterone secretion from the zona glomerulosa. Through its action on the distal convoluted tubule, aldosterone has a negative feedback effect on the juxtaglomerular apparatus.

Potassium has a direct stimulatory effect on the zona glomerulosa cells to release aldosterone.

Table 1
Effects of glucocorticoids on different body systems

Liver	Increased gluconeogenesis Increased glycogen stores Induction of certain enzymes
Muscle	Increased protein catabolism — muscle wasting and weakness
Bone	Osteoporosis associated with increased protein catabolism and negative calcium balance
Skin	Increased protein catabolism — thin skin, poor wound healing and poor scar formation.
Blood	Erythrocytosis Decrease in circulating lymphocytes Decrease in circulating eosinophils Increase in circulating neutrophils
Kidney	Increased glomerular filtration rate or interference with ADH release or action — polyuria Increased calcium excretion
Immune system	Diminished inflammatory response Reduced immune response
Adipose tissue	Increased lipolysis Redistribution of fat deposits
Pituitary and hypothalamus	Suppression of ACTH and CRH secretion

ACTH and sodium play a less significant role in aldosterone secretion. ACTH is necessary to maintain normal aldosterone output. In the absence of ACTH, the zona glomerulosa partially atrophies, causing mild to moderate aldosterone deficiency, compared with almost total atrophy of the other zones.

FUNCTIONS OF MINERALOCORTICOIDS

The main function of aldosterone is to protect against hypotension and potassium intoxication. Aldosterone promotes sodium, chloride and water reabsorption as well as potassium excretion in many epithelial tissues including the intestinal mucosa, salivary glands, sweat glands and kidneys. Its main site of action is the renal tubule where it promotes sodium and chloride reabsorption in the proximal convoluted tubule and sodium reabsorption by exchange with potassium in the distal convoluted tubule. It is one of the complex systems for the regulation of extracellular fluid electrolyte concentrations, extracellular fluid volume, blood volume and arterial pressure.

PHYSIOLOGY OF THE ADRENAL MEDULLA

The interlacing cords of cells in the adrenal medulla are modified postganglionic sympathetic neurons that release the catecholamines, adrenaline and noradrenaline, into the circulation. Thus, any stimulus that activates the sympathetic nervous system will cause release of adrenaline and noradrenaline from the adrenal medulla. Circulating adrenaline and noradrenaline have almost the same effects on different organs as those caused by direct sympathetic nervous stimulation, except that the effects last 5 to 10 times as long.

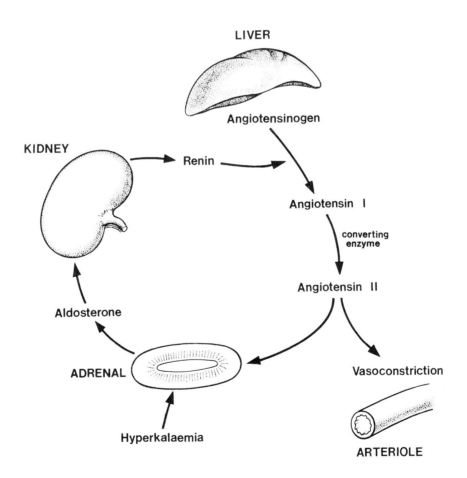

Figure 2
Regulation of mineralocorticoid release.
The renin-angiotensin-aldosterone system.

In normal adult dogs, about 20 to 25 per cent of adrenal medullary secretion is noradrenaline, whereas in the cat about 40 per cent is noradrenaline. However, the relative proportions of adrenaline and norandrenaline may vary in response to different stimuli. Noradrenaline excites mainly α receptors, whereas adrenaline excites both α and β receptors. Table 2 summarises the most important α and β adrenergic effects. The main differences between adrenaline and noradrenaline are that adrenaline has a greater effect on cardiac activity and on metabolic rate and that noradrenaline is a far more potent vasoconstrictor of blood vessels to muscle.

Table 2
Summary of α and β adrenergic effects

	α	β
Heart		
Force of contraction		Increased (β_1)
Heart rate		Increased (β_1)
Blood vessels		
Skeletal muscle vasculature	Constricted	Dilated (β_2)
Coronary arteries		Dilated (β_1)
Lung		
Bronchial smooth muscle	Bronchoconstriction	Bronchodilation (β_2)
Smooth muscle		
Uterine	Contraction	Relaxation (β_2)
Gastrointestinal	Relaxation	Relaxation
G.I. sphincter tone	Increased	Increased
Metabolism		
Gluconeogenesis	Stimulated	
Glycogenolysis	Stimulated (liver)	Stimulated (in heart and skeletal muscle)
Lipolysis		Stimulated
Hormone secretion		
Glucagon		Stimulated (β_2)
Insulin	Inhibited	Stimulated (β_2)
Parathormone		Stimulated
Renin		Stimulated (β_1)

HYPERADRENOCORTICISM (CUSHING'S DISEASE)

Hyperadrenocorticism is associated with excessive production or administration of glucocorticoids and is one of the most commonly diagnosed endocrinopathies in the dog. Hyperadrenocorticism is rare in the cat and will be dealt with separately at the end of this section.

CAUSES OF HYPERADRENOCORTICISM

Hyperadrenocorticism can be spontaneous or iatrogenic. Spontaneously occurring hyperadrenocorticism may be associated with inappropriate secretion of ACTH by the pituitary (*pituitary-dependent hyperadrenocorticism)* or associated with a primary adrenal disorder (*adrenal-dependent hyperadrenocorticism)* (Figure 3).

Figure 3

a) The hypothalamic-pituitary-adrenal axis in
   pituitary-dependent hyperadrenocorticism

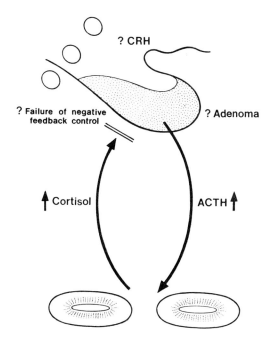

? CRH

? Failure of negative
feedback control

? Adenoma

↑Cortisol

ACTH↑

b) The hypothalamic-pituitary-adrenal axis in
   adrenal-dependent hyperadrenocorticism

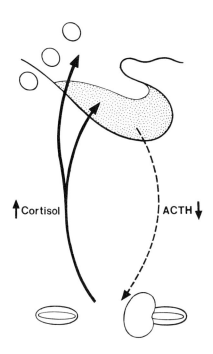

↑Cortisol

ACTH↓

PITUITARY—DEPENDENT HYPERADRENOCORTICISM

Pituitary-dependent hyperadrenocorticism accounts for 80 per cent of dogs with naturally occurring hyperadrenocorticism. Excessive ACTH secretion results in bilateral adrenocortical hyperplasia and excess cortisol secretion. There is a failure of the negative feedback mechanism of cortisol on ACTH. However, episodic secretion of ACTH results in fluctuating cortisol levels that may at times be within the normal range. The presence of excess cortisol secretion can be confirmed by measuring urine cortisol excretion over a 24-hour period.

Pathological changes in pituitary-dependent hyperadrenocorticism

Microadenomas — less than 1 cm diameter. The incidence of chromophobe adenomas associated with pituitary-dependent hyperadrenocorticism varies widely probably because detection of small tumours requires careful microdissection, experience and special stains.

In one study using immunocytochemical staining, more than 80 per cent of dogs with pituitary-dependent hyperadrenocorticism were positive for pituitary adenomas (Peterson *et al.,* 1982a).

Macroadenomas — greater than 1 cm diameter. Only a small percentage of dogs have large chromophobe adenomas. These may compress the remaining pituitary gland and extend dorsally into the hypothalmus (Plate 4:1). However, they are generally slow growing and may not produce neurological signs. Malignant pituitary tumours are rare.

Primary failure of the feedback response — The defect responsible for pituitary-dependent hyperadrenocorticism unassociated with pituitary neoplasia is unknown. A primary failure of the negative feedback response by cortisol has been proposed. Others suspect an overproduction of CRH from the hypothalamus, which may cause diffuse hyperplasia of ACTH-producing cells in the anterior pituitary.

From a clinical point of view the precise pituitary pathology is not of great importance unless neurological signs are present at the time of diagnosis or become apparent during the initial treatment.

ADRENAL-DEPENDENT HYPERADRENOCORTICISM

The remaining 15—20 per cent of spontaneous cases of hyperadrenocorticism are caused by unilateral or bilateral adrenal tumours, which can be benign or malignant.

Adrenocortical adenomas

These are small, well-circumscribed tumours that do not metastasize and are not locally invasive. Approximately 50 per cent are partially calcified.

Adrenocortical carcinomas

These are usually large, locally invasive, haemorrhagic and necrotic. Tumour calcification also occurs in 50 per cent of dogs. Carcinomas, especially of the right adrenal, frequently invade the phrenicoabdominal vein and caudal vena cava and metastasize to the liver, lung and kidney (Plate 4:2).

In dogs, adrenocortical adenomas and carcinomas occur in approximately equal proportions. The cortex contiguous to the tumour and that of the contralateral gland atrophy in the presence of functional adenomas and carcinomas (Plate 4:3). This is important if the tumour is removed surgically as post-operatively the animal may not be able to secrete glucocorticoids. The function of the zona glomerulosa should not be affected.

BREED, SEX AND AGE PREDISPOSITION

Breed

Any breed can develop hyperadrenocorticism but poodles, dachshunds and small terriers, Yorkshire terrier, Jack Russell terrier and Staffordshire bull terrier, appear more at risk of developing pituitary-dependent hyperadrenocorticism. Adrenocortical tumours occur more frequently in larger breeds of dog.

Age

Pituitary-dependent hyperadrenocorticism is usually a disease of the middle-aged to older dog, with an age range of 2 to 16 years and a median age of 7 to 9 years. Dogs with adrenal-dependent hyperadrenocorticism tend to be older, ranging between 6 and 16 years with a median age of 10 to 11 years (Meijer, 1980; Feldman and Nelson, 1987).

Sex

There is no significant difference in sex distribution in pituitary-dependent hyperadrenocorticism. However, female dogs are three times more likely to develop adrenal tumours than males (Meijer, 1980).

CLINICAL SIGNS

Affected dogs usually develop a classic combination of clinical signs associated with increased glucocorticoid levels and these are listed in Table 3 in approximate decreasing order of frequency. However, larger breeds of dogs may not show all the classic signs and are thus more difficult to diagnose.

Hyperadrenocorticism has an insidious onset and is slowly progressive over many months or even years. Many owners consider the early signs as part of the normal ageing process of their dog. In a few cases, clinical signs may be intermittent, with periods of remission and relapse (Peterson *et al.,* 1982 b) and in others there may be apparent rapid onset and progression of clinical signs.

Table 3
Clinical signs of hyperadrenocorticism in approximate decreasing order of frequency

Polydipsia and polyuria
Polyphagia
Abdominal distension
Liver enlargement
Muscle wasting/weakness
Lethargy, poor exercise tolerance
Skin changes
Alopecia
Persistent anoestrus or testicular atrophy
Calcinosis cutis
Myotonia
Neurological signs

Polydipsia and polyuria

Polydipsia, defined as water intake in excess of 100 ml/kg body weight/day and polyuria, defined as urine production in excess of 50 ml/kg body weight/day, are seen in nearly all cases of hyperadrenocorticism. Excessive thirst, nocturia and/or urination in the house are usually noted by owners.

The polydipsia occurs secondary to the polyuria, which is only partially responsive to water deprivation. The precise cause of the polyuria remains obscure, but may be due to increased glomerular filtration rate, inhibition of the release of antidiuretic hormone (ADH), inhibition of the action of ADH on the renal tubules and possibly accelerated inactivation of ADH.

Polyphagia

Increased appetite is common but owners often assess this as a sign of good health. A voracious appetite, scavenging or stealing food, however, may give rise to concern especially if the dog previously had a poor appetite.

Polyphagia is assumed to be a direct effect of glucocorticoids.

Abdominal distension

The pot-bellied appearance is very common in hyperadrenocorticism but may be so gradual that owners fail to recognise its significance (Plate 4:4).

The abdominal distension is associated with redistribution of fat to the abdomen, liver enlargement and abdominal muscle wasting and weakness. The weakness of the abdominal muscles makes palpation of the pendulous abdomen easier and more rewarding.

Muscle wasting/weakness

The gradual onset of lethargy and poor exercise tolerance are usually considered by most owners to be compatible with ageing. Only when muscle weakness is severe as reflected by an inability to climb stairs or jump into the car does the owner become concerned. Lethargy, excessive panting and poor exercise tolerance are an expression of muscle wasting and weakness. Apart from the development of a pendulous abdomen, decreased muscle mass may be noted around the limbs, over the spine or over the temporal region. Muscle weakness is the result of muscle wasting caused by protein catabolism.

Occasionally, dogs with hyperadrenocorticism develop myotonia, characterised by persistent active muscle contractions that continue after voluntary or involuntary stimuli. All limbs may be affected, but the signs are usually more severe in the hindlegs. Animals with myotonia walk with a stiff, stilted gait. The affected limbs are rigid and rapidly return to extension after being passively flexed. Spinal reflexes are difficult to elicite because of the rigidity, but pain sensation is normal. The muscles are usually slightly hypertrophied rather than being atrophic and a myotonic dimple can be elicited by percusssion of the affected muscles. Bizarre, high frequency discharges are noted on electromyography (Duncan *et al.,* 1977).

Skin changes

The skin, particularly over the ventral abdomen, becomes thin and inelastic. Elasticity can be assessed clinically by tenting the skin between the thumb and forefinger (Plate 4:5). In the normal dog the skin will flow back to a smooth contour but in hyperadrenocorticism it remains tented (Plate 4:6). Striae can form as a result of this inelasticity. The abdominal veins are prominent and easily visible through the thin skin. There is often excessive surface scale and comedomes caused by follicular plugging are seen especially around the nipples (Plate 4:7). Hyperpigmentation of the skin is rare in canine hyperadrenocorticism.

Protein catabolism causes atrophy of collagen which leads to excessive bruising following either venepuncture or other minor trauma. Wound healing is extraordinarily slow, presumably because of inhibition of fibroblast proliferation and collagen synthesis. Healing wounds often undergo dehiscence and even old scars may start to breakdown (Plate 4:8).

Calcinosis cutis is a frequent finding in biopsy material from the skin. However, clinical evidence of calcinosis cutis is less common. The gross appearance can vary but the predilection sites are the neck, axillae, ventral abdomen and inguinal areas (Plates 4:9 and 4:10). Calcinosis cutis usually appears as a firm, slightly elevated, white or cream plaque surrounded by a ring of erythema. Large plaques tend to crack, become secondarily infected and develop a crust containing white powdery material. The exact pathogenesis is unknown but plasma calcium and phosphorus levels are usually normal.

Mineralisation may be seen at other sites, for example the bronchial walls and kidneys on radiographic examination (see below).

Haircoat changes

Thinning of the haircoat leading to bilaterally symmetrical alopecia is frequently seen with hyper-adrenocorticism and occurs because of the inhibitory effect of cortisol on the anagen or growth phase of the hair cycle. The remaining hair is dull and dry because it is in the telogen or resting phase of the hair cycle. The alopecia is non-pruritic and affects mainly the flanks, ventral abdomen and chest, perineum and neck. The head, feet and tail are usually the last areas to be affected (Plate 4:4). The coat colour is often lighter than normal.

Anoestrus/testicular atrophy

Entire bitches with hyperadrenocorticism usually cease to cycle. The length of anoestrus, often years, indicates the duration of the disease process. In the intact male both testes become soft and spongy.

Anoestrus and testicular atrophy occur due to the negative feedback effect of high levels of cortisol on the pituitary, which also suppresses secretion of gonadotrophic hormones.

Neurological signs

Although uncommon at the time of presentation, a few cases will develop neurological signs associated with a large functional pituitary tumour. The most common clinical signs are dullness, depression, loss of learned behaviour, anorexia, aimless wandering, head pressing, circling, ataxia, blindness, anisocoria and seizures. More often, however, neurological signs develop during initial treatment of pituitary-dependent hyperadrenocorticism with mitotane. This is thought to occur due to the sudden reduction in cortisol levels which can allow some pituitary tumours to enlarge rapidly.

ROUTINE LABORATORY FINDINGS

The main haematological, biochemical and urinalysis findings are listed in Table 4.

Haematology

The most consistent haematological finding is a stress leukogram with a relative and absolute lymphopenia ($< 1500/mm^3$) and eosinopenia ($< 200/mm^3$). Lymphopenia is most likely the result of steroid lympholysis and eosinopenia results from bone marrow sequestration of eosinophils (Feldman and Feldman, 1977). A mild to moderate neutrophilia and monocytosis may be found and is thought to result from decreased capillary margination and diapedesis associated with excess glucocorticoids.

Table 4
Routine laboratory findings in hyperadrenocorticism

Haematology	Lymphopenia ($<1500/mm^3$)
	Eosinopenia ($<200/mm^3$)
	Neutrophilia
	Monocytosis
	Erythrocytosis
Biochemistry	Increased alkaline phosphatase (often markedly elevated)
	Increased ALT
	High normal fasting blood glucose. Rarely diabetic.
	Decreased blood urea.
	Increased cholesterol (>8 mmol/l)
	Lipaemia
	Increased BSP retention
	Increased bile salt levels
Urinalysis	Urine specific gravity <1.015
	Glycosuria (< 10 per cent of cases)
	Urinary tract infection
Other findings	Low T_4 levels
	Subnormal response to TSH

The red cell count is usually normal, although mild polycythaemia may occasionally be noted. Platelet counts may also be elevated. These findings are thought to result from stimulatory effects of glucocorticoids on the bone marrow.

Biochemistry

Alkaline phosphatase — Glucocorticoids, both endogenous or exogenous, induce a specific hepatic isoenzyme of alkaline phosphatase. The increase in serum alkaline phosphatase is commonly 5 to 40 times the normal level and is perhaps one of the most reliable indicators of hyperadrenocorticism.

Measurement of the specific steroid-induced isoenzyme of alkaline phosphatase has been used for more accurate assessment of elevated serum alkaline phosphatase activity (Oluju *et al.,* 1984).

Alanine aminotransferase (ALT) — ALT is commonly elevated in hyperadrenocorticism, but the increase is usually only mild and is believed to result from liver damage caused by swollen hepatocytes due to glycogen storage.

Blood glucose — Blood glucose is usually in the high normal range. About 10 per cent of cases may develop overt diabetes mellitus which is caused by antagonism to insulin from the gluconeogenic effect of glucocorticoids, and subsequent development of pancreatic islet cell exhaustion.

Blood urea — Blood urea is usually below normal due to the continual urinary loss associated with glucocorticoid-induced diuresis. Serum creatinine concentration also tends to be in the low to normal range.

Cholesterol and lipaemia — Cholesterol and lipid levels are usually increased due to glucocorticoid stimulation of lipolysis. Cholesterol is usually greater than 8 mmol/l but this is not a specific finding as cholesterol is also raised in hypothyroidism, diabetes mellitus, chronic liver disease and chronic renal disease, all of which may be differential diagnoses. Lipaemia is important in that it can interfere with the accurate assessment of a number of laboratory parameters.

Serum electrolytes — Sodium, potassium, calcium and phosphorus are usually in the normal range.

Bromsulphthalein (BSP) retention test — BSP retention is mildly to moderately elevated in hyperadrenocorticism and therefore cannot be used to differentiate it from primary liver disorders.

Bile salt levels — Bile salt levels also usually show a mild to moderate elevation in hyperadrenocorticism.

Urinalysis

Urine specific gravity — The specific gravity of the urine is usually less than 1.015 and is often hyposthenuric (< 1.010) provided water has not been witheld. Dogs with hyperadrenocorticism can concentrate their urine if water is deprived, but their concentrating ability is usually reduced.

Urine glucose — Glycosuria is present in the 10 per cent of cases with diabetes mellitus.

Urinary tract infection — The urine should be analysed for infection, because urinary infections occur in about half the cases of hyperadrenocorticism.

Other laboratory findings

Thyroxine (T$_4$) — Basal thyroxine levels are decreased in about 70 per cent of dogs with hyperadrenocorticism (Peterson et al, 1984). This is, in part, due to inhibition of thyrotropin-releasing hormone (TRH) and reduced pituitary secretion of thyroid-stimulating hormone (TSH). Excess cortisol, however, may also alter thyroid hormone binding to plasma proteins and enhance the metabolism of thyroid hormone. The response to a TSH stimulation test usually parallels normal but thyroxine levels both pre- and post-TSH are subnormal.

RADIOGRAPHIC FINDINGS

Radiographic examination of the thorax and abdomen is advisable in all cases. Although positive diagnostic information is only obtained in the small number of cases in which adrenal enlargement can be detected, the number and frequency of radiological changes consistent with hyperadrenocorticism provides a useful aid to diagnosis. In addition, survey radiographs may reveal significant intercurrent disease. The radiological signs of hyperadrenocorticism have been reviewed (Huntley et al., 1982) and the common changes are listed below.

Abdominal radiographs

There is good radiographic contrast because of the large deposits of intra-abdominal fat. This permits easy identification of the abdominal structures.

Radiological signs of note are:-

Pot-bellied appearance — This is usually very obvious on recumbent lateral projection (Figure 4)

Hepatomegaly — This is the most consistent finding in hyperadrenocorticism. It may be mild to severe and the ventral lobe borders vary between sharply wedge-shaped and distinctly rounded.

Adrenal enlargement/calcification — Adrenomegaly is the least common finding on radiographs. Gross enlargement is suggestive, though not diagnostic, of an adrenal carcinoma.

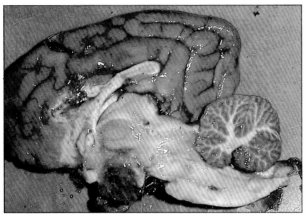

Plate 4:1
A chromophobe adenoma found at post-mortem examination
of a 13-year-old golden retriever, which had been successfully
treated with mitotane for five years. No neurological signs had
been associated with the presence of this tumour.

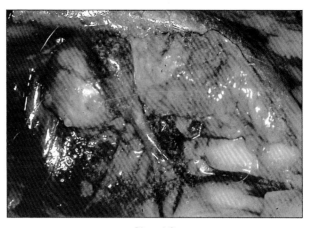

Plate 4:2
An adrenocortical carcinoma of the right adrenal
gland invading the phrenicoabdominal vein.
The caudal vena cava can be seen at the top
of the photograph.

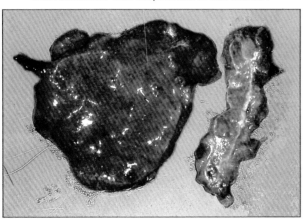

Plate 4:3
The cut surface of both the adrenal glands from the case
shown in Plate 4:2. There are large areas of necrosis
in the adrenocortical carcinoma. Note the severe cortical
atrophy (pale rim) of the contralateral adrenal.

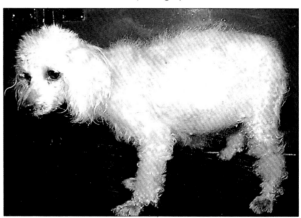

Plate 4:4
A six-year-old poodle bitch with pituitary-dependent
hyperadrenocorticism showing abdominal distension,
muscle wasting and alopecia.

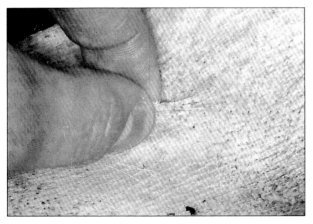

Plate 4:5
Tenting the skin of the ventral abdomen
to assess elasticity.

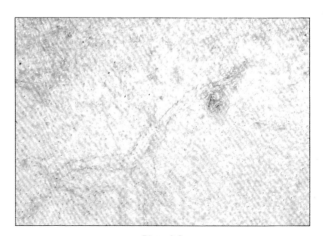

Plate 4:6
In hyperadrenocorticism, the skin is thin, inelastic and
remains tented after release. An abdominal vein
is visible through the thin skin.

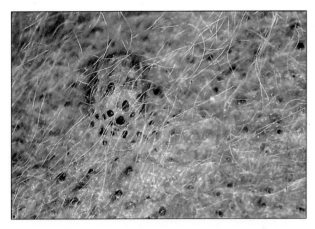

Plate 4:7
Comedomes are seen around the nipple of a dog
with hyperadrenocorticism. The skin is thin and
abdominal veins are prominent.

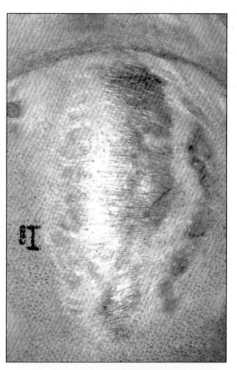

Plate 4:8
Partial breakdown of an
abdominal incision in a boxer
with hyperadrenocorticism.
Note the striae to the right
at the cranial end of the incision.
The mark to the left
represents 1 cm.

Plate 4:9
Skin in the inguinal region of a
poodle with hyperadrenocorticism.
Focal areas of calcinosis cutis
can be seen eroding through
the epidermis.
Comedomes are also present.

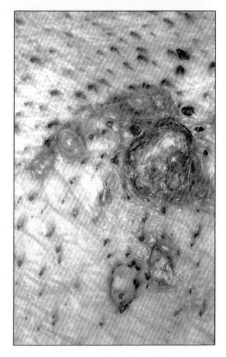

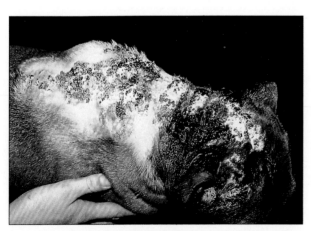

Plate 4:10
Diffuse calcinosis cutis involving the dorsal aspect
of the neck of a Staffordshire bull terrier
with hyperadrenocorticism. The skin is ulcerated
and secondarily infected.

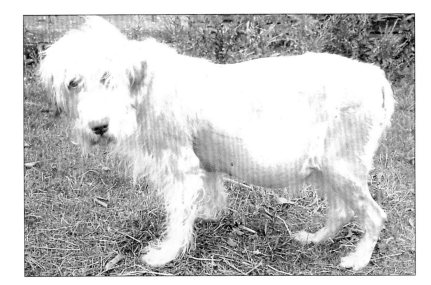

Plate 4:11a
A 10-year-old crossbred dog with pituitary-dependent hyperadrenocorticism before treatment

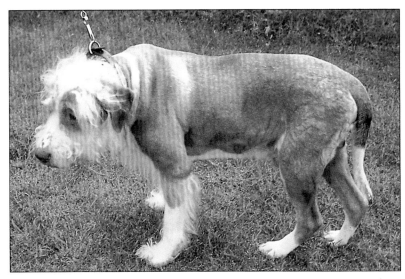

Figure 4:11b
The same dog eight weeks after commencing treatment with mitotane.

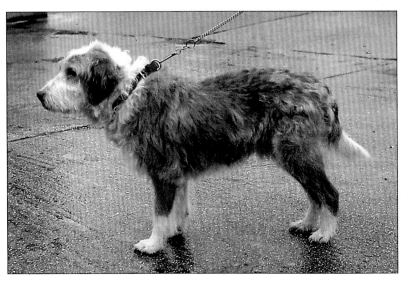

Plate 4:11c
The same dog six months later.

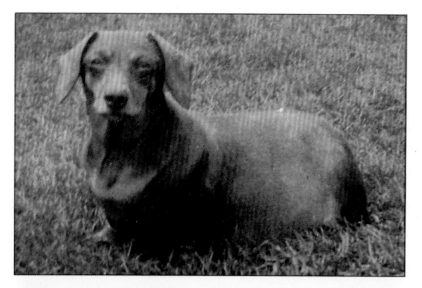

Plate 4:12a
A 7-year-old dachshund bitch with pituitary-dependent hyperadrenocorticism before treatment

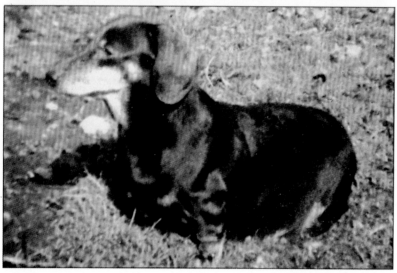

Plate 4:12b
The same dog four months after commencing mitotane therapy. Note the marked change in coat colour following successful treatment.

Unilateral mineralisation in the region of an adrenal gland suggests an adrenal tumour. Both adrenocortical adenomas and carcinomas can become calcified.

Calcinosis cutis and soft tissue mineralisation — Calcinosis cutis tends to have a nodular mineralisation pattern, whereas calcification in the fascial planes, for example just dorsal to the thoracolumbar spine, tends to be linear (Figure 4). Mineralisation may also be seen in the renal pelvis, liver, gastric mucosa, abdominal aorta and hindlimb muscles.

Distended bladder/cystic calculi — A grossly distended urinary bladder may be seen radiographically even when the animal has been allowed to urinate prior to radiography. Cystic calculi may also be present and are usually associated with urinary tract infection.

Osteoporosis — Objective evaluation of skeletal mineralisation is notoriously difficult. However, occasionally the impression of osteoporosis is gained from a distinct reduction in radiographic density of the lumbar vertebral bodies relative to the vertebral end plates (Figure 4).

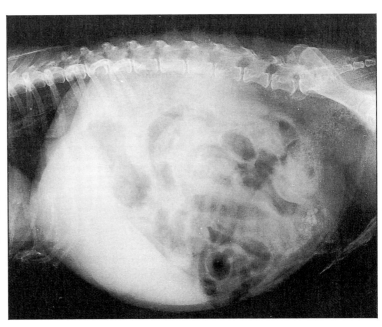

Figure 4
A lateral abdominal radiograph of a Cairn terrier with pituitary-dependent hyperadrenocorticism. The radiological signs include hepatomegaly, abdominal distension, an enlarged bladder with cystic calculi, calcinosis cutis, dystrophic calcification in the soft tissues along the spine and osteoporosis.

Thoracic radiographs

Radiological signs of note are:-

Tracheal and bronchial wall calcification — This is frequently seen in cases of hyper-adrenocorticism. However, calcification of these structures occurs normally in ageing animals and is not considered highly significant.

Pulmonary metastases from adrenocortical carcinoma

Osteoporosis of the thoracic spine

Congestive heart failure (rare)

Pulmonary thromboembolism — another rare complication which may be suspected when radiographic signs include evidence of pleural effusion, increased diameter and blunting of the pulmonary arteries, decreased vascularity of the affected lobes and overperfusion of the unobstructed pulmonary vasculature. However, in some cases of pulmonary thromboembolism, the radiographs may reveal no abnormalities.

Calcinosis cutis and soft tissue mineralisation — This may also be noticed on thoracic radiographs.

Skull radiographs

Plain radiographs of the skull are usually unrewarding. Cavernous sinus venography, however, may be used to identify large pituitary tumours (Lee and Griffiths, 1972) which can cause pituitary-dependent hyperadrenocorticism.

Other imaging techniques

Abdominal ultrasonography has been used to detect large adrenocortical tumours (Kantrowitz *et al.*, 1986).

Computer tomography (CT) has proved helpful in the diagnosis of adrenal tumours, adrenal hyperplasia and large pituitary tumours but is expensive and not widely available (Voorhout *et al.*, 1988).

Gamma camera imaging of the adrenal glands has also been reported (Mulnix *et al.*, 1976).

CONFIRMATION OF DIAGNOSIS

A presumptive diagnosis of hyperadrenocorticism can be made from clinical signs, physical examination, routine laboratory tests and radiographic findings, but the diagnosis must be confirmed by either an ACTH stimulation test or a low-dose dexamethasone suppression test. The practical details of these tests are given in Chapter 14, and only the relative merits of each test will be discussed here.

ACTH stimulation test

Advantages — The ACTH stimulation test is the best screening test for distinguishing spontaneous from iatrogenic hyperadrenocorticism and reliably identifies more than 50 per cent of dogs with adrenal-dependent hyperadrenocorticism and about 85 per cent of dogs with pituitary-dependent hyperadrenocorticism. It is a simple test to perform and the only one that documents excessive production of glucocorticoids by the adrenal cortex. The information gained is also helpful to provide a baseline for monitoring mitotane therapy.

Disadvantages — The ACTH stimulation test does not reliably differentiate adrenal-dependent from pituitary-dependent hyperadrenocorticism. A diagnosis of hyperadrenocorticism should not be excluded on the basis of a normal ACTH response if the clinical signs are compatible with the disease. Occasionally, an animal under chronic stress may develop some degree of adrenal hyperplasia, which produces an abnormal ACTH response. The author has seen this with diabetes mellitus and pyometra and documented a normal ACTH response after treatment in each case.

Interpretation — It is essential to use absolute values for pre- and post- ACTH plasma cortisol levels rather than a ratio or percentage increase in post-ACTH cortisol levels over the basal concentration. Regardless of the pre-ACTH cortisol value, a diagnosis of hyperadrenocorticism depends on the demonstration of a post-ACTH cortisol concentration higher than 600 nmol/l (Figure 5).

Low-dose dexamethasone suppression test

Advantages — The low-dose dexamethasone suppression test is more reliable that the ACTH stimulation test in confirming hyperadrenocorticism, since the results are diagnostic in all adrenal-dependent cases and in 90 to 95 per cent of dogs with pituitary-dependent hyperadrenocorticism.

Disadvantages — It is not as useful as the ACTH stimulation test for the detection of iatrogenic hyperadrenocorticism. It is also affected by more variables, takes 8 hours to complete and does not provide pretreatment information that may aid in monitoring the effects of mitotane therapy. The low-dose dexamethasone suppression test does not reliably differentiate pituitary-dependent from adrenal-dependent hyperadrenocorticism.

Interpretation — Interpretation of the results of a low-dose dexamethasone suppression test must be based on the laboratory's normal range for the dose and preparation of dexamethasone administered. If the dose of dexamethasone fails to adequately suppress circulating cortisol concentrations in a dog with compatible clinical signs, a diagnosis of hyperadrenocorticism is confirmed. While basal and 8-hour post-dexamethasone samples are most important for interpretation of the test (Figure 6), one or more samples taken at intermediate times (for example, 2, 4, or 6, hours) during the test period may also prove helpful. If a plasma cortisol concentration determined two to six hours after dexamethasone injection is suppressed normally or near-normally (to below 40 nmol/l), while the 8-hour sample shows escape from cortisol suppression, then a diagnosis of pituitary-dependent hyperadrenocorticism is indicated (Peterson, 1984).

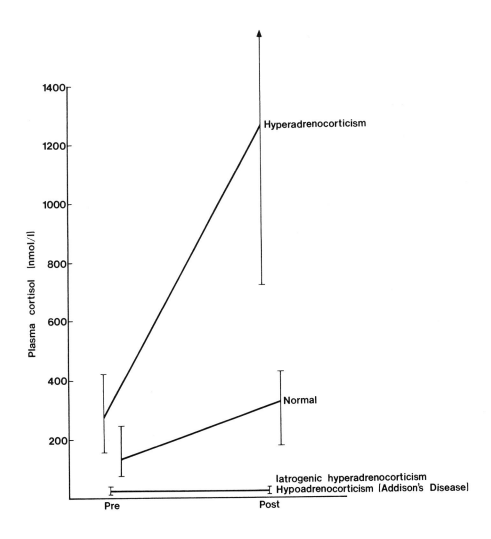

Figure 5
The ACTH stimulation test.
Interpretation of plasma cortisol concentrations
determined before and after administration of synthetic ACTH.

Other screening tests

Evaluation of urinary corticoid/creatinine ratio rather than the more laborious 24-hour urinary corticoid excretion has been shown to be a simple and valuable screening test (Rijnberk *et al*, 1988). This test is not yet routinely available in veterinary laboratories in the United Kingdom.

TESTS TO DIFFERENTIATE PITUITARY-DEPENDENT AND ADRENAL-DEPENDENT HYPERADRENOCORTICISM

Although the determination of plasma ACTH concentrations would provide a reliable test for differentiating pituitary and adrenal causes of hyperadrenocorticism, canine ACTH assays are not readily available. The high-dose dexamethasone suppression test is most commonly used for differentiating the cause of hyperadrenocorticism.

High-dose dexamethasone suppression test

The high dose dexamethasone suppression test is indicated in those cases where the diagnosis of hyperadrenocorticism has been established by a screening test, but the differentiation of adrenal-dependent and pituitary-dependent hyperadrenocorticism has not been determined. The high dose of dexamethasone inhibits pituitary ACTH secretion through negative feedback in pituitary-dependent hyperadrenocorticism thus suppressing cortisol levels. Adrenocortical tumours are autonomous and thus cortisol is not suppressed. Approximately 15 per cent of pituitary-dependent cases, however, will not suppress with this test. The test does not differentiate adrenocortical adenomas from adreno-cortical carcinomas.

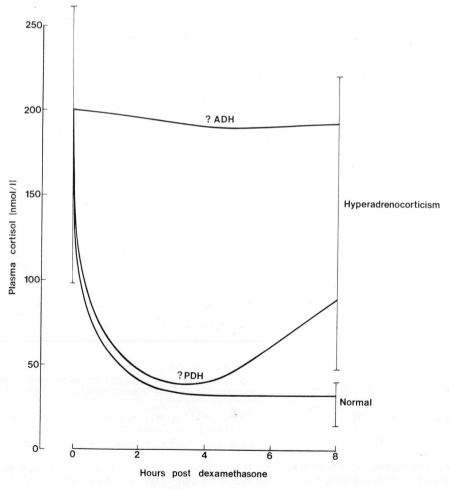

Figure 6

The low-dose dexamethasone suppression test.

Interpretation of plasma cortisol concentrations determined during low-dose dexamethasone screening.
?ADH represents the type of response seen in most cases of adrenal-dependent hyperadrenocorticism.
?PDH represents a possible response in pituitary-dependent cases

TREATMENT OF PITUITARY-DEPENDENT HYPERADRENOCORTICISM

Mitotane therapy

Mitotane* is the treatment of choice for pituitary-dependent hyperadrenocorticism. During its evaluation as an insecticide, mitotane was discovered to have adrenocorticolytic effects. It selectively destroys the zona fasciculata and zona reticularis while tending to preserve the zona glomerulosa.

Pre-treatment assessment — Mitotane therapy should only be considered once the diagnosis of hyperadrenocorticism has been confirmed. Because of its powerful effects, it should never be used empirically. Before treatment is instigated, the patient's daily water consumption should be measured over at least two consecutive 24-hour periods. If the water intake and appetite are not increased then baseline lymphocyte counts and cortisol levels, pre- and post- ACTH stimulation, are required in order that the effects of treatment can be monitored. In cases with concomitant diabetes mellitus, the diabetes should be stabilised with insulin prior to treatment with mitotane.

Initial treatment — The author prefers to have his patients hospitalised for the initial course of treatment, although many clinicians have dogs treated by their owners at home, with the owners doing the necessary monitoring.

Mitotane is given orally at a dose rate of 50 mg/kg/day and should be administered with food. Concomitant glucocorticoid treatment is not advised, although if the dog is being treated at home, the owner should be given a small supply of prednisolone tablets to used in an emergency. Daily mitotane therapy should be continued until one of the following changes is noted:

1. the water intake of a polydipsic dog drops to below 60 ml/kg/day
2. the dog takes longer to consume its meal than before treatment or stops eating completely
3. the dog vomits or has diarrhoea
4. the dog becomes listless and depressed.

The initial mitotane course is then stopped and the dog put on maintenance therapy (see below). The importance of close monitoring of the patient during this period cannot be over emphasised.

Table 5

Possible problems that may be encountered during mitotane therapy and their management

PROBLEM	MANAGEMENT
Vomiting or anorexia within the first 3 days of treatment (gastric irritation).	Discontinue mitotane and reassess patient. Divide dose and give 2 to 4 times a day.
Profound weakness, depression and anorexia on 4th or 5th day of treatment.	Discontinue mitotane and reassess patient. Check sodium and potassium levels and institute prednisolone (0.2 mg/kg/day). Start maintenance therapy with mitotane or reassess ACTH stimulation test.
Acute onset of neurological signs.	Reassess patient. Continue mitotane unless the dog is anorexic, vomiting or depressed. Give prednisolone 2.0 mg/kg/day or dexamethasone 0.1 mg/kg/day and decrease dose slowly once neurological signs have resolved.
Failure to resume normal water intake.	Recheck urinalysis and blood urea. Reassess ACTH stimulation test. Increase mitotane dose by 50% if post ACTH cortisol level is greater than 300 nmol/l.
Failure to regrow hair.	Reassess ACTH stimulation test. Determine baseline T_4. Increase mitotane by 50% if post ACTH cortisol level is greater than 300 nmol/L. (If <200 nmol/l perform a TSH stimulation test).
Excessive depression or weakness related to weekly maintenance therapy.	Reassess patient. Check sodium and potassium levels. Repeat ACTH stimulation test. If cortisol level post ACTH is less than 50 nmol/l reduce maintenance dose or give dose every other week.

*Currently available from Idis Limited, 51 High Street, Kingston-upon-Thames, Surrey KT1 1LQ.

Mitotane therapy is comparatively safe and the side effects which commonly occur — anorexia, vomiting and diarrhoea — are rarely serious providing they are noticed early so that mitotane can be withheld. Some of the problems occasionally encountered during treatment are summarised in Table 5 with their suggested management.

The majority of dogs with pituitary-dependent hyperadrenocorticism require between 7 and 14 days treatment with an average of 10 days before water consumption drops below 60 ml/kg/day. If the dog is not polydipsic or polyphagic then treatment should continue until the lymphocyte count is above 1000/mm^3 or until the cortisol levels both pre- and post-ACTH are below 200 nmol/l. A few dogs respond in 2 to 3 days, and occasionally others require more than 60 consecutive days of treatment. It is important to emphasise that each dog must be treated as an individual if the treatment is to be successful.

Maintenance therapy — Having produced sufficient adrenocortical damage with daily mitotane treatment, it is important to continue therapy, albeit at a lower dose, otherwise the zona glomerulosa will regenerate a hyperplastic zona fasciculata and zona reticularis and the clinical signs will recur.

Mitotane is given at a dose of 50 mg/kg/week with food. Cases that are well controlled may sleep for a few hours after the weekly dose and for that reason it is often recommended that the treatment be given in the evening. More profound depression or weakness requires re-evaluation and possibly a reduction of the maintenance dose. Failure to control the polydipsia may require an increased maintenance dose of mitotane (Table 5).

Re-examination — Treated dogs should be re-examined 6 to 8 weeks after completion of the initial therapy, unless there are any problems. Marked improvement should be noted at this time. The most obvious and rapid response is a reduction in water intake, urine output and appetite and this is usually obvious at the end of the initial course of therapy. Muscle strength and exercise tolerance improve over the first 3 to 4 weeks. Skin and hair coat changes take longer and the progress variable. The skin and alopecia may deteriorate markedly before improving. Alternatively, there may be gradual and noticeable resolution of the clinical signs. Although improvement should be noted at 8 weeks, the skin and haircoat may not return to normal for 3 to 6 months. (Plate 4:11). A few dogs have dramatic changes in coat colour following successful therapy (Plate 4:12).

Re-evaluation every 3 to 6 months is recommended for the remainder of the animal's life. Relapses and episodes of overdose may occur. Relapses may require a short course of daily mitotane therapy or an increase in the maintenance dosage. Overdosage requires reassessment by an ACTH stimulation test and a reduction of the maintenance dose.

In one study the life expectancy was 23.4 months with a range of 18 days to over 7 years. (Feldman and Nelson, 1987.)

Other treatments

Hypophysectomy has been successfully performed in the dog for treatment of pituitary-dependent hyperadrenocorticism, but the operation is technically difficult and very few surgeons are able to carry it out.

Bilateral adrenalectomy has been employed successfully but involves the risk of putting an ill animal with a compromised immune system and poor wound healing, through a difficult surgical procedure. Dogs treated by this approach require life long treatment for hypoadrenocorticism.

Ketoconazole (Nizoral, Janssen), an imidazole derivative used primarily for its antifungal properties, has a reversible inhibitory effect on glucocorticoid synthesis whilst having negligible effects on mineralocorticoid production. It promises to be an attractive alternative to mitotane in the management of canine hyperadrenocorticism (Feldman and Nelson, 1987). A dose of 5 mg/kg should be given twice daily with food for 7 days increasing to 10 mg/kg twice daily thereafter. An ACTH stimulation test should be performed after 10 days on this higher dosage. If the cortisol level exceeds 300 nmol/l, the dose should be increased to 15 mg/kg twice daily and the ACTH stimulation test repeated. Twice daily therapy must be maintained long-term because the inhibitory effect of ketoconazole only is transient. Side effects include anorexia, vomiting, diarrhoea and, in some cases, administration of ketoconazole may result in hepatotoxicity and jaundice. The main disadvantage of this treatment at present is the high cost of the drug.

Cyproheptadine (Periactin, MSD), a serotonin and histamine antagonist with anticholinergic properties, may reduce the secretion of ACTH in some dogs with pituitary-dependent hyper-adrenocorticism. However, the response to treatment is variable with only a very low success rate reported.

Bromocriptine (Parlodel, Sandoz) is a potent dopamine receptor agonist which may also decrease the secretion of ACTH in some dogs with pituitary-dependent hyperadrenocorticism. It appears to have limited utility in the treatment of hyperadrenocorticism because of the small percentage of cases that respond, the high frequency of side-effects (vomiting, anorexia, depression and behavioural changes) and the frequency with which relapses occur.

Pituitary irradiation has been used successfully in the treatment of hyperadrenocorticism associated with large pituitary tumours. Computed tomography or magnetic resonance imaging is essential for diagnosis of the tumour and for treatment planning. Facilities capable of delivering megavoltage radiation are required to penetrate to the depth of the pituitary gland without seriously injuring the overlying soft tissues.

TREATMENT OF ADRENAL-DEPENDENT HYPERADRENOCORTICISM

Dogs diagnosed as having adrenal-dependent hyperadrenocorticism carry the best prognosis if the tumour can be removed surgically, although mitotane therapy may also be tried (Chastain and Ganjam, 1986).

Unilateral adrenalectomy requires considerable experience and expertise because of the complex anatomy. The technique is well-described using the paracostal, flank approach (Johnston 1977, 1983), but should only be performed by experienced surgeons. Mitotane or ketoconazole may be useful as preoperative preparation for surgical adrenalectomy, since control of hyperadrenocorticism may reduce the anaesthetic risks and help to minimise such complications as thromboembolism, sepsis and poor wound healing. Post-operative support is important as the contralateral adrenal cortex will be atrophic and unable to respond to the stress.

FELINE HYPERADRENOCORTICISM (CUSHING'S DISEASE)

Feline hyperadrenocorticism is rare but resembles the canine disorder in many respects. The majority of cases are pituitary-dependent although adrenal-dependent cases have been reported (Nelson *et al.,* 1988).

The clinical signs are similar to those in the dog. The cat, however, appears more prone to developing hyperglycaemia and overt diabetes mellitus. In contrast to the dog where polydipsia and polyuria are amongst the earliest clinical signs of hyperadrenocorticism, the onset of polydipsia and polyuria is delayed and coincides with the development of moderate to severe hyperglycaemia and glycosuria in the cat. Hyperadrenocorticism should be suspected in any cat which requires high daily insulin doses to control the hyperglycaemia and glycosuria.

In contrast to the dog, routine laboratory tests on cats with hyperadrenocorticism give variable and inconsistent results. The most common and striking abnormality is severe hyperglycaemia and glycosuria. A marked increase in serum alkaline phosphatase is rarely seen in cats with hyperadrenocorticism, because they have the ability to clear serum of excess alkaline phosphatase rapidly. Radiography of the abdomen not infrequently demonstrates calcification of the adrenal glands in normal older cats that is not associated with any functional abnormality. Hepatomegaly and a pendulous abdomen are the most consistent radiographic findings in cats with hyperadrenocorticism.

The ACTH stimulation test is a valuable screening test for hyperadrenocorticism in the cat, provided samples are taken before, and at 120 and 180 minutes after, administration of ACTH so as to detect peak cortisol response (Sparkes *et al.,* 1990). The test does not appear to help differentiate pituitary-dependent from adrenal-dependent causes of hyperadrenocorticism. Low- and high-dose dexamethasone suppression tests have not been well-standardised for the cat and should be interpreted with caution.

A number of different treatment protocols have been attempted in the treatment of feline hyperadrenocorticism with vaying degrees of success. Mitotane therapy has not proved effective in controlling the clinical signs of hyperadrenocorticism. Some improvement was reported in one cat with metyrapone, an enzyme inhibitor that blocks adrenal synthesis of glucocorticoids, but the cat was lost to follow up (Feldman and Nelson, 1987). At present, adrenalectomy appears to be the most successful means of treating feline hyperadrenocorticism. Unilateral adrenalectomy should be performed on cats with an adrenocortical tumour and bilateral adrenalectomy, followed by mineralocorticoid and glucocorticoid replacement therapy, should be used for cats with pituitary-dependent hyperadrenocorticism. The surgery, however, is technically difficult and should only be performed by surgeons with considerable experience.

PRIMARY ALDOSTERONISM

Increased production of aldosterone by an abnormal zona glomerulosa appears to be very rare in dogs and cats. In humans, primary aldosteronism is associated with marked muscle weakness, sometimes progressing to flaccid paralysis, polyuria, polydipsia, headache, paraesthesia and hypertension. The condition is caused by an abnormally high level of circulating aldosterone, whose source is usually a benign, unilateral adrenal adenoma or benign bilateral adrenocortical hyperplasia. In a few cases these tumours are malignant and metastasise to the liver.

Aldosterone excess leads to increased sodium and water retention, potassium depletion and suppression of the renin-angiotensin system. Two cases have been reported in the veterinary literature, one in a cat (Eger *et al.,* 1983) and one in a dog (Breitschwerdt *et al.,* 1985). The cat was aged and presented with a history of chronic relapsing weakness and depression. Profound hypokalaemia was detected in association with increased serum aldosterone levels and marginally subnormal plasma renin activity. Creatinine phosphokinase (CPK) was raised but blood urea levels were normal which distinguishes it from the more commonly occurring hypokalaemic polymyopathy of older cats (Dow *et al.,* 1987; Herrtage and McKerrell, 1989). Treatment of primary aldosteronism with potassium supplementation and spironolactone, an aldosterone antagonist, was sucessful in that cat. The case report of primary aldosteronism in the dog was more vague and less conclusive.

HYPOADRENOCORTICISM

Hypoadrenocorticism is a syndrome that results from a deficiency of both glucocorticoid and mineralocorticoid secretion from the adrenal cortices. Destruction of more than 95 per cent of both adrenal cortices causes a clinical deficiency of all adrenocortical hormones and is termed *primary hypo-adrenocorticism* (Addison's disease). *Secondary hypoadrenocorticism* is caused by a deficiency in ACTH which leads to atrophy of the adrenal cortices and impaired secretion of glucocorticoids. The production of mineralocorticoids, however, usually remains adequate.

PRIMARY HYPOADRENOCORTICISM (ADDISON'S DISEASE)

Primary hypoadrenocorticism occurs more frequently in the dog than is recognised but it is still much less common than hyperadrenocorticism (Cushing's disease). Hypoadrenocorticism is rare in the cat and will be dealt with separately at the end of this section.

CAUSES OF PRIMARY HYPOADRENOCORTICISM

Primary hypoadrenocorticism in the dog has been associated with the following conditions:

1. Idiopathic adrenocortical insufficiency

This is the commonest cause in the dog and is thought to result from immune-mediated destruction of the adrenal gland. The presence of anti-adrenal antibodies in two dogs and characteristic histopathological findings in another support this hypothesis (Schaer *et al.,* 1985). In humans, hypoadrenocorticism has been found to be associated with other immune-mediated disorders such as thyroiditis, diabetes mellitus, hypoparathyroidism, primary gonadal failure and atrophic gastritis.

2. Mitotane-induced adrenocortical necrosis

Although mitotane usually spares the zona glomerulosa, and therefore mineralocorticoid secretion, cases of complete adrenocortical failure can occasionally occur. When hypoadrenocorticism occurs, it most commonly develops several weeks or months after the beginning of maintenance therapy with mitotane.

3. Bilateral adrenalectomy

4. Haemorrhage or infarction of the adrenal glands.

Rare but can cause acute adrenocortical insufficiency.

5. Mycotic or neoplastic involvement of the adrenal gland.

Rare.

The adrenocortical pathology leads to mineralocorticoid and glucocorticoid deficiency. Aldosterone is the major mineralocorticoid and deficiency causes impaired ability to conserve sodium and water and failure to excrete potassium leading to hyponatraemia and hyperkalaemia. Hyponatraemia induces lethargy, depression and nausea and leads to the development of hypovolaemia, hypotension, reduced cardiac output and decreased renal perfusion. Hyperkalaemia causes muscle weakness, hyporeflexia and impaired cardiac conduction. Glucocorticoid deficiency causes decreased tolerance of stress, loss of appetite and a normocytic, normochromic anaemia.

BREED, AGE AND SEX PREDISPOSITION

Breed

There are no breed predilections but a recent report suggests the possibility of an hereditary factor in standard poodles (Shaker et al., 1988). Bearded collies may also be over-represented.

Age

Hypoadrenocorticism appears to be a disease of the young and middle-aged dog with an age range of 3 months to 9 years and a median age of 4 to 5 years.

Sex

Approximately 70 per cent of reported cases are female.

CLINICAL SIGNS

The progression of adrenocortical insufficiency may be acute or chronic. In the dog, chronic hypoadrenocorticism is far more common than the acute disease.

Acute primary hypoadrenocorticism

The clinical appearance of the acute form is that of hypovolaemic shock (adrenocortical crisis). The animal is usually found in a state of collapse or collapses when stressed. Other signs include weak pulse, profound bradycardia, abdominal pain, vomiting, diarrhoea, dehydration and hypothermia. The condition is rapidly progressive and life-threatening. Aggressive fluid therapy will help most patients and allow more time to make a diagnosis.

Chronic primary hypoadrenocorticism

The clinical signs in the chronic form are often vague and non-specific (Table 6). The diagnosis should be considered in any dog with a waxing and waning type of illness or that shows episodic weakness and collapse (Herrtage and McKerrell, 1989). The most consistent clinical signs include anorexia, vomiting, lethargy, depression and/or weakness. The severity of each sign can vary during the course of the disease and may be interspersed with periods of apparent good health often following non-specific veterinary therapy, usually consisting of corticosteroid medication and/or fluid administration. Hypoadrenocorticism can easily be mistaken for chronic renal insufficiency, primary neuromuscular disorders and various other causes for signs such as weight loss, weakness, anorexia, vomiting and diarrhoea.

Common findings on physical examination apart from depression and weakness, include dehydration, bradycardia and weak femoral pulses. The electrocardiographic (ECG) findings are described below.

Table 6
Clinical signs of primary
hypoadrenocorticism
(Addison's Disease)

Anorexia
Lethargy/depression
Weakness, usually episodic
Waxing and waning illness
Periodic vomiting
Periodic diarrhoea or constipation
Weight loss or failure to gain weight
Polydipsia and/or polyuria
Dehydration
Bradycardia
Syncope
Restlessness/shaking/shivering
Abdominal pain

ROUTINE LABORATORY FINDINGS

The commonest findings are listed in Table 7.

Haematology

Haematological changes may include lymphocytosis, eosinophilia and mild normocytic, normochromic, non-regenerative anaemia. However, these findings are not as consistent as those changes seen in hyperadrenocorticism. Normal or elevated eosinophil and lymphocyte counts in an ill animal with signs compatible with hypoadrenocorticism are significant, because the expected response to stress would result in eosinopenia and lymphopenia. Mild anaemia may not be obvious until the dog has been rehydrated because of the haemoconcentration effect of dehydration.

Biochemistry

The most consistent laboratory findings in hypoadrenocorticism are prerenal uraemia, hyponatraemia and hyperkalaemia. However, approximately 10 per cent of dogs with hypoadrenocorticism have normal electrolyte levels.

Blood urea is increased secondary to reduced renal perfusion and decreased glomerular filtration rate. Reduced renal perfusion results from hypovolaemia, reduced cardiac output and hypotension, which in turn result from chronic fluid loss through the kidneys, acute fluid loss through vomiting and/or diarrhoea and inadequate fluid intake.

Table 7

Routine laboratory findings in primary hypoadrenocorticism (Addison's Disease)

Haematology	Lymphocytosis
	Eosinophilia
	Relative neutropenia
	Normocytic, normochromic, non-regenerative anaemia
Biochemistry	Increased blood urea
	Hyponatraemia (< 135 mmol/l)
	Hyperkalaemia (> 5.5 mmol/l)
	Reduced sodium: potassium ratio (< 25:1)
	Hypercalcaemia
	Hypoglycaemia
Urinalysis	Specific gravity (usually > 1.025)

Pre-renal uraemia is usually associated with concentrated urine (specific gravity > 1.030) whereas the urine in primary renal failure is often isothenuric or only mildly concentrated (1.008 to 1.025). Some severe cases of hypoadrenocorticism, however, may develop impaired concentrating ability because of chronic sodium loss reducing the renal medullary concentration gradient. Either way with adequate fluid therapy, the blood urea will return to normal in cases of hypoadrenocorticism.

Sodium is usually less than 135 mmol/l.

Potassium is usually greater than 5.5 mmol/l.

The ratio of sodium to potassium may be more reliable than the absolute values. The normal ratio varies between 27:1 and 40:1, whereas in patients with hypoadrenocorticism, the ratio is commonly less than 25:1 and may be below 20:1. However, 10 per cent of cases may have normal electrolyte levels at the time of presentation.

Calcium — Mild to moderate hypercalaemia is seen in about a third of cases of hypo-adrenocorticism, usually those dogs which are most severely affected by the disease. Hypercalcaemia is caused by haemoconcentration, increased renal tubular reabsorption and decreased glomerular filtration.

Blood glucose — Cases of hypoadrenocorticism have a tendency to develop hypoglycaemia because glucocorticoid deficiency reduces glucose production by the liver and peripheral cell receptors become more sensitive to insulin. Hypoglycaemia is uncommon (Willard *et al.,* 1982) but the potential should remain a concern for the clinician.

ELECTROCARDIOGRAPHIC FINDINGS

Hyperkalaemia impairs cardiac conduction which can be assessed by electrocardiography (ECG) (Figure 7). Although the ECG changes do not correlate directly with serum potassium levels, the following guidelines have proved helpful:

> 5.5 mmol/l — peaking of the T wave, shortening of the Q-T interval

> 6.5 mmol/l — increased QRS duration

> 7.0 mmol/l — P wave amplitude decreased, P-R interval prolonged

> 8.5 mmol/l — P wave absent, severe bradycardia

Electrocardiography can also be used for monitoring the patient during treatment.

Figure 7.
Electrocardiograms from a 4-year-old bearded collie dog with primary hypoadrenocorticism
taken a) before and b) after supplementation with glucocorticoids and mineralocorticoids (I mV/cm, 25mm/sec).

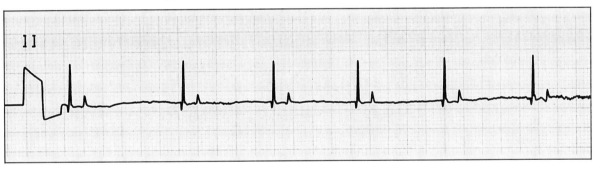

a. The P waves are absent, the T waves are peaked and there is a profound bradycardia.
The plasma sodium was 138 mmol/l and the plasma potassium 9.5 mmol/l.

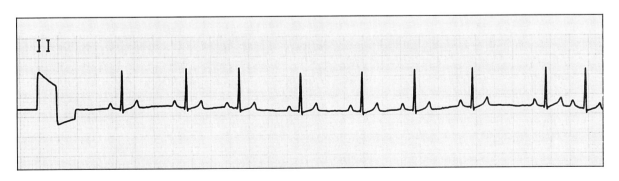

b. ECG after treatment showing sinus arrhythmia.
The plasma sodium was 142 mmol/l and the plasma potassium 5.4 mmol/l.

RADIOGRAPHIC FINDINGS

Dogs with hypoadrenocorticism may show radiographic signs of hypovolaemia which include: microcardia, decreased size of pulmonary vessels and reduced size of the caudal vena cava. The changes are not specific and only represent hypovolaemia and dehydration irrespective of the cause. A few dogs with hypoadrenocorticism develop oesophageal dilation as a result of generalised muscle weakness and this can be seen on thoracic radiographs (Burrows, 1987).

CONFIRMATION OF DIAGNOSIS

ACTH stimulation test

The ACTH stimulation test is commonly used to confirm the presence of hypoadrenocorticism. The intravenous preparation of ACTH, tetracosactin (Synacthen, Ciba), should be used as absorption of ACTH gel (Acthar Gel, Rorer) cannot be relied on if the patient is in a collapsed state with severe hypotension. In hypoadrenocorticism, the resting cortisol level will be low with a subnormal or negligible response to ACTH (Figure 5, page 91). The ACTH stimulation test, however, does not distinguish between primary and secondary hypoadrenocorticism. Plasma ACTH levels, if available, would differentiate primary and secondary hypoadrenocorticism.

TREATMENT OF PRIMARY HYPOADRENOCORTICISM

Acute primary hypoadrenocorticism

Intravenous saline — Hyperkalaemia is life-threatening in the acute crisis but can be reliably treated with aggressive intravenous fluid therapy using normal saline. The response to treatment is often dramatic and glucose and insulin therapy or calcium administration are not required for the treatment of hyperkalaemia due to hypoadrenocorticism. The serum potassium falls because of the dilution effect of the saline and the improvement in renal perfusion. The increased renal blood flow allows further excretion of potassium into the urine.

Glucocorticoid therapy — Glucocorticoid therapy should be used early in the treatment of the acute crisis. Once the animal has improved with saline and glucocorticoids, maintenance therapy with mineralocorticoids can be instigated (see below). Glucocorticoids of choice in the acute crisis include:

hydrocortisone sodium succinate	10 mg/kg i/v
prednisolone sodium succinate	5 mg/kg i/v
dexamethasone sodium phosphate	0.5 mg/kg i/v

If plasma cortisol levels are to be measured for diagnosis, then dexamethasone should be used to avoid interference with the assay.

Chronic primary hypoadrenocorticism (maintenance therapy)

Fludrocortisone acetate (Florinef, Squibb) — This is an oral synthetic adrenocortical steroid with mineralocorticoid effects and is the treatment of choice for maintenance therapy in the dog. An initial dose of 0.1 mg/10kg/day of fludrocortisone is given and serum electrolytes checked after 5 to 7 days. The dose rate should then be adjusted until sodium and potassium levels are within the normal range. The daily maintenance dose required is usually between 0.1 and 0.5 mg. The dose often needs increasing during the first 6 to 18 months of therapy and may be required twice daily in a few cases.

Glucocorticoids. The majority of cases do not require daily glucocorticoid supplementation after initial treatment. However, the owners should be given a supply of prednisolone tablets to be given if the patient appears unwell. Prednisolone at a dose of 0.1 to 0.2 mg/kg daily should be sufficient for those cases that do require glucocorticoid replacement therapy.

Salt supplementation. Salt tablets or salting the food should be instigated initially to help correct hyponatraemia but can be phased out and is not required long-term in most cases. Dogs requiring unusually high doses of fludrocortisone, however, may respond to oral salt and fewer fludrocortisone tablets.

The prognosis with hypoadrenocorticism is excellent when oral therapy has been used providing owner education is adequate.

FELINE PRIMARY HYPOADRENOCORTICISM (ADDISON'S DISEASE)

Spontaneous primary hypoadrenocorticism is rare in the cat and only 10 cases have been reported (Peterson *et al.,* 1989). The clinical signs and routine laboratory findings are essentially similar to those seen in the dog. Diagnosis is by ACTH stimulation testing (see page 95). The findings of a low basal plasma cortisol concentration with a subnormal or negligible response to ACTH is indicative of hypoadrenocorticism (Figure 5). In interpreting results of an ACTH stimulation test, it is important to remember that the protocol is different from the dog in that at least 3 samples must be collected to ensure detection of the peak cortisol response. In addition, because cats tend to respond to ACTH with a lower rise in plasma cortisol concentrations than do dogs, it is imperative to compare test results to reference values obtained in normal cats.

Treatment of primary hypoadrenocorticism in the cat follows the same principles as those for the dog. The long-term prognosis with proper replacement therapy is good.

SECONDARY HYPOADRENOCORTICISM

Secondary hypoadrenocorticism is associated with a deficiency of glucocorticoids caused by a deficiency in ACTH production and/or release. The production of mineralocorticoids, although reduced, generally remains adequate. Secondary hypoadrenocorticism occurs in both dogs and cats. (See also Pituitary chapter.)

CAUSES OF SECONDARY HYPOADRENOCORTICISM

Secondary hypoadrenocorticism can be associated with destructive lesions, for example non-functional tumours, in the hypothalamus or anterior pituitary. More commonly, however, it is iatrogenic and associated with prolonged suppression of ACTH by drug therapy with glucocorticoids. In the cat, secondary hypoadrenocorticism is seen following prolonged megestrol acetate therapy.

CLINICAL SIGNS

The clinical signs are variable and may include depression, anorexia, occasional vomiting or diarrhoea, weak pulse and sudden collapse when stressed. If it is associated with glucocorticoid therapy, then clinical signs of iatrogenic hyperadrenocorticism (Cushing's disease) are usually present.

DIAGNOSIS AND TREATMENT

The diagnosis is based on a failure of the animal's cortisol levels to respond to ACTH stimulation (Figure 5). Glucocorticoid replacement, using prednisolone at a dose of 0.1 to 0.2 mg/kg daily is indicated for immediate correction of the clinical signs. Further treatment and the prognosis depend on the cause and whether it can be eliminated.

PHAEOCHROMOCYTOMA

Tumours of the adrenal medulla (phaeochromocytomas) are rare in dogs and have not been reported in cats. Phaeochromocytomas are usually unilateral, benign, slow growing tumours that may reach a considerable size. Rarely, they are malignant and may invade the caudal vena cava or metastasise to lung, liver or bone (White and Cheyne, 1977). Phaeochromocytomas may secrete excessive amounts of catecholamines.

CLINICAL SIGNS

Clinical signs of a phaeochromocytoma may relate to an abdominal mass compressing adjacent structures or to the secretion of catecholamines.

Clinical signs related to tumour size might include a palpable abdominal mass, ascites and hindlimb weakness. Secretion of catecholamines may be intermittent or persistent and can cause hypotension or hypertension, tachycardia, tachyarrhythmias with weakness and trembling, head pressing or seizures. Epistaxis and retinal haemorrhages may also be noted. The clinical signs vary depending on whether an excess of adrenaline or noradrenaline is predominant (see section on 'Physiology of the Adrenal Medulla', page 77).

DIAGNOSIS AND TREATMENT

The diagnosis should be suspected in any unexplained case of episodic weakness (Herrtage and McKerrell, 1989). Radiographic and ultrasonographic examinations will often reveal a mass in the adrenal area. Confirmation, however, requires quantification of the urinary excretion of catecholamines and their metabolites, which is not widely available.

Surgical removal is the treatment of choice, but should only be performed by experienced surgeons since excessive handling of the tumour during surgery may provoke massive secretion of catecholamines. Phentolamine (Rogitine, Ciba) an α-blocker for intravenous use, can be used at a dose of 0.02 to 0.1 mg/kg to lower blood pressure while manipulating the tumour and lignocaine or propranolol can be administered intravenously as necessary during surgery to control tachycardia or tacharrhythmias.

REFERENCES AND FURTHER READING

BLAXTER, A. C. and GRUFFYDD-JONES, T. J. (1990). Concurrent diabetes mellitus and hyperadrenocorticism in the dog: Diagnosis and management of eight cases. *J. small Anim. Pract.* **31**, 117.

BREITSCHWERDT, E. B., MEUTEN, D. J., GREENFIELD, C. L., ANSON, L. W., COOK, C. S. and FULGHUM, R. E. (1985). Idiopathic hyperaldsteronism in a dog. *J. Am. vet. med. Ass.* **188**, 841.

BURROWS, C. F. (1987). Reversible mega-oesophagus in a dog with hypoadrenocorticism. *J. small Anim. Pract.* **28**, 1073.

CHASTAIN, C. B. and GANJAM, V. K. (1986). *Clinical Endocrinology of Companion Animals.* p. 329. Lea and Febiger, Philadelphia.

DOW, S. W., LECOUTEUR, R. A., FETTMAN, M. J. and SPURGEON, T. L. (1987). Potassium depletion in cats: hypokalaemic polymyopathy. *J. Am. vet. med. Ass.* **191**, 1563.

DUNCAN, I. D., GRIFFITHS, I. R. and NASH, A. S. (1977). Myotonia in canine Cushing's disease. *Vet. Rec.* **100**, 30.

EGER, C. E., ROBINSON, W. F. and HUXTABLE, C. R. R. (1983). Primary aldosteronism (Conn's syndrome) in a cat: a case report and review of comparative aspects. *J. small Anim. Pract.* **24**, 293.

FELDMAN, B. F. and FELDMAN, E. C. (1977). Routine laboratory abnormalities in endocrine disease. *Vet. Clin. North Am.* **7**, 443.

FELDMAN, E. C. and NELSON, R. W. (1987). Hyperadrenocorticism. In: *Canine and Feline Endocrinology and Reproduction.* p. 137. W. B. Saunders, Philadelphia.

FLUCKIGER, M. A. and GOMEZ, J. A. (1984). Radiographic findings in dogs with spontaneous pulmonary thrombosis or embolism. *Vet. Radiol.* **25**, 124.

GRUFFYDD-JONES, T. J. (1989). Medical management of Cushing's syndrome in dogs. *Vet. Rec.* **124**, 317.

HERRTAGE, M. E. and McKERRELL, R. E. (1989). Episodic weakness. In: *Manual of Dog and Cat Neurology* (ed. S. L. Wheeler) p. 223. British Small Animal Veterinary Association, Cheltenham.

HUNTLEY, K., FRAZER, J., GIBBS, C. and GASKELL, C. J. (1982). The radiological features of canine Cushing's syndrome: a review of forty-eight cases. *J. small Anim. Pract.* **23**, 369.

JOHNSTON, D. E. (1977). Adrenalectomy via retroperitoneal approach in dogs. *J. Am. vet. med. Ass.* **170**, 1092.

JOHNSTON, D. E. (1983). Adrenalectomy in the dog. In: *Current Techniques in Small Animal Surgery.* (ed. M.J. Bojrab) p. 386. Lea and Febiger, Philadelphia.

KANTROWITZ, C. M., NYLAND, T. G. and FELDMAN, E. C. (1986). Adrenal ultrasonography in the dog: detection of tumours and hyperplasia in hyperadrenocorticism. *Vet. Radiol.* **27**, 91.

KEMPPAINEN, R. J. and SARTIN, J. L. (1984). Evidence for episodic but not circadian activity in plasma concentrations of adrenocorticotropin, cortisol and thyroxine in dogs. *J. Endocrinol.* **103**, 219.

LEE, R. and GRIFFITHS, I. R. (1972). A comparison of cerebral arteriography and cavernous sinus venography in the dog. *J. small Anim. Pract.* **13**, 225.

MEIJER, J. C. (1980). Canine hyperadrenocorticism. In: *Current Veterinary Therapy VII* (ed. R.W. Kirk) p. 975. W. B. Saunders, Philadelphia.

MULNIX, J. A., VAN DEN BROM, W. E., LUBBERINK, A. A. M. E., DE BRUIJNE, J. J. and RIJNBERK, A. (1976). Gamma camera imaging of bilateral adrenocortical tumours in the dog. *Am. J. Vet. Res.* **37**, 1467.

NELSON, R. W., FELDMAN, E. C. and SMITH, M. C. (1988). Spontaneous hyperadrenocorticism in cats: 6 cases (1978-1986). *J. Am. vet. med. Ass.* **193**, 245.

OLUJU, M. P., ECKERSALL, P. D. and DOUGLAS, T. A. (1984). Simple quantitative assay for canine steroid-induced alkaline phosphatase. *Vet. Rec.* **115**, 17.

OWENS, J. M. and DRUCKER, W. D. (1977). Hyperadrenocorticism in the dog: Canine Cushing's syndrome. *Vet. Clin. North Am.* **7**, 583.

PETERSON, M. E. (1984). Hyperadrenocorticism. *Vet. Clin. North Am: Small Anim. Pract.* **14**, 731.

PETERSON, M. E., KRIEGER, D. T., DRUCKER, W. D. and HALMI, N. S. (1982a). Immunocytochemical study of the hypophysis in 25 dogs with pituitary-dependent hyperadrenocorticism. *Acta Endocrinol.* **101**, 15.

PETERSON, M. E., GILBERTSON, S. R. and DRUCKER, W. D. (1982b). Plasma cortisol response to exogenous ACTH in 22 dogs with hyperadrenocorticism caused by an adrenocortical neoplasia. *J. Am. vet. med. Ass.* **180**, 542.

PETERSON, M. E., FERGUSON, D. C., KINTZER, P. P. and DRUCKER, W. D. (1984). Effects of spontaneous hyperadrenocorticism on serum thyroid hormone concentrations in the dog. *Am. J. Vet. Res.* **45**, 2034.

PETERSON, M. E., KEMPPAINEN, R. J. and GRAVES, T. K. (1988). Episodic but not circadian activity in plasma concentrations of ACTH, cortisol and thyroxine in the normal cat. p.721. *American College of Veterinary Internal Medicine Scientific Proceedings, Washington, D.C. (abstract).*

PETERSON, M. E., GRECO, D. S. and ORTH, D. N. (1989). Primary hypoadrenocorticism in 10 cats. *J. Vet. Int. Med.* **3**, 55.

RIJNBERK, A., VAN WEES, A. and MOLL, J. A. (1988). Assessment of two tests for the diagnosis of canine hyperadrenocorticism. *Vet. Rec.* **122**, 178.

SCHAER, M. (1980). Pheochromocytoma in a dog: a case report. *J. Am. Anim. Hosp. Ass.* **16**, 583.

SCHAER, M., RILEY, W. J., BUERGELT, C. D., BOWEN, D. J., SENIOR, D. F., BURROWS, C. F. and CAMPBELL, G. A. (1985). Autoimmunity and Addison's disease in the dog. *J. Am. Anim. Hosp. Ass.* **22**, 789.

SHAKER, E., HURVITZ, A. J. and PETERSON, M. E. (1988). Hypoadrenocorticism in a family of standard poodles. *J. Am. vet. med. Ass.* **192**, 1091.

SPARKES, A. H., ADAMS, D. T., DOUTHWAITE, J. A. and GRUFFYDD-JONES, T. G. (1990). Assessment of adrenal function in cats: Response to intravenous synthetic ACTH. *J. small Anim. Pract.*, **31**, 2.

VOORHOUT, G., STOLP, R., LUBBERINK, A. A. M. E. and VAN WAES, P. F. G. M. (1988). Computed tomography in the diagnosis of canine hyperadrenocorticism not suppressible by dexamethasone. *J. Am. vet. med. Ass.* **192**, 641.

WILLARD, M. D., SCHALL, W. D., McCAW, D. E. and NACHREINER, R. F. (1982). Canine hypoadrenocorticism: Report of 37 cases and review of 39 previously reported cases. *J. Am. vet. med. Ass.* **180**, 59.

WHITE, R. A. S. and CHEYNE, I. A. (1977). Bone metastases from a phaeochromocytoma in the dog. *J. small Anim. Pract.* **18**, 579.

CHAPTER 5

THE ISLETS OF LANGERHANS

Elspeth M. Milne, B.V.M.& S., M.R.C.V.S., Ph.D.

ANATOMY

The pancreas is a 'V' shaped lobulated organ lying in the upper anterior abdomen. The right lobe extends from the concave surface of the duodenal loop to the pylorus of the stomach and the left lobe extends from the pylorus along the greater curvature of the stomach. Two pancreatic ducts discharge exocrine secretions into the duodenum.

HISTOLOGY

The pancreas is a mixed exocrine and endocrine gland, the exocrine portion consisting of a compound acinar gland. The islets of Langerhans, which form the endocrine pancreas, consist of clusters of cells interspersed among the acini (Figure 1). The main cell types in the islets are the α and β cells and a small number of δ cells. The β cells predominate and are mainly found in the centre of the islet with the α cells at the periphery.

ENDOCRINE SECRETION

The α and β cells synthesize two polypeptide hormones, glucagon and insulin respectively, while the δ cells produce somatostatin which is involved in controlling the release of insulin and glucagon. Insulin and glucagon are involved in the control of carbohydrate, lipid and protein metabolism, and are particularly important in blood glucose homeostasis.

Figure 1.
Section of pancreas showing islet of Langerhans surrounded by acini.
a = acinar tissue
i = islet

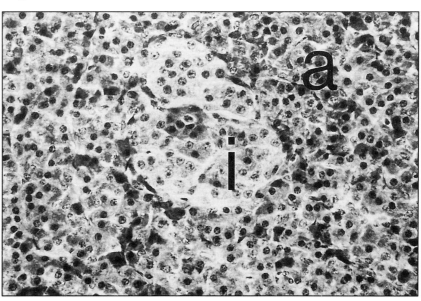

PROPERTIES OF INSULIN AND GLUCAGON

Insulin

1. Secreted in response to hyperglycaemia.
2. Facilitates uptake of glucose, amino acids, fatty acids, potassium and magnesium from the blood into peripheral tissues and therefore *decreases* blood glucose.
3. Stimulates glycogen synthesis in the liver.
4. Inhibits the production of glucose by inhibiting glycogenolysis and gluconeogenesis.
5. Inhibits lipolysis, ketogenesis and protein catabolism.
6. The effects of insulin stimulate glucagon release to maintain glucose homeostasis.

Glucagon

1. Secreted in response to hypoglycaemia.
2. Opposes the action of insulin (2—5, above) and therefore *increases* blood glucose.
3. The effects of glucagon stimulate insulin release.
   Several other hormones have an opposing effect to insulin i.e. growth hormone, progesterone, oestrogen, androgens, glucocorticoids, thyroxine and catecholamines although these are less important than glucagon in maintaining euglycaemia.

ABNORMALITIES OF PANCREATIC ENDOCRINE FUNCTION
DIABETES MELLITUS

AETIOLOGY

Diabetes mellitus is characterised by disturbances of carbohydrate, lipid and protein metabolism and an abnormal response to glucose load. It may be due to an absolute lack of insulin or a relative lack with respect to hormones antagonistic to insulin.

In diabetes mellitus, the relative or absolute lack of insulin results in impairment of glucose uptake by peripheral tissues. Gluconeogenesis and glycogenolysis are stimulated to increase the supply of glucose to the tissues, triglycerides are oxidised to release fatty acids with the concomitant production of ketones, and protein catabolism is increased to release amino acids, some of which are precursors in gluconeogenesis. The overall effect is an increase in glucose production and a decrease in its utilisation leading to hyperglycaemia and eventually to glycosuria (and sometimes ketonuria) with osmotic diuresis and polydipsia. Diuresis will also result in urinary loss of sodium and potassium which may result in hyponatraemia and hypokalaemia.

Diabetes mellitus is not usually due simply to a lack of insulin and a wide variety of factors are now known to initiate or exacerbate the diabetic state.

Aetiology of diabetes mellitus in dogs

Factors thought to be involved in the aetiology of canine diabetes mellitus are shown in Table 1.

Table 1.
Aetiology of canine diabetes mellitus

1. Primary diabetes mellitus	(a) congenital hypoplasia of islets (b) senile atrophy of islets
2. Secondary diabetes mellitus	(a) following pancreatitis (b) excessive secretion of hormones antagonistic to insulin i.e. glucagon, growth hormone, glucocorticoids, progesterone, oestrogen, androgens, catecholamines or thyroxine (c) iatrogenic due to long-term progestagen or glucocorticoid therapy (d) obesity (e) immune-mediated insulin resistance?

Secondary diabetes mellitus associated with hormone antagonism or obesity appears to be the commonest form in dogs. High progesterone levels may contribute since progesterone stimulates growth hormone production (Eigenmann, *et al.,* 1983), the latter being a powerful insulin antagonist in dogs. Thus entire bitches are predisposed during pregnancy or dioestrus, as are females to whom certain progestagens such as medroxyprogesterone acetate have been administered. Initially, high progesterone levels may result in a compensatory hyperinsulinaemia but this will be followed by hypoinsulinaemia due to β cell exhaustion. Hyperadrenocorticism or chronic exogenous glucocorticoid administration can also induce diabetes mellitus in some cases as glucocorticoids are also antagonistic to insulin. In one survey, overt diabetes mellitus occurred in 8% of dogs with hyperadrenocorticism (Peterson, *et al.,* 1984). Obesity is known to predispose to diabetes as it modulates glucose and insulin homeostasis (Mattheeuws, *et al.,* 1984). The greater the degree of obesity, the higher the blood insulin levels will be and eventually, β cell depletion and frank diabetes mellitus may occur.

Aetiology of diabetes mellitus in cats

In cats, the aetiology is less certain. Deposition of amyloid in islet cells is a frequent finding in diabetic cats (and some apparently normal cats) and is associated with impaired glucose tolerance (Yano *et al.,* 1981). The presence of the amyloid is thought to be a secondary event and indicates the presence of β cell dysfunction of unknown aetiology. Other factors which have been incriminated in cats are pituitary tumours, hyperadrenocorticalism, hyperthyroidism, obesity and megoestrol acetate therapy. The relationship between recent oestrus and the onset of diabetes is less clear in cats and entire queens are not predisposed.

INCIDENCE

The incidence of diabetes mellitus is approximately 1 in 200 in dogs and 1 in 800 in cats. The disease is more common in small breeds of dog, particularly dachshunds, poodles and terriers; of the larger breeds, samoyeds and rottweilers may be predisposed. Siamese cats may also have a breed predisposition. The peak age of onset is 7—9 years in both species, although occasional congenital cases occur. Before puberty, there is no significant sex predisposition. In mature canines, however, entire bitches constitute two-thirds of cases, while males and spayed bitches contribute equally to the remaining one-third. Mature male and female cats are affected equally.

HISTORY

There is usually a history of sudden or gradual onset of polyuria, polydipsia, polyphagia and weight loss although the animal may be obese. Bitches have often been in oestrus recently and the owner may report episodes of transient polyuria and polydipsia following previous oestrus periods. Poor vision or blindness due to cataract formation may be present in dogs even when first presented but in some cases these will be senile rather than diabetic cataracts.

CLINICAL SIGNS

Cases fall into three main categories according to their presenting signs, i.e. uncomplicated diabetes mellitus, ketoacidotic diabetes mellitus and diabetic coma, in descending order of frequency in dogs (Chastain and Nichols, 1984). Most cats are ketoacidotic at presentation.

Typical signs in uncomplicated diabetes mellitus are polyuria, polydipsia of more than 60 ml/kg/day, polyphagia, weight loss, mild dehydration, hepatomegaly (50% of cases) and there may be uni-or bilateral stellate cataracts in dogs.

In diabetic ketoacidosis there is also likely to be mental depression, anorexia, vomiting with or without diarrhoea, tachypnoea, a ketotic breath and in cats, icterus may be present. Oliguria or anuria may replace polyuria. Dehydration is more severe in ketoacidosis and usually results in a loss of between 10—12% of body weight. In diabetic coma, the animal shows severe stupor or loss of consciousness and in ketoacedotic coma this will be accompanied by signs referable to the ketoacidosis.

DIAGNOSIS

The history and clinical signs of polyuria, polydipsia, polyphagia and weight loss are not pathognomonic for diabetes mellitus and although the additional presence of stellate cataracts in dogs and a ketotic smell to the breath are suspicious, it is essential to confirm the tentative diagnosis by laboratory tests.

Laboratory findings in diabetes mellitus

1. **Specific tests**

   a. **Blood glucose** — fasting hyperglycaemia consistently >8.5 mmol/l at least 8 hours after the last meal. Remember that 'stress' hyperglycaemia is a common finding in cats with various illnesses and should not be confused with overt diabetes mellitus. In these cases blood glucose may reach 8.5—12.5 mmol/l.

   b. **Blood ketones** — may be elevated.

   c. **Urine analysis** — glycosuria occurs if the blood glucose exceeds the renal threshold of 8—11 mmol/l. Before treatment, the urine glucose is usually >0.5% and is often >2%. Ketonuria is also present in some cases. Despite polydipsia, urine specific gravity may be normal due to glycosuria.

   d. **Intravenous glucose tolerance test** — this is of great value in mild hyperglycaemia where the diagnosis is uncertain. The oral glucose tolerance test is unsuitable as the result depends partly on the absorptive capacity of the small intestine. To carry out the intravenous test 1g of glucose per kg of body weight is administered as a 40% or 50% solution over 30 seconds. Blood samples are taken into tubes containing fluoride/oxalate before and immediately after glucose administration, and subsequently at intervals of 10, 15, 20, and 40 minutes. In normal dogs the immediate post-injection level of blood glucose is approximately 30 mmol/l, falling to about 25,15 and 7 mmol/l at 10,20 and 40 minutes respectively. In diabetics there will be a slower return to resting values (Doxey, 1983.) Note that the blood should be collected from a different vein to that used for glucose administration.

2. **Non-Specific tests**

   The following are of some value in forming a pre-treatment prognosis and assessing response to treatment.

   a. Liver enzymes — serum alkaline phosphatase (dogs only) and to a lesser extent γ-glutamyl transpeptidase and alanine aminotransferase may be elevated due to fatty liver.

   b. Serum lipids — the serum may be visibly milky due to hyperlipidaemia. Serum cholesterol and triglycerides may be elevated due to lipolysis and failure of clearance of lipoproteins.

   c. Blood urea — may be normal or moderately elevated (up to 20 mmol/l) due to dehydration and protein catabolism. Elevated levels following rehydration suggest concurrent renal disease.

   d. Serum electrolytes — sodium, potassium, bicarbonate and blood pH may be low especially in ketoacidosis.

Differential diagnosis of diabetes mellitus

Table 2
Differential diagnosis of diabetes mellitus

Renal disease
Hyperadrenocorticalism
Pyometra
Diabetes insipidus
Psychogenic polydipsia
Hepatic failure
Stress glycosuria
Fanconi syndrome

Hyperadrenocorticism and stress glycosuria may precipitate the diabetic state. Hyperadrenocorticism and diabetes mellitus may exist concurrently.

Mild hyperglycaemia and glycosuria may sometimes occur in hyperadrenocorticism, hepatic failure or stress glycosuria.

In Fanconi syndrome (a rare disorder in which there is failure of the renal tubules to reabsorb glucose) glycosuria is present without hyperglycaemia.

TREATMENT

Immediately upon confirmation of the diagnosis, it should be explained to the owner that daily insulin injections and monitoring of urine glucose will almost certainly be required for the rest of the animal's life. The owners must accept this or further treatment is pointless as euthanasia due to unwillingness of the owner to continue treatment is the major cause of death after stabilisation.

Treatment of diabetic ketoacidosis

If ketonuria is present but is not associated with signs of diabetic ketoacidosis, the case can be treated as one of uncomplicated diabetes mellitus. However, if clinical signs and laboratory findings suggesting ketoacidotic diabetes mellitus are present, emergency treatment is required.

1. **Aims of treatment in ketoacidosis:**
   a. Correction of fluid deficit.
   b. Correction of acid-base balance.
   c. Correction of electrolyte disturbances.
   d. Reduction of blood glucose and ketone levels.

2. **Procedure for treatment of ketoacidosis (conscious or comatose)**
   a. **First considerations**

      Ensure a clear airway, especially if comatose, then cannulate the cephalic or jugular vein and place an indwelling catheter into the bladder to allow monitoring of urine output.

   b. **Correction of fluid deficit**

      Assess the degree of dehydration by clinical examination and if possible, by PCV and total serum protein estimations. Calculate the total fluid deficit to be corrected (usually 10−12% of body weight). Blood volume must be restored quickly so start fluid administration at a rate of 20−40 ml/kg body-weight/hour (not more than 90 ml/kg/hour) for the first two hours. Decrease the rate thereafter so that 50% of the deficit has been restored by 12 hours. Over the subsequent 36 hours, give the remainder of the deficit, **plus** the animal's daily maintenance requirement of 40 ml/kg/day. If in doubt and serum electrolyte levels cannot be measured, lactated Ringer's solution (Hartmann's solution) is the safest fluid as it will also help to correct acidosis.

   c. **Correction of acid-base balance**

      Determine blood pH and bicarbonate deficit, if possible, before correcting acid-base imbalance. Bicarbonate deficit is likely to be moderate to severe, requiring 6−9 mM lactate or bicarbonate per kg body weight (i.e. 0.50−0.76g $NaHCO_3$/kg).

      This should be added as a sterile solution to the intravenous infusion. If lactated Ringer's solution is being given, only 4 mM/kg is required (i.e. 0.34g $NaHCO_3$/kg) and this should be added evenly to the lactated Ringer's solution required. Never give alkalinising solutions as a bolus as paradoxical acidosis of cerebro-spinal fluid (CSF),which may itself cause coma, might occur. Acid-base correction should be carried out over 48 hours. Bicarbonate is probably preferable to lactate as lactate will not act as an alkalinising agent if lactic acidosis is complicating the ketoacidosis, although there is no evidence that it will greatly exacerbate the lactic acidosis.

d. **Correction of electrolyte disturbances**

Serum sodium and potassium may be low in some cases and potassium may fall further to reach a critical level when insulin therapy is started. Ideally, serum sodium and potassium levels should be monitored before and during initial insulin therapy. 30mM KCl can be added per litre of lactated Ringer's solution (2.24g KCl/l) to give a total of 34 mM/l. Do *not* add potassium to intravenous fluids until the fluid administration rate has been decreased from the initial rapid rate and never give potassium chloride at a rate faster than 0.5 mM/kg body weight/hour, (i.e. 0.037g KCl/kg/hour).

e. **Reduction of blood glucose and ketone levels**

Soluble insulin must be used in ketoacidosis (see Table 3) and should be given intravenously or intramuscularly as dehydration will result in poor absorption from subcutaneous sites. The insulin can be given as repeated intravenous boluses at a rate of 1 unit/kg for large dogs, 2 units/kg for small dogs and 0.5 unit/kg for cats (as they are more insulin-sensitive). The bolus should be repeated every two hours together with blood glucose estimations until blood glucose is approximately half the original level. Wait a further two hours before more insulin is given, if necessary.

Alternatively, slow intravenous soluble insulin infusion can be given. This is preferable to boluses of insulin as hypokalaemia and hypoglycaemia are less likely to occur. 5 units of soluble insulin is added to 500 ml lactated Ringer's and is given at a rate of 0.5—1 unit/hour using a pediatric infusion set. Non-insulin containing fluid must be given simultaneously to correct dehydration. The insulin infusion is stopped when blood glucose, again measured 2-hourly, is less than 11 mmol/l. This infusion rate allows for the fact that some of the insulin will adhere to the plastic infusion apparatus.

Once the appropriate blood glucose level is reached, treatment for uncomplicated diabetes mellitus can be commenced.

Table 3
Types of insulin available

Insulin	peak activity[+] (hours)	duration[+] (hours)	route of administration
Short acting (soluble, regular or crystalline) e.g. Hypurin soluble® (CP)	½—6	1—10	i/v, i/m or s/c
Intermediate-acting (isophane or insulin zinc suspension) e.g. Insulatard® (Nordisk Wellcome)	4—12	8—24	s/c
Long-acting (protamine zinc insulin) e.g. Hypurin Protamine Zinc® (CP)	5—14	8—30	s/c

All insulins are now U100 i.e. the concentration is 100 units/ml.

+ The figures given are for dogs and are usually lower in cats which metabolise insulin more rapidly.

Treatment of hyperosmolar coma

If the animal is presented in a non-ketotic coma which cannot be attributed to over-zealous correction of acidosis leading to paradoxical CSF acidosis, a hyperosmolar coma is likely to be present. This is caused by hyperglycaemia which results in the development of an osmotic gradient between the extracellular and intracellular compartments in the brain followed by efflux of water from brain cells. Therapy is as for ketoacidotic coma except that hypotonic solutions e.g. 0.45% NaCl, should be used for rehydration. Avoid solutions containing glucose or alkalinising agents as acidosis is not likely to be present.

Treatment of uncomplicated diabetes mellitus

Stabilisation is much more easily carried out if the animal is hospitalised. It may take from a few days to a few weeks.

1. **Procedure for treatment of uncomplicated diabetes mellitus**

   a. **Oral hypoglycaemic therapy**

      There are only two indications for oral hypoglycaemics in diabetes mellitus, (a) to reduce the amount of insulin required by animals on high insulin doses and (b) in the rare case of mild glucose intolerance associated, for example, with obesity in the absence of other precipitating causes. For these purposes the biguanide, metformin (Glucophage®, Lipha) has been used in dogs at a rate of 250-500 mg twice daily with food. Glucophage is not licensed for veterinary use. The use of the sulphonylureas is not recommended (see Table 4).

Table 4.
Oral Hypoglycaemics

Group	Examples	Action
Biguanide	Metformin	Increases peripheral utilisation of glucose
Sulphonylurea	Tolbutamide	Stimulate insulin secretion
	Chlorpropamide	Hepatotoxic

It should be re-emphasised that the vast majority of canine and feline diabetics are already insulin-dependent when first presented.

   b. **Stabilisation on insulin**

      Animals can be stabilised on the basis of their blood or urine glucose levels. It is more practicable to use urine glucose as this is the parameter the owner must measure when the patient is discharged. It is, of course, useful to measure both parameters during stabilisation but urine glucose should be used to decide how much insulin is required. Collect a fasting urine sample first thing in the morning. If possible, in the case of dogs, allow the animal to urinate, discard this sample and 30 minutes later, collect a fresh sample for analysis. This will give a better reflection of blood glucose levels than an overnight sample. It is more difficult to collect urine samples from cats but special collection trays with non-absorbable litter are now available. The urine is tested for glucose and ketones using a dipstick e.g. Ames Ketodiastix® .These are interpreted as follows;

0% glucose — give 2 units less than the previous day's insulin dose. If urine glucose is negative, the blood glucose level is below the renal threshold and could be dangerously low.

$\frac{1}{10}$ — ½% glucose — this is the ideal level and indicates that the renal threshold is just exceeded. Keep the insulin dose the same as the previous day.

1—2% glucose — increase the insulin dose by 2 units in dogs or 1 unit in cats.

Commence insulin therapy with an intermediate-acting insulin which should be given subcutaneously once daily unless there is a specific reason for twice-daily dosage (see section on investigation of instability). Since there is an individual variation in the response to a given dose of insulin, it is not given on a weight basis so start with an arbitrary dose of 1 unit for a cat, 2 units for a small dog under 10 kg and 4 units for a dog over 10 kg body weight. Ideally, the insulin should be given 30 minutes before the morning meal but if the animal is a poor feeder, it is safer to give the insulin immediately after feeding to avoid the risk of hypoglycaemia if the food is refused after the insulin has been given. If the morning meal is refused, only half the daily insulin dose should be given. Cats tend to metabolise insulin more rapidly than dogs and may sometimes require twice-daily injections of an intermediate-acting insulin or once-daily injections of a long-acting insulin.

c. **Diet**

The animal should be weighed and the total daily food intake calculated on the basis of 30g/kg body weight, with modifications if it is above or below its ideal body weight. The calculated requirements should be divided into a small morning meal and a larger afternoon meal, 8 hours later (see Table 5). Cats or dogs which are on twice-daily insulin, should have half the daily food every 12 hours, just before each insulin injection. It is more important to be consistent with the amount and content of the diet than it is to feed any particular type of diet. However, high fibre diets which are low in absorbable carbohydrate and high in protein are recommended. The fibre can consist of soluble, unabsorbable carbohydrate (e.g. guar gum, pectin) or insoluble fibre (e.g. cellulose), both of which are said to be beneficial in diabetic cats and dogs (Nelson, 1988). Dietry fibre delays absorption of glucose from the small intestine and therefore blunts post-prandial increases in blood glucose and lowers insulin requirements. Rather than concocting diets, it is much easier to feed a specially designed proprietary diet such as Hill's Canine or Feline r/d® or w/d® , the latter having a higher fibre content. If the animal is overweight, canine or feline r/d can be used; if at, or below, optimal weight, canine or feline w/d. If a diabetic dog has difficulty in maintaining body weight, canine g/d is preferable.

Table 5.
Suggested daily schedule for once-daily insulin therapy

8.00 a.m. — collect urine and test for glucose and ketones
8.30 a.m. — give ¼ — ⅓ of daily food
8.35 a.m. — inject insulin (only half the dose if food is not eaten)
4.00 p.m. — give remaining ¾ — ⅔ of daily food

d. **Water**

Water should, of course, be freely available and intake should be measured as it gives a good indication of response to therapy. If the animal has mild ketonuria at the start of treatment, sodium bicarbonate can be added to the water at a rate of one teaspoonful to 500 ml for the first few days.

e. **Other therapy**

Diabetics are predisposed to infections, particularly cystitis, and this should be investigated and treated if necessary.

*The litter tray is called the Mikki® urine collector tray for cats, made by M D Components, Hamelin House, 211/213 High Town Road, Luton, Beds.

Discharging the stabilised diabetic

When the signs of polydipsia, polyuria and polyphagia have resolved, the animal is bright, and has required approximately the same daily dose of insulin for 3 to 4 consecutive days, it can be discharged. It is essential to supply the owner with an instruction sheet which should be discussed before they leave the surgery. The sheet should contain the following information;

1. A brief description of the disease and why insulin therapy is required.

2. A description of how to store insulin and inject it. If some insulin is spilt during injection, they should not 'top it up' as there is a risk of overdosage.

3. Exact details of the diet and the ideal body weight for the individual animal.

4. How to collect urine.

5. How to store, use and interpret urine test strips.

6. The amount of exercise to be given.

7. A daily timetable (see Table 5), with slight modifications of timing to suit the owner's circumstances.

8. How to recognise instability e.g. continuing polydipsia or episodes of hypoglycaemia including hypoglycaemic coma.

9. How to give emergency treatment for hypoglycaemia i.e. if conscious, feed or give oral powdered glucose or if unconscious, smear syrup on the tongue. (The use of intravenous glucose in hypoglycaemia is discussed in the section on insulinoma, under 'Acute hypoglycaemic crisis' page 118).

10. Instructions to keep a book to be completed daily. This should record morning urine glucose and ketone levels, insulin dose given and time of injection, amount of morning feed, amount of afternoon feed and, weekly, body weight.

Having discussed the sheet, allow the owner to try the urine dipstick test and practice filling a syringe and giving a subcutaneous injection using sterile water. Warn them that as the animal has been stabilised in the hospital, it is stabilised on a regime of little or no exercise and it is important that exercise is severely restricted initially, gradually increasing it over the next few days in order to avoid hypoglycaemic episodes. Make sure the owner is supplied with insulin syringes suitable for the type of insulin being used.

Finally, arrange to check the patient one week later and, if all is well, at three-monthly intervals thereafter. Emphasise that if hypoglycaemic coma or ketonuria occur, immediate veterinary advice should be sought.

Investigation of instability

Signs of instability are continuing polydipsia, polyuria and polyphagia, persistent morning glycosuria or signs of hypoglycaemia. Most causes of instability result from misunderstandings about management and include:

1. Improper feeding, especially feeding tit-bits.

2. Inability to administer insulin properly.

3. Inadequate or too vigorous mixing of insulin.

4. Out-of-date or wrongly stored insulin.

5. Using the wrong syringe for the type of insulin.

6. Out-of-date urine dipsticks.

7. Improper interpretation of urine dipsticks.

Having eliminated these factors as being the cause of the instability, the patient should be hospitalised for further investigation. The management regime used by the owner should be followed, and samples should be taken for blood glucose at intervals for 24 hours starting prior to insulin administration and morning feeding. Ideally, the samples should be taken every two hours but four hour intervals have been found to be satisfactory. The resulting graph of blood glucose against time for 24 hours is very useful in sorting out the problem. Three of the more complex causes of instability will now be discussed.

1. **Insulin-induced hyperglycaemia**

    Paradoxically, excessive insulin administration can lead to hyperglycaemia. A large dose causes blood glucose to fall precipitously, stimulating the release of hormones antagonistic to insulin. Blood glucose quickly starts to rise again and because endogenous insulin is insufficient, this rise in blood glucose cannot be damped. The following morning, the urine will contain more than 1 per cent glucose, so the owner will increase the insulin dose still further. Diagnosis is by demonstration of hypoglycaemia (less than 3.5 mmol/l) followed by hyperglycaemia (more than 16.5 mmol/l) within a 24 hour period (Figure 2) and therapy involves halving the insulin dose and restabilising. It may be safer to put animals susceptible to this problem on a fixed dose of insulin once they are sent home.

2. **Rapid metabolism of insulin.**

    In some cases, the exogenous insulin is more rapidly metabolised than usual, resulting in considerable periods of hyperglycaemia during the day, persistent morning glycosuria and perhaps evening polydipsia and polyuria. This is very common in cats, which metabolise insulin more rapidly than dogs. The diagnosis is based on hyperglycaemia (more than 11 mmol/l) within 18 hours of insulin administration with a minimum blood glucose of 4.5—5.5 mmol/l (Figure 3). There are two ways of treating this problem. If the effect of insulin lasts 12-18 hours, protamine zinc insulin can be tried. Theoretically, this has a longer duration of effect than intermediate-acting insulins, but it may be found that the animals will metabolise protamine zinc insulin rapidly as well. If the duration of the intermediate-acting insulin is less than 12 hours, protamine zinc insulin once daily can be tried, or alternatively, the intermediate-acting insulin can be given twice daily at 12 hour intervals. Urine glucose should be tested before each dose is given. However, care must be taken with twice-daily injections as there is a danger of a cumulative effect.

3. **Insulin resistance.**

    Persistence of hyperglycaemia despite insulin therapy may occur where there is peripheral antagonism to the effects of exogenous insulin, e.g. hyperadrenocorticism or hyperprogesteronism. The importance of antibody production against exogenous insulin is uncertain but changing from bovine to porcine insulin sometimes appears to be beneficial. This may be because it has an identical amino-acid sequence to canine insulin and is therefore less likely to stimulate antibody production. Insulin resistance is diagnosed by demonstrating a persistent hyperglycaemia throughout the day (more than 16.5 mmol/l), depsite high doses of insulin (Figure 4). Clearly, it is imperative to investigate the cause of the resistance before it can be treated rationally.

Management of the diabetic during surgery

Elective surgery is best avoided with the exception of spaying entire bitches to prevent instability during dioestrus. The day before surgery, the normal routine should be followed but no food should be given after midnight. On the morning of surgery, half the daily dose of insulin is administered. During surgery, a 5% glucose intravenous infusion is given and this is maintained during recovery and until the animal is eating again. Blood glucose and urine glucose and ketones should be monitored post-operatively and if hyperglycaemia is present, small doses of soluble insulin can be given every 4-6 hours.

Prognosis and long-term complications

With careful management, approximately 70% of diabetic dogs can be stabilised successfully. Sixty-five per cent of those stabilised should survive for at least one year with some surviving for five years or more (Doxey, Milne and Mackenzie, 1985). These figures are lower in cats. The major long-term complications are diabetic cataracts in dogs and repeated bouts of cystitis. Glomerulonephritis is a frequent post-mortem finding in diabetic dogs but is less often associated with signs of renal faliure. Rare complications are diabetic retinopathy and peripheral neuropathies.

Figure 2 *(right)*
Insulin-induced hyperglycaemia. Blood glucose concentration in the same dog after 20 units (solid line) and four units (broken line) of an intermediate-acting insulin at 8.00 a.m.
After Nelson and Feldman, 1983.

Figure 3 *(below)*
Rapid metabolism of insulin. Blood glucose concentration in the same dog after five units of an intermediate-acting insulin at 8.00 a.m. (solid line) and after five units at 8.00. a.m. and 8.00. p.m. (broken line).
After Nelson and Feldman, 1983.

Figure 4 *(below right)*
Resistance to exogenous insulin. Blood glucose concentration in the same dog after 49 units of an intermediate-acting insulin during dioestrus (solid line) and after 49 units during anoestrus (broken line).
After Nelson and Feldman, 1983.

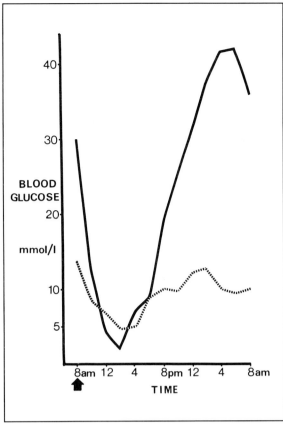

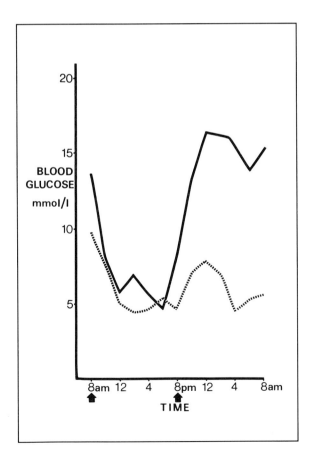

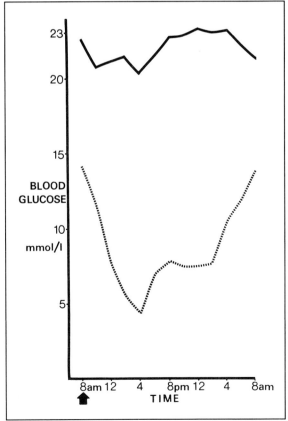

INSULINOMA

AETIOLOGY

Insulinoma is a rare endocrine disease of dogs and cats associated with functional tumours of the pancreatic β cells. It is also known as insulin-secreting tumour, islet cell tumour, β-cell carcinoma or hyperinsulinism. Very few cases have been described in cats (McMillan *et al.,* 1985) and the following discussion on the disease and its management refers to the dog.

Insulinomas are insulin-secreting adenomas or adenocarcinomas of the β cells. Approximately 90 per cent are malignant in dogs whereas in humans, 80 to 90 per cent are benign. The gross appearance (if they are visible to the naked eye) is of single, or more often multiple, firm nodules within the pancreas. The tumours range from microscopic to over 10 cm in diameter. Most are small but are either visible or palpable. On histopathology the neoplastic cells occur in cords or groups surrounded by collagenous stroma. The tumour may be well or poorly encapsulated. The cells do not stain consistently for β cell granules (Mattheeuws *et al.,* 1976). Mitotic figures are rarely seen and degree of encapsulation is a better guide to degree of malignancy. Metastases occur early, particularly to the regional lymph nodes and liver but the mesentery and lungs may also be affected (Njoku *et al.,* 1972).

Excessive secretion of biologically active insulin results in a raised blood insulin and low blood glucose level which is not under control of the negative feedback mechanisms for glucose homeostasis. Thus, clinical signs of hypoglycaemia develop in an episodic manner at times of glucose utilisation or stimulation of insulin secretion.

INCIDENCE

Large breeds are more commonly affected, especially Irish setters, boxers, golden retrievers, standard poodles and German shepherd dogs. The age range is from 5—14 years (Mehlhaff *et al.,* 1985), i.e. middle aged—elderly dogs. There is no sex predilection.

HISTORY AND CLINICAL SIGNS

The clinical signs are mainly referable to the effect of low blood glucose levels on the autonomic and central nervous system. The history is usually one of gradual onset of several signs including grand mal seizures, collapse, weakness, ataxia, exercise intolerance, muscle tremors or twitching (especially of facial muscles), nervousness, hysteria, mental confusion, poor vision, polyphagia with weight gain, hypothermia and sometimes polydipsia and polyuria. Initially the signs will last only a few minutes at a time and the dog will be clinically normal between episodes but as the disease progresses, the episodes become more frequent and prolonged, and death may result during hypoglycaemic coma or status epilepticus from depression of the respiratory centre. The episodes occur during times of blood glucose uptake e.g. fasting, excitement or exercise, or during stimulation of insulin secretion e.g. after feeding.

DIFFERENTIAL DIAGNOSIS

The differential diagnosis is that of episodic collapse or weakness. This is summarised in Table 6. (See also Chapter 12, page 189)

DIAGNOSIS

History and clinical examination

A detailed history including a description of the signs during episodes of hypoglycaemia and their time of onset in relation to feeding and exercise are very important as the dog may be clinically normal when presented for examination. Most animals will have a history of showing several of the clinical signs although a few will be presented for one complaint, usually epileptic fits.

Radiography

Radiography is unhelpful in confirming the diagnosis due to the small size of the tumours in most cases.

Table 6.
Differential diagnosis of insulinoma

1. Functional CNS disease   (a) epilepsy
   (b) narcolepsy (instantaneous sleep attacks)

2. CNS hypoxia   (a) cardiac insufficiency especially episodic problems e.g. some bradydysrhythmias

   (b) severe respiratory disease

   (c) vascular disorders e.g. venous thrombosis

   (d) vasomotor syncope

   (e) anaemia

3. Chronic primary CNS disease e.g tumours, encephalitis due to distemper

4. Chronic metabolic disease (a) other causes of hypoglycaemia e.g. hypoadrenocorticism or hepatic failure

   (b) hyperkalaemia e.g hypoadrenocorticism

   (c) hypocalcaemia e.g. hypoparathyroidism

   (d) uraemia in renal failure

   (e) hyperammonaemia in hepatic failure

5. Neuromuscular disease e.g. myaesthenia gravis

6. Idiopathic syncope

Laboratory findings

1. Blood glucose and insulin

The most accurate means of diagnosis is to demonstrate inappropriately high blood insulin levels for the level of blood glucose. Insulin and glucose must therefore be measured simultaneously. This can be done in two ways:

a. A raised blood insulin when blood glucose is low or normal may occur when clinical signs of hypoglycaemia are present, either spontaneously or after fasting. Usually an overnight fast is sufficient but in some cases fasts of 24 to 72 hours are required. Great care should be taken to ensure that an acute hypoglycaemic crisis does not develop during fasting.

b. If hypoglycaemia is accompanied by normal blood insulin levels, the amended insulin/glucose ratio (AIGR) should be calculated as follows:

$$\text{AIGR} = \frac{\text{plasma insulin } (\mu U/ml) \times 100}{\text{plasma glucose } (mg/100\ ml) - 30}$$

Note that old units rather than SI units are used in the calculation. To convert SI units for glucose (mmol/l) to old units (mg/100 ml), multiply the old units by 18.02. This is a sensitive indicator of the presence of an insulinoma but is subject to false positive results.

2. Tolerance tests

A number of tolerance tests can be used when blood glucose and insulin results are equivocal. These include glucagon, glucose and tolbutamide tolerance tests. In all three tests insulin release is stimulated and there is a risk of inducing severe, prolonged hypoglycaemia. They are also expensive and in most cases have no diagnostic advantage over blood glucose and insulin levels.

TREATMENT

Surgical management

Unless there is good reason not to do so, surgical removal should be attempted as it is likely to increase survival time (Leifer *et al.*, 1986). Early surgery is desirable but time should be taken for proper pre-operative preparation.

1. **Pre-operative treatment**
   a. **Control of blood glucose**
      — feed small meals high in protein and low in simple sugars, 5—6 times daily.
      — administer oral glucocorticoids (0.5—1 mg/kg in two divided doses daily *or* oral diazoxide (Eudemine® , Allen and Hanbury's, 10—40 mg/kg in 3 divided doses daily) (see section below on medical treatment).
      — give an intravenous infusion of balanced electrolyte solutions containing 5% glucose before and during surgery.
   b. **Control of pancreatitis** — the risk of iatrogenic pancreatitis can be reduced by giving parasympatholytics e.g. propantheline bromide (Pro-Banthine® , Gold Cross) at a dose rate of 15 mg t.i.d. or q.i.d., and antibiotic cover, starting before surgery. Pro-Banthine® is available in 15 mg tablets and is not licensed for veterinary use.

2. **Surgery**

   Surgery involves removal of all visible or palpable pancreatic tumours. The drainage lymph nodes (duodenal, hepatic, splenic and greater mesenteric lymph nodes) and liver should be examined and if possible, metastases removed. Surgery is not easy, particularly if the left lobe of the pancreas is affected as it is difficult to visualise. Occasionally the tumours are not visible or palpable but even if this is the case, or if the tumours are not all resectable, euthanasia need not necessarily be undertaken at this stage as medical management is likely to be of benefit.

3. **Post-operative treatment**
   a. Nothing should be given orally for 24—48 hours.
   b. The intravenous infusion of balanced electrolyte solutions containing 5% glucose should be continued until the dog is eating again.
   c. Parasympatholytics and antibiotics should be continued for a few days.
   d. Blood glucose should be monitored every 4 hours for the first few days.

Post-operative complications include persistent seizures, iatrogenic pancreatitis or peritonitis, and diabetes mellitus. The latter is usually transitory and does not usually require insulin therapy unless it persists for more than 4—5 days.

Medical Treatment

1. **Acute hypoglycaemic crisis**

   Acute hypoglycaemia is an emergency which should be treated by administering 2—10 ml of 40—50% glucose solution (Polyfusor Dextrose solution, 50% (Boots Co. plc.), Astrocalc No. 8 (BK Vet Products Ltd.) by slow intravenous injection. If it occurs at home, the owner should feed the dog a meal containing glucose or, if the dog is unconscious, should smear syrup on the tongue. Glucose administration must be regarded as an emergency measure only and cannot be used for long-term control as it will stimulate further insulin secretion.

2. **Long-term management**

   This will be required if the owner does not agree to surgery; if surgery only partially controls hypoglycaemia or if signs of hypoglycaemia recur after remission following surgery.
   a. Exercise — this should be strictly limited.
   b. Diet — see section on pre-operative treatment.
   c. Hyperglycaemic agents — Short acting glucocorticoids e.g. prednisone or prednisolone can be used at a dose rate of 0.5—1 mg/kg bodyweight/day in 2 divided doses but in

in some cases they are ineffective or only effective for a short time. Since long-term therapy is required, there is a risk of producing signs of iatrogenic hyperadrenocorticalism. The drug of choice for long-term therapy is diazoxide (Eudemine®, Allen & Hanbury's), although it is not licensed for veterinary use. Diazoxide is a non-diuretic compound related to the thiazide diuretics which inhibits insulin secretion, stimulates glucose production from the liver and inhibits tissue utilisation of glucose. 10–40 mg/kg bodyweight in three divided doses daily is the recommended rate starting with a dose of 10 mg/kg divided tid. The exact dose required depends on the response. Diazoxide is relatively safe, the major side effect being vomiting, but it can cause diabetes mellitus and bone marrow suppression. Streptozotocin, a cytotoxic agent, may cause temporary remission but its highly nephrotoxic properties preclude its use in practice (Meyer, 1977).

Prognosis and long-term complications

Surgery is of benefit in controlling the disease but the fact that most insulinomas are malignant, together with the difficulty in finding and removing all neoplastic tissue, makes the long-term prognosis poor. Almost inevitably, signs of hypoglycaemia will return a variable time after surgery. The mean survival time in dogs treated by a combination of surgical and medical therapy was 14 months in one survey (Mehlhaff et al., 1985). As time goes on, the response to medical therapy tends to become poorer and euthanasia due to uncontrollable hypoglycaemia may eventually be required.

ACKNOWLEDGEMENTS

Figure 1. was supplied by Mr J. S .D. Ritchie.
Figures 2., 3. and 4. are reproduced by kind permission
of the Journal of the American Veterinary Medical Association.

REFERENCES

DIABETES MELLITUS

CHASTAIN, C. B. and NICHOLS, C. E. (1984). Current concepts on the control of diabetes mellitus. *Vet clins. N. Am.* **14**, 859.

DOXEY, D. L. (1983). *Clinical Pathology and Diagnostic Procedures.* 2nd edn. Balliere Tindall, London, p 74.

DOXEY, D. L., MILNE, E. M. and MACKENZIE, C. P. (1985). Diabetes mellitus: a retrospective survey. *J. small Anim. Pract.* **26**, 555.

EIGENMANN, J. E., EIGENMANN R. Y., RIJNBERK, A., VAN DER GAAG, I., ZAPF, J. and FROESCH, E. R. (1983). Progesterone controlled growth hormone overproduction and naturally occurring diabetes mellitus and acromegaly. *Acta Endocrin.* **104**, 167.

MATTHEEUWS, D., ROTTIERS, R., KANEKO, J. J. and VERMEULEN, A. (1984). Diabetes mellitus in dogs: relationship of obesity to glucose tolerance and insulin response. *Am. J. vet. Res.* **45**, 98.

NELSON, R. W. and FELDMAN, E. C. (1983). Complications of insulin therapy in canine diabetes mellitus. *J. Am. vet. med. Ass.* **182**, 1321.

PETERSEN, M. E., ALTSZULER, N. and NICHOLS, C. E. (1984). Decreased insulin sensitivity and glucose tolerance in spontaneous canine hyperadrenocorticism. *Res. in Vet. Science,* **36**, 177.

YANO, B. L., HAYDEN, D. W. and JOHNSON K. H. (1981). Feline insular amyloid: association with diabetes mellitus. *Vet. Pathol.* **18**, 621.

INSULINOMA

LEIFER, C. E., PETERSON, M. E. and MATUS, R. E. (1986). Insulin secreting tumour: diagnosis and medical and surgical management in 55 dogs. *J. Am. vet. med. Ass.* **188**, 60.

MATTHEEUWS, D., ROTTIERS, R., RIJCKE. J., De RICK, A. and De SCHEPPER, J. (1976). Hyperinsulinism in the dog due to pancreatic islet-cell tumour: a report on three cases. *J. small Anim. Pract.* **17**, 313.

McMILLAN, F. D., BARR, B. and FELDMAN, E. C. (1985). Functional pancreatic islet cell tumour in a cat. *J. Am. Anim. Hosp. Ass.* **21**, 741.

MEHLHAFF, C. J., PETERSON, M. E., PATNAIK, A. K. and CARRILLO, J. M. (1985). Insulin-producing islet cell neoplasms: surgical considerations and general management in 35 dogs. *J. Am. Anim. Hosp. Ass.* **21**, 607.

MEYER, D. J. (1977). Temporary remission of hypoglycaemia in a dog with an insulinoma after treatment with streptozotocin. *Am. J. vet. Res.* **38**, 1201.

NELSON, R. W. (1988). Dietary therapy for diabetes mellitus. *Comp. Contin. Ed. Pract. Vet., Small Animal Section.* **10**, 1387.

NJOKU, C. O., STRAFUSS, A. C. and DENNIS, S. M. (1972). Canine islet cell neoplasia: a review. *J. Am. Anim. Hosp. Ass.* **8**, 284.

FURTHER READING

MILNE, E. M. (1987). Diabetes melittus: an update. *J. small Anim. Pract.* **28**, 727;

MILNE, E. M. (1989). Diabetes mellitus. *In Practice.* **11**, 105.

CHAPTER 6

REPRODUCTIVE ENDOCRINOLOGY OF THE DOG

W. Edward Allen, M.V.B., Ph.D., F.R.C.V.S.
and Gary C .W. England, B.Vet.Med., M.R.C.V.S.

The testes of the dog descend to a superficial scrotal position and are situated in an outpouching of the peritoneal cavity, the vaginal process. They are supported by a mesentery called the mesorchium. Testicular function is controlled by two gonadotrophins secreted from the anterior pituitary gland under the influence of gonadotrophin releasing hormone (GnRH).

Luteinising hormone (interstitial cell stimulating hormone, ICSH) stimulates the interstitial cells of Leydig to produce testosterone and dihydrotestosterone.

Follicle stimulating hormone (FSH) acts on the seminiferous tubules together with endogenous testosterone to promote spermatogenesis. FSH allows spermatid development by promoting Sertoli cell function. Testosterone is necessary for the development of the ductal system, the growth and maintenance of the prostate gland, the development of secondary sexual characteristics and the maintenance of libido. Testosterone suppresses hypothalamic release of FSH. There is, however, only a single releasing hormone for both FSH and LH, and it is believed that regulation of FSH may be achieved by a substance called inhibin which is secreted by the Sertoli cells.

REPRODUCTIVE HORMONES

ANDROGENS

		ANDROGENS	
AGENT	PREPARATION	FORMULATION	MANUFACTURER
Methyltestosterone	Orandrone	Tabs. 5mg	Intervet
Testosterone	Testosterone	Implant 25mg	Intervet
Testosterone phenylpropionate	Androject	Inj. 10mg/ml	Intervet
Testosterone propionate			
phenyl-proprionate	Durateston	Inj.	Intervet
isocaproate		total 50 mg/ml	
deconoate			

Androgens are divided into those with virilising actions and those with anabolic actions. The virilising effects include the development of secondary sexual characteristics, including physical changes and the promotion of libido and spermatogenesis. The anabolic effect promotes protein synthesis, muscle deposition and the retention of certain elements including nitrogen, potassium, phosphorus and calcium, as well as stimulating appetite. High doses will inhibit gonadotrophin release.

Adverse effects

The anabolic component of androgens will cause the retention of both sodium and water, such that these compounds are contra-indicated in nephrotic conditions. Liver dysfunction has been recorded following their use and androgens should not be administered to animals with hepatic dysfunction. Androgens may produce premature growth plate closure in prepubertal dogs and aggression in older animals.

PROGESTAGENS

PROGESTAGENS			
AGENT	PREPARATION	FORMULATION	MANUFACTURER
Delmadinone acetate	Tardak	Inj. 10mg/ml	Norden Labs
Megestrol acetate	Ovarid	Tabs. 5mg, 20mg	Pitman-Moore Ltd
Medroxyprogestorone acetate	Perlutex	Inj. 25mg/ml	Leo

Although widely used in the bitch, other preparations are not specifically licenced for use in the male animal.

Progestagens inhibit gonadotrophin release and therefore may be used for their anti-androgenic effect.

Adverse effects

Progestagens may produce transient side effects such as increased appetite and weight gain, lethargy, mammary enlargement and occasional lactation, hair and coat changes and temperament changes. Progestagens may also be diabetogenic and can produce hair discolouration or loss following subcutaneous injection, so that they should be administered in an inconspicuous site.

Progestagens suppresss spermatogenesis, an effect which is reversed when therapy is stopped; careful consideration should thus be given to the use of progestagens in stud dogs.

OESTROGENS

Oestrogens in high doses will inhibit gonadotrophin release. Oestrogens also increase osteoblastic activity and cause the retention of calcium and phosphorus; they cause an increase in total body protein and metabolic rate and affect skin texture and vascularity.

Adverse effects

Oestrogens produce a dose-related bone marrow suppression resulting in a severe anaemia and thrombocytopenia which may be fatal. In the dog, prolonged oestrogen therapy may produce a syndrome similar to that seen with Sertoli cell tumour. Signs exhibited include bilaterally symmetrical alopecia, epidermal hyperpigmentation, gynaecomastia and squamous metaplasia of the prostate gland. The latter may lead to prostatic enlargement which would worsen the effects of prostatic hyperplasia.

GONADOTROPHINS

Both equine chorionic gonadotrophin (Folligon, Intervet UK Ltd.) and human chorionic gonadotrophin (Chorulon, Intervet UK Ltd) are available for use in the UK.

Human chorionic gonadotrophin (hCG) is mainly LH-like in effect, and LH has been successfully used to increase the secretion of testosterone from Leydig cells.

Equine chorionic gonadotrophin (eCG) is mainly FSH-like in action and should, in theory, promote spermatogenesis.

Adverse effects

Anaphylactoid reaction and antibody formation may be induced following the injection of these protein preparations.

CLINICAL CONDITIONS OF THE PREPUBERTAL DOG

CRYPTORCHIDISM

Cryptorchidism is a failure of one or both testes to descend into the scrotum. It is believed to be a sex-linked autosomal recessive trait with a definite breed prediposition, the risk being greater in smaller breeds. Cryptorchid dogs should not be used for breeding because of the hereditary nature of the disorder. Castration should be advised because of the increased risk of testicular neoplasia and testicular torsion. Medical therapy with hCG and testosterone is empirical and is contraindicated in dogs.

TESTICULAR HYPOPLASIA

In some dogs the abnormal development of the germinal epithelium causes the formation of degenerate spermatocytes resulting in oligospermia or azoospermia. The condition may be congenital and possibly hereditary. Treatment with gonodotrophins and gonadotrophin releasing hormones is not successful and it is pointless to attempt it.

CLINICAL CONDITIONS OF THE ADULT DOG

ANTISOCIAL AND OTHER BEHAVIOURAL PROBLEMS

Problems such as aggression, roaming, territory marking, copulatory activity, destruction and excitability exhibited by both entire and castrated dogs may be controlled, in some cases, by hormonal therapy.

Progestagens

Progestagens have both anti-androgenic properties and a central effect on the cerebral cortex. Depot progestagen therapy such as delmadinone acetate (Tardak, Norden Laboratories) and medroxyprogesterone acetate (Perlutex Injection, Leo Laboratories Ltd) may be used but need to be repeated every month (Tardak) or six months (Perlutex). Oral preparations such as megestrol acetate (Ovarid, Pitman-Moore Ltd.) have been shown to be effective and have the advantage that the dose may be adjusted to effect. With oral preparations drugs are usually given at a high dose (2mg/kg) for two weeks with a gradual reduction over subsequent months. *Behaviour modification training is an essential adjunct to progestagen therapy.*

Oestrogens

Oestrogens (Oestradiol Benzoate, Intervet UK Ltd.) may also be used to control libido and other testosterone-stimulated conditions in the dog. However, due to the possible side effects of long term oestrogen therapy and the superior action of progestagens, the latter are more commonly used in practice.

In the instance of aggressive behaviour towards man, owners should be cautioned over the risks in attempting to treat such dogs, and referral to an animal behaviour consultant or euthanasia may be necessary.

DEFICIENT LIBIDO AND POOR SEMEN QUALITY

There is no evidence that impotence in the dog is caused by low circulating concentrations of testosterone; the condition is more likely to be psychological or due to musculoskeletal pain during copulation. Although androgen therapy in the form of testosterone (Testosterone Implant, Intervet UK Ltd.) and testosterone esters (Androject, Intervet UK Ltd.; Durateston, Intervet UK Ltd.) have been advocated, they should be used with care because they may cause suppression of pituitary function and thus inhibit spermatogenesis. An analogue of dihydrotestosterone, mesterolone (Pro-Viron, Schering Health Care Ltd.) is available in the UK for human use and is unusual in that at therapeutic doses, it does not significantly suppress the release of pituitary gonodotrophins and has been used to treat infertility in man; it has not, as yet, been evaluated in the dog.

Theoretically, eCG should stimulate spermatogenesis, and both eCG and hCG should increase the production of testosterone but their value in impotent and subfertile male dogs has not been proven. Neither is effective in reversing spermatogenic arrest.

EPILEPSY

Castration and/or progestagen therapy have been used for the control of some epileptiform seizures. Delmadinone acetate (Tardak, Norden Laboratories) is recommended at 1—2 mg/kg every three to four weeks and medroxyprogesterone acetate (Perlutex, Leo Laboratories Ltd.) at 20 mg/kg every two weeks.

CLINICAL CONDITIONS OF THE AGEING DOG

BENIGN PROSTATIC HYPERPLASIA

Glandular enlargement may encroach on the structures within the pelvic canal producing dysuria and constipation. Ribbon-like faeces and haematuria are frequently seen.

Progestagen therapy

Depot therapy with delmadinone acetate (Tardak, Norden laboratories) given at 1—2 mg/kg usually causes remission of clinical signs within four days although a second treatment one week later may be necessary; effects generally last at least three months. Oral therapy should be similarly effective.

Oestrogen therapy

Repeated parenteral oestrogen (1mg Ostradiol Benzoate daily or 5 mg weekly) therapy will cause a reduction in prostate size although oral therapy with diethlystilboestrol (0.5—1.0 mg/day for 5 days) may be more convenient. Oestrogen therapy may also provide temporary improvement in some cases of prostatic neoplasia although prolonged treatment may cause prostatic squamous metaplasia.

CIRCUM-ANAL ADENOMATA

These benign tumours which occur in the perineal region of older male dogs respond to anti-androgen therapy and have been treated with progestagens, oestrogens and castration.

TESTICULAR TUMOURS

Testicular tumours are frequently found in the old dog at post-mortem examination.

The three types of testicular tumour seen in the dog all have a similar frequency of occurrence. There is a considerably greater risk of tumour development in abdominal testes.

Sertoli cell tumours

Sertoli cell tumours are usually discrete, unilateral slow growing tumours, being more common on the right side. They have a firm consistency and may be nodular due to the presence of fluid-filled cysts. They may be malignant and metastasise to local lymph nodes as well as pulmonary tissue. Sertoli cell tumours secrete increased amounts of oestrogen which accounts for the clinical signs produced.

Clinical signs;

- — Feminisation.
- — Mammary gland development.
- — Preputial swelling.
- — Attractiveness to other males.
- — Adoption of female squatting posture during urination.
- — Bilaterally symmetrical non-pruritic alopecia.
- — Atrophy of the non-neoplastic testis induced by negative feedback effect on the pituitary/hypothalamus, with decreased libido and oligospermia.
- — Prostatic metaplasia may develop.
- — Oestrogen-induced bone marrow suppression.
- — Low incidence of peri-anal adenomata.

Whilst these signs are characteristic of Sertoli cell tumours they are not pathognomonic since similar effects are recorded with seminomas (although this may be due to the presence of Sertoli cells within the seminoma).

The feminising effect of Sertoli cell tumours may be suppressed by the anti-oestrogenic properties of various androgens, although the treatment of choice is castration. Testosterone esters (Androject, Intervet UK Ltd.) 5—10 mg every 14 days have been used to reverse the oestrogenic effects after castration, although these should subside naturally provided that there are no metastases.

Interstitial cell tumours

These tumours arise from Leydig cells which are found between the seminiferous tubules. They may be single or multiple and occur in one or both testicles. They are often small and frequently produce no change in testicular size although the testicle may be firmer than normal. They are discrete, being brown/yellow in colour and are friable due to central areas of necrosis. They are very rarely malignant and are generally endocrinologically inactive, although testosterone may be secreted which produces a higher incidence of prostatic dysfunction and peri-anal adenomata.

Seminomas

Seminomas arise from the spermatogenic tissue of the tubular epithelium. They are unilateral and generally conform to the shape of the testicle. They are palpably soft with fibrous tissue dividing the tumour into white or grey/white lobulations. They are generally benign although metastasis occasionally occurs.

Feminisation may be seen, although signs believed to be due to androgen secretion have also been described, including a higher incidence of prostatic problems and peri-anal adenomata.

AGEING AND DEBILITY

Various androgens have been used for their anabolic effects in ageing and debilitated dogs. Repeated parenteral or oral therapy is recommended.

DIAGNOSTIC USE OF HORMONES IN THE DOG

CRYPTORCHIDISM

Dogs with functional testicular tissue, whether intra- or extra-abdominal, have higher resting plasma concentrations of testosterone (3—30 nmol/l) than castrated dogs (<0.5 nmol/l). However, positive confirmation of testicular tissue, is achieved by obtaining a plasma sample, giving an intravenous injection of hCG (e.g. 750 I.U. for a 15 kg dog) and obtaining a second plasma sample 1 hour later; a significant rise in plasma testosterone is diagnostic.

SERTOLI CELL TUMOUR

Dogs with intra-abdominal and scrotal Sertoli cell tumours have raised plasma oestrogen concentrations. However, diagnosis from clinical signs is usually straightforward.

ANTISOCIAL AND AGGRESSIVE BEHAVIOUR

These conditions are not accompanied by raised circulating testosterone concentrations.

POOR LIBIDO

Dogs that are unwilling to copulate have not been shown to have low plasma testosterone concentrations.

FURTHER READING

BURKE, T. J. (1986). *Small Animal Reproduction and Infertility, A Clinical Approach to Diagnosis and Treatment.* Lea and Febiger, Philadelphia.

CHRISTIANSEN, Ib. J. (1984). *Reproduction in the Dog and Cat.* Bailliere Tindall, London.

CHAPTER 7

REPRODUCTIVE ENDOCRINOLOGY OF THE BITCH

W. Edward Allen, M.V.B., Ph.D., F.R.C.V.S.
and Gary C. W. England B. Vet. Med., M.R.C.V.S.

The ovaries of the bitch are located mid-abdominally, caudal to the kidneys at the level of the third or fourth lumbar vertebra. Each ovary is supported by the mesovarium with an extension of this, the mesosalpinx which contains the fallopian tube and encircles the ovary to create the ovarian bursa.

The ovary produces oestrogens, progesterone and small amounts of androgens, the theca interna and granulosa layers of the Graafian follicle being of major endocrine importance. The control of ovarian hormone secretion is achieved via the release of the gonadotrophins, luteinizing hormone (LH) and follicle stimulating hormone (FSH), from the anterior pituitary gland.

DEVELOPMENT OF THE FOLLICLE

The development of the ovarian follicle is initiated by the production of gonadotrophin releasing hormone (GnRH) by the hypothalamus. This induces the release of FSH and LH which cause the follicles to develop into several distinct layers. Theca cells have the capacity to synthesise androgens from cholesterol under the influence of LH, and granulosa cells utilise these androgens to produce oestrogens under the influence of FSH. Thus, following the rise of plasma gonadotrophins, plasma oestrogen concentrations increase. The oestrogens promote a negative feedback on the hypothalamus so that gonadotrophin values now fall. At this point the maturing follicles develop an antrum and accumulate FSH and LH so that oestrogen production is maintained, whilst follicles that are not going to mature become atretic due to falling levels of FSH and LH. Antral follicles increase in size until a point is reached where oestrogen concentrations are very high and gonadotrophin values are very low. This induces a switch from a negative to a positive hypothalamic feedback, producing a massive release of GnRH and causing the anterior pituitary to secrete LH (the so called 'LH surge'). These high levels of LH cause the granulosa cells to produce progesterone (i.e. luteinize). Follicle rupture subsequently occurs with the release of the ovum. Corpora lutea develop within the follicular cavities and continue to produce progesterone.

THE OESTROUS CYCLE AND PREGNANCY

The bitch is monoestrous (one oestrus per breeding season) and polyovular, generally reaching puberty 2—3 months after adult bodyweight is attained. The interoestrus period is usually 5—10 months. A schematic representation of the major hormonal events is shown in Figure 1.

The oestrous cycle may be divided into four phases;

Proestrus

Proestrus commences with the first signs of vulval oedema and blood-tinged vaginal discharge, and terminates with the first acceptance of the male. This period lasts for nine days on average (range 3—16 in the normal bitch), and it is the influence of oestrogens which brings about both the behavioural and physical changes.

Oestrus

Oestrus is limited to the period of acceptance of the male and often lasts for a similar period to that of proestrus (nine days with a range of 4—12 in normal bitches). Oestrogen concentrations usually peak prior to the onset of oestrus and during oestrus follicles begin to luteinize and secrete progesterone.

The LH surge is commonly observed at the onset of standing oestrus and most ovulations occur within the next three days; however, the LH surge and the onset of oestrus are not closely related in some bitches. Oestrogen and LH concentrations vary within and between bitches. The measurement of circulating values of these hormones to predict ovulation is impractical as samples would need to be taken 3 to 4 times daily and there would be a delay in obtaining results. However, there is a more consistent increase of progesterone production during pre-ovulatory luteinization and plasma concentrations >10ng/ml tend to indicate impending ovulation. Samples can be taken daily or every two days and semi-quantitative results can be obtained rapidly using enzyme-linked assays. (See page 214 for further details).

Figure 1

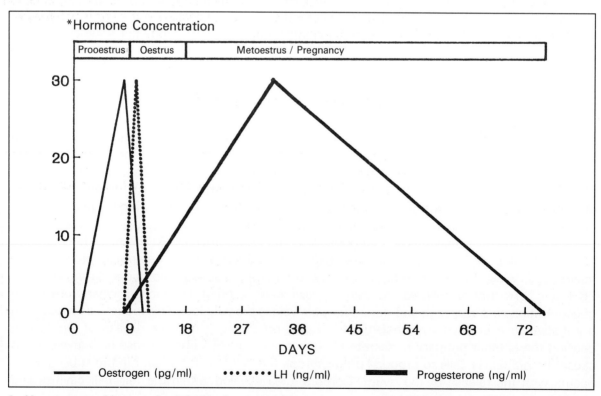

* Measurements of hormone levels in this chapter are given in mass units. The following conversion factors are used to convert to S.I. units:

progesterone	x 3.18
oestradiol	x 3.67
testosterone	x 3.46

Metoestrus

Metoestrus commences with the last acceptance of the male, and ends with the regression of the corpora lutea; during this period progesterone concentrations are increased. Metoestrus averages seventy-five days with a range of 60 – 90 days; it then gradually merges into anoestrus which is characterised by ovarian inactivity. If fertilisation has occurred progesterone levels are maintained by the corpora lutea as in metoestrus. Statistically, however, pregnant bitches have higher progesterone concentrations than non-pregnant bitches, although the individual variation is so great that this is not useful for pregnancy diagnosis. A plasma progresterone concentration greater than 1ng/ml, 14 to 21 days after the end of oestrus indicates that luteinization and presumably ovulation has occurred.

Anoestrus

Anoestrus is the variable period between the end of metoestrus and the beginning of proestrus; it lasts for 210 days on average with a range of 120 – 390 days.

HORMONAL CONTROL OF PARTURITION

The hormonal control of parturition has not been fully defined in the bitch, but it is thought to be similar to that in other species. The major change is the alteration of the progesterone/oestrogen ratio. Progesterone concentrations rapidly fall 24 to 36 hours before parturition, whilst there is a slight elevation of oestrogen concentration in late pregnancy. The changing ratio causes relaxation of the cervix and vagina and allows the uterus to become more active. Maternal cortisol concentrations are elevated 24 hours prior to parturition; these are probably foetal in origin and may promote the release of prostaglandin from the placenta and thus induce lysis of the corpora lutea. Lowered progesterone values increase myometrial sensitivity to oxytocin; however, concentrations of oxytocin and relaxin have not been reported for the bitch. Prolactin values increase to a peak around parturition and remain high for another 10 to 14 days. The significance of this hormone in parturition is unclear, although its action to promote lactation is well recognised. Elevated concentrations are also found in non-pregnant bitches with mammary development (pseudopregnancy).

REPRODUCTIVE HORMONES

PROGESTAGENS

AGENT	PREPARATION	FORMULATION	MANUFACTURER
Medroxyprogestorone acetate	Anoestrolin	Inj. 50mg/ml	Berk
	Perlutex	Tabs. 5mg	Leo
		Inj. 25mg/ml	Leo
	Promone E	Inj. 50mg/ml	Upjohn
Megestrol acetate	Ovarid	Tabs. 5mg, 20mg	Pitman-Moore
Progesterone	Progesterone	Inj. 25mg/ml	Intervet
	Progesterone	Implant 50mg 100mg	Intervet
Proligestone	Covinan	Inj. 100mg/ml	Intervet
	Delvosteron	Inj. 100mg/ml	Mycofarm

Two other synthetic agents; delmadinone acetate (Tardak, Norden Laboratories) and norethisterone acetate (Micronor, Ortho Cilag Pharmaceuticals Ltd.) have also been used.

Progesterone suppresses spontaneous myometrial activity and stimulates endometrial growth. It also induces mammary glandular development. Progestagens (compounds with progesterone-like activity) are widely used to control reproduction since they exert a powerful negative feedback effect upon the hypothalamus/anterior pituitary gland, inhibiting gonadotrophin and prolactin release.

Adverse effects

Many transient effects have been noted with progestagen therapy. These include increased appetite and weight gain, lethargy, mammary enlargement with occasional lactation, hair and coat changes and temperament changes. These adverse effects vary in incidence between the different progestagens although in general they are less frequent in the more recently developed ones such as megestrol acetate and proligestone.

The greatest concern over progestagen usage is that cystic endometrial hyperplasia, mucometra and pyometra might be induced. The risk is related to both the amount of progestagen and the duration of administration, the latter being most important. For this reason the depot preparations of progesterone and medroxyprogesterone acetate are recommended only for use for oestrus *prevention* i.e. during deep anoestrus. The other depot preparations, proligestone and delmadinone have been shown to be safe when given at practically any stage of the cycle, although delmadinone is licensed only for use in the male dog. Oral therapy with both megestrol acetate and medroxyprogesterone acetate has been shown to produce only a low incidence of such effects, and as yet there are no recorded problems with norethisterone although this drug is not widely used in dogs.

There are no preparations recommended for use in the first oestrous period or in prepubertal dogs.

Benign mammary nodules can be induced by progestagen therapy and it has been suggested that progestagens may induce mammary neoplasia, although this does not appear to be the case with proligestone. This is paradoxical since progestagens are used to control some cases of neoplasia, which may be explained by the fact that low doses of progestagens are stimulatory whilst high doses are inhibitory.

Progesterone acts as a potent insulin antagonist and there are several reports of progestagens being diabetogenic.

Progestagens may induce acromegaly in entire female bitches; clinical signs are inspiratory stridor, excess skin fold formation, abdominal enlargement, polydipsia/polyuria, hyperglycaemia, fatigue and in some cases enlargement of the interdental spaces. (See 'Pituitary' chapter.

Progestagen therapy during pregnancy may produce masculinised female and cryptorchid male puppies.

The subcutaneous administration of some progestagens may produce hair discolouration and local alopecia; it is therefore recommended by the manufacturers that injections should be given in an inconspicuous site (although this is usually impractical).

Progestagens are not recommended for use where there is concurrent systemic infection.

OESTROGENS

AGENT	PREPARATION	FORMULATION	MANUFACTURER
Oestradiol benzoate	Oestradiol benzoate	Inj. 5mg/ml	Intervet
Ethinyl oestradiol	Sesoral	Tabs. 0.005mg	Intervet
(and methyltestosterone)		(4.0mg)	

The naturally occurring oestrogen, oestradiol (Oestradiol benzoate, Intervet UK Ltd.) is only effective parentrally, since partial inactivation occurs in the gut. However, diethlystilboestrol (Stilboestrol, APS Ltd.) is available in an oral formulation and ethinyloestradiol is thought to be effective orally; the latter is one constituent of Sesoral (Intervet UK Ltd.) and is also available as a medical preparation.

Oestrogens are responsible for the development of the female sexual characteristics, including uterine growth, signs of proestrus and mammary development. They also increase osteoblastic activity and cause the retention of calcium and phorphorus; cause an increase in total body protein and metabolic rate and affect skin texture and vascularity. Oestrogens in high doses inhibit the output of gonadotrophins, whilst in very low doses there is an enhancement of FSH output.

Adverse effects

Oestrogens should be used with caution since they may produce severe side effects. They do not stimulate cystic endometrial hyperplasia or pyometra *per se* but they may potentiate the stimulatory effect of progesterone on the uterus and may also cause cervical relaxation, thus allowing vaginal bacteria to enter the uterus.

Oestrogens have been shown to produce a dose related bone marrow suppression which results in a severe and possibly fatal anaemia and thrombocytopenia. There is considerable individual variation to the toxic dose — which may lie within the manufacturer's normal recommended dose range. Toxic effects are generally dose-related with toxicity being less likely if low doses are given over a period of time. The toxic dose cannot be determined due to individual variation: however, a maximum suggested dose is 1mg/kg or a total dose of 20mg, although toxicity occurred when 15mg stilboestrol was given over nine days to a corgi (Reed and Thornton, 1982). Oral therapy should be prescribed whenever possible.

If oestrogens are administered during pregnancy cervical relaxation and abortion may occur; they may also cause congenital defects in developing foetuses.

Prolonged oestrogen therapy may produce non-pruritic bilaterally symmetrical alopecia and skin hyperpigmentation (see Chapter 10, page 174). Large doses stimulate signs of oestrus in the bitch.

ANDROGENS

AGENT	PREPARATION	FORMULATION	MANUFACTURER
Drostanolone propionate	Masteril	Inj. 100mg/ml	Syntex
Methyltestosterone	Orandrone	Tabs. 5mg	Intervet
Methyltestosterone (and Ethinyl oestradiol)	Sesoral	Tabs. 4mg (0.005mg)	Intervet
Testosterone	Testosterone	Implant 25mg	Intervet
Testosterone phenylpropionate	Androject	Inj. 10mg/ml	Intervet
Testosterone propionate			
Testosterone phenylpropionate	Durateston	Inj. total esters	Intervet
Testosterone isocaproate		50 mg/ml	
Testosterone deconoate			

The naturally occurring androgens testosterone and dihydrotestosterone are produced by the interstitial cells of the testis. Their duration of activity is related to the nature of the synthetic ester (propionate, phenylpropionate etc.). Androgens may be divided into those with primarily virilising actions and those with primarily anabolic actions. The virilising effects include the development of the secondary sexual characteristics. The anabolic effect promotes protein synthesis, muscle deposition and the retention of certain elements including nitrogen, potassium, phosphorus and calcium, as well as stimulating appetite. Androgens will inhibit the hypothalamic/pituitary release of gonadotrophins in a similar manner to oestrogens.

Adverse effects

Androgen therapy may produce virilising effects such as aggression, clitoral hypertrophy and vaginitis; in prepubertal animals premature epiphyseal growth plate closure may also occur.

Androgens are contraindicated in nephrotic conditions since the anabolic component causes both sodium and water retention and liver dysfunction has been recorded following androgen therapy.

Severe urogenital abnormalities may develop in female puppies if androgens are administered to pregnant bitches.

GONADOTROPHINS

Both equine chorionic gonadotrophin (Folligon, Intervet UK) and human chorionic gonadotrophin (Chorulon, Intervet UK Ltd.) are licensed and available for use in the bitch in the United Kingdom.

Equine chorionic gonadotrophin (eCG) is produced by the mare during pregnancy. It is mainly FSH-like in action but does have LH-like activity so that it promotes the growth and maturation of ovarian follicles. Human chorionic gonadotrophin (hCG) is extracted from the urine of pregnant women and is primarily LH-like in effect. It causes final maturation and ovulation of follicles and the formation of corpora lutea in the female.

Adverse effects

The LH-like activity of eCG may cause luteinisation of follicles before the onset of behavioural oestrus or ovulation. Hyperstimulation of the ovary may also occur resulting in cystic follicles or prolonged oestrous behaviour.

There is a risk of inducing both anaphylactoid reactions and antibody formation following the injection of these protein preparations.

PROSTAGLANDINS

There are no naturally occurring or synthetic prostaglandin analogues specifically licensed for use in the dog in the United Kingdom. There are, however, several preparations available, including the naturally occurring prostaglandin $F_2\alpha$, dinaprost (Lutalyse, Upjohn Ltd.) and the analogues: alfaprostol (Alphacep, Beechams Animal Health), cloprostenol (Estrumate, Coopers Animal Health Ltd.; Planate, Coopers Animal Health Ltd.), luprostiole (Prosolvin, Intervet UK Ltd.), fenprostalene (Synchrocept B, Syntex Animal Health Ltd.), and tiaprost (Iliren, Hoechst Animal Health).

The reproductive prostaglandins are synthesised in the endometrium and are considered to be luteolytic in nature. However, bitch corpora lutea are not very responsive to prostaglandin action so their uses are related to their presumed ability to produce myometrial contraction and relaxation of the cervix.

Adverse effects

Prostaglandin administration may be followed by restlessness, hypersalivation, vomiting, abdominal pain, fever, tachycardia and diarrhoea. These effects are seen soon after injection and may last for up to three hours. There is a suggestion that these effects may be controlled by the prior administration of atropine.

OXYTOCIN

AGENT	PREPARATION	FORMULATION	MANUFACTURER
Oxytocin	Oxytocin S	Inj. 10 I.U./ml	Intervet
Pituitary extract	Hyposton	Inj. 10 I.U./ml	Paines & Byrne
	Pituitary (post. lobe)	Inj. 10 I.U./ml	Arnolds
	Pituitary (post. lobe)	Inj. 10 I.U./ml	Univet
	Pituitary extract	Inj. 10 I.U./ml	Vet Drug

Oxytocin is administered at a dose rate of 0.5—10.0 I.U. per dog by intramuscular or subcutaneous injection.

Oxytocin stimulates myoepithelial cells within the mammary gland and thus induces the milk let-down reflex. It also causes contraction of the uterine smooth muscle during parturition. Posterior pituitary extract contains both oxytocin and antidiuretic hormone.

Adverse effects

There is a low incidence of skin sloughing or abscess formation recorded by some manufacturers following the subcutaneous administration of oxytocin. Therefore it is best given by the intramuscular route.

ERGOT PREPARATIONS

There are no preparations licensed for use in the dog although both parenteral and oral preparations of ergometrine maleate (Ergometrine maleate, Evans Medical Ltd.; Syntometrine, Sandoz Pharmaceuticals) are available.

Ergotamines are, like oxytocin, ecbolic drugs. However, they produce a prolonged spasm of uterine muscle. Relaxation occurs only after one to two hours when the uterus then contracts rhythmically in a similar manner to that produced by oxytocin.

Adverse effects

Ergot alkaloids may produce emesis and slight stimulation of the central nervous system.

BROMOCRIPTINE

Bromocriptine (Parlodel, Sandoz Pharmaceuticals) is a synthetic ergot alkaloid which inhibits prolactin secretion. It is not licensed for use in the bitch although it is available as an oral formulation. The dose required varies although on average 0.01mg/kg/day is used.

Adverse effects

The most commonly reported side effect in the dog is vomiting. This can be reduced by using the minimum effective dose (0.01—0.1 mg/kg/day) and mixing the drug with food or by using specific anti-emetics such as metoclopramide (Emequell, Beecham Animal Health). Administration of bromocriptine during pregnancy can cause abortion.

TOCHOLYTIC AGENTS

There is a variety of compounds with uterine spasmolytic properties including hyoscine (Buscopan Compositum Injection, Boehringer Ing. Ltd.), monzaldon (Monzaldon, Boehringer Ing. Ltd.) and proquamezine fumarate (Myspamol, RMB Animal Health Ltd.). The drugs clenbuterol (Planipart, Boehringer Ing. Ltd.; Ventipulmin, Boehringer Ing. Ltd.) and isoxsuprine (Duvadilan Injection, Duphar Laboratories Ltd.) are also available although not licensed for use in the dog.

Adverse effects

There are few side effects of these drugs; proquamezine may produce mild sedation.

NON-HORMONAL ABORTIFACIENTS

There are several reports concerning the use of agents which can terminate pregnancy in the bitch. Drugs such as derivatives of methoxphenyltriazaloisoquinolines (L12717 and others) have actions which are unclear but they appear to affect the utero-placental unit, slowing embryonic development and causing a degeneration of foetal and placental tissue; they are not available at present in the UK but L12717 is available in Europe.

Drugs which inhibit progesterone synthesis (e.g. epostane), and thus terminate pregnancy, are being evaluated.

Adverse effects

L12717 has been reported to produce septic necrotic metritis and several bitches have died following its administration; the drug has recently been withdrawn from the market in Germany.

Epostane produces severe abcessation following intramuscular injection which precludes its use in general practice.

Note: the therapeutic use of some hormone preparations, particularly the oestrogens, is mainly empirical in the dog and bitch; dose rates appear to have been defined more by trial and error than experimental design.

CONTROL OF OESTRUS

The oestrous cycle may be controlled with a variety of reproductive hormones. There has been some confusion concerning the terminology used to describe the control of the oestrous cycle. The term 'prevention' is used to describe the administration of agents to an anoestrous bitch to prevent the occurrence of oestrus, whilst the term 'suppression' is used to describe the administration of agents during pro-oestrus or oestrus to abolish the signs of that particular oestrus.

PROGESTAGEN THERAPY

There several different ways in which progestagens can be used to control oestrus;

Depot Injections

The subcutaneous injection of long-acting preparations (medroxyprogesterone acetate, proligestone) provides a slow release of progestagen. They may be administered during anoestrus to prevent the subsequent oestrus. Progesterone and delmadinone acetate have been used in a similar manner. Repeated regular dosing (every 3—6 months) will achieve long-term prevention, although the risk of inducing adverse effects (e.g. acromegaly, diabetes mellitus) is increased and it is thought inadvisable to extend anoestrus for more than two years. Proligestone may also be given in early pro-oestrus to suppress the signs of that oestrus. When using injections it is necessary to consider the variable time of action, so that the prediction of the next oestrus or the timing of subsequent injections may be difficult. Following the use of depot preparations, bitches will eventually return to a fertile oestrus, although some manufacturers do not recommend drug usage in breeding animals.

Oral Administration During Anoestrus

The oral administration of low doses of medroxyprogesterone acetate and megestrol acetate during anoestrus will prevent the subsequent oestrus for as long as oral administration is continued.

The necessity for constant oral medication is a disadvantage although anoestrus is ensured during treatment and there is the option to stop medication should side effects occur.

Progestagens should preferably be given in late anoestrus so that treatment coincides with the next expected oestrus. However, if the animal enters oestrus during the first few days of medication (i.e. the course was started too late in anoestrus) the dose can be increased to that required for suppression. Oestrus usually returns within six months after the end of medication but to some extent this depends on the stage of anoestrus when therapy was initiated.

Progestagens cannot be used to prevent oestrus indefinitely because the risk of adverse effects increases with the duration of therapy.

Oral Administration During Pro-oestrus

The administration of high doses of orally active progestagen (medroxyprogesterone acetate, megestrol acetate) starting early in pro-oestrus will suppress the signs of that oestrus. The correct timing of treatment is essential, for late dosing is often inadequate to cause follicular atresia whilst early dosing is similarly ineffective. In both situations a fertile oestrus may reappear soon after the termination of treatment.

Therapy is administered for eight days at a dose rate of 2mg/kg, or for sixteen days if the dosage is reduced to 0.5 mg/kg after the first four days. This regime will usually suppress the signs of pro-oestrus within five days. Oestrus usually recurs four to six months after the termination of therapy.

The authors prefer the use of orally active progestagens and do not advocate the use of injectable preparations during pro-oestrus. Proligestone is the only suitable progestagen for oestrus prevention in greyhounds (D.A. Poulter, personal communication).

Table 1. Oestrus Prevention and Suppression

OESTRUS PREVENTION

A. Depot injections

Medroxyprogesterone acetate	Perlutex 25mg/ml	<15kg 2ml 15—25kg : 2—3ml 25—35kg : 3—4ml 35—50kg : 4—6ml	Leo Laboratories Ltd
	Promone E 50mg/ml	50mg per animal	Upjohn Ltd
Proligestone	Covinan 100mg/ml	<5kg : 1.0—1.5ml 5—10kg : 1.5—2.5ml 10—20kg : 2.5—3.5ml 20—30kg : 3.5—4.5ml 30—45kg : 4.5—5.5ml 45—60kg : 5.5—6.0ml Thereafter 10mg/kg	Intervet UK Ltd
	Delvosterone 100mg/ml	as above	Mycofarm

Progesterone and delmadinone have been used in a similar manner.

B. Oral preparations

Medroxyprogesterone acetate	Perlutex 5mg	<25kg : 5mg/day >25kg : 10mg/day	Leo Laboratories Ltd
Megestrol acetate	Ovarid 5mg/20mg	0.5mg/kg/day up to 40 days 0.1—0.2mg/kg/twice weekly if over 40 days	Glaxovet Ltd

OESTRUS SUPPRESSION

A. Oral preparations

Medroxyprogesterone acetate	Perlutex 5mg	<25kg—10mg/day for 4 days then 5mg for 12 days >25kg—2x above regime	Leo Laboratories Ltd
Megestrol acetate	Ovarid 5mg/20mg	2mg/kg/day for 8 days or 2mg/kg/day for 4 days then 0.5mg/kg/day for 16 days	Glaxovet Ltd

B. Depot injections

Proligestone	Covinan 100mg/ml	dose as above	Intervet UK Ltd
	Delvosterone 100mg/ml	dose as above	Mycofarm

ANDROGEN THERAPY

Androgens suppress gonadotrophin release and can, therefore, be used for oestrus prevention.

Testosterone implants and repeated parental and/or oral administration have been used, especially in the greyhound. A suggested regime is to use 25mg Androject (Intervet UK Ltd.) and 125mg Durateston (Intervet UK Ltd.) in two different intramuscular sites, followed by the daily administration of 10mg methyltestosterone (Orandrone, Intervet UK Ltd.) (D.A. Poulter, personal communication). Although this is successful, the possibility of androgen-induced side effects (e.g clitoral hyperplasia) is not acceptable to some owners.

A synthetic androgen, mibolerone (Cheque Drops, Upjohn Ltd.) is available in the USA and elsewhere but not in the United Kingdom, and is approved for the effective long term prevention of oestrus in the bitch. The drug may produce mild adverse effects similar to the other androgens.

OTHERS

Research is being undertaken to evaluate the efficacy of LHRH agonists and antagonists (such as nafarelin and detirelix) to prevent oestrus, ovulation and fertilisation. These drugs are not available at this stage.

CLINICAL CONDITIONS OF THE PREPUBERTAL BITCH

JUVENILE VAGINITIS

Vaginal discharge (which may become purulent), with frequent licking, attractiveness to male dogs and perivulval dermatitis is sometimes seen after eight weeks of age. The condition usually regresses after the first oestrus but some control may be achieved by the daily administration of 0.5—1mg diethylstilboestrol for 5 days. Antibiotics rarely give more than temporary relief.

DELAYED PUBERTY

Some bitches, especially those of the larger breeds, do not enter oestrus at the anticipated age (6—18 months). In those bitches that are not cycling by two years of age hormone therapy may be attempted to induce oestrus (see 'Oestrus induction').

FIRST OESTRUS

Some bitches exhibit little sign of pro-oestrus in their first cycle so that it is not noticed by the owner (so-called 'silent oestrus'). Other bitches have prolonged or recurrent periods of pro-oestrus, which do not appear to culminate in ovulation. Efforts to stimulate ovulation with hCG are rarely effective and ovarian activity is best suppressed with an eight day course of megestrol acetate (2mg/kg). The ensuing oestrus is usually normal.

CLINICAL CONDITIONS OF THE MATURE BITCH

OESTRUS-INDUCTION

Periods of prolonged anoestrus are occasionally seen in some mature bitches after they have had one or more cycles. In such circumstances there have been attempts to induce oestrus using oestrogens, eCG, hCG, FSH, LH, GnRH and combinations of these. However, it is best to wait for a normal heat if time allows.

The use of eCG (Folligon, Intervet) (50—200 I.U. daily, subcutaneously, for up to three weeks) in cases of prolonged anoestrus or delayed puberty in the bitch gives variable results and if ovulatory oestrus is achieved it may be followed by a short luteal phase. Repeated dosing with eCG to induce oestrus can be followed by hCG on the next two or three days to stimulate ovulation.

Small doses of oestradiol (0.1—0.5mg) repeated two to four times at intervals of two to three days followed by eCG therapy has also been used to induce ovulation. Drugs which may be useful in the dog, but have not been evaluated, are gonadotrophin releasing hormone and clomiphene, which stimulate the secretion of gonadotrophins.

IRREGULARITIES OF THE OESTROUS CYCLE

Prolonged pro-oestrus or oestrus and ovarian cysts have all been treated with many different dose regimes of a variety of progestagens (progesterone, megestrol acetate, medroxyprogesterone acetate, proligestone, delmadinone acetate and norethisterone); the results have been variable, but in some cases signs disappear with a return to normal cyclical activity. However, pyometra may develop.

MISALLIANCE

After the unwanted mating of a bitch, nidation may be prevented by the oral or parental administration of high doses of oestrogens. Oestrogens interfere with progesterone dominance during the tubular phase of development of the fertilised ova which may alter oviducal transport time, and create a hostile uterine environment. Generally, oestrogens are effective when administered up to five days after mating.

Until recently the intramuscular administration of diethylstilboestrol post-mating was used to prevent nidation. Oestradiol benzoate is now used in a similar manner up to four days post-mating, although Christiansen (1984) suggests that treatment before three days after mating may fail to prevent pregnancy. Oestrogens may cause animals to continue to show signs of oestrus or they may return to oestrus and thus may be remated. A subsequent mating may be fertile, but this is unlikely unless treatment was given in pro-oestrus (i.e. there will not be a second crop of ovulations). Oestrogens should only be administered once to avoid toxicity.

Daily oral diethylstilboestrol has been suggested for seven days after mating, although this may be unreliable.

If a bitch is not required for breeding purposes, ovariohysterectomy two weeks following oestrus is a safe alternative.

PSEUDOPREGNANCY

Since endocrinologically the events of metoestrus and pregnancy are similar in the bitch it is not surprising that the signs of pregnancy are exhibited by non-pregnant bitches. Many show mild signs so that treatment is not indicated. However, when the condition becomes clinically significant treatment aimed at inhibiting or antagonising the action of prolactin may be attempted.

Oestrogens

The negative feedback of steroids on the hypothalamic/pituitary axis means that oestrogens are effective in the treatment of pseudopregnancy. Both parenteral and oral diethylstilboestrol and parenteral oestradiol benzoate have been used although neither is specifically licensed for this purpose. A preparation of ethinyl oestradiol combined with methyltestosterone (Sesoral, Intervet UK Ltd.) is available although the dose suggested seems arbitary and the large numbers of tablets required make it unsuitable for the anorexic bitch.

Progestagens

Both megestrol acetate (2 mg/kg for 5 days) and proligestone (single dose 33 mg/kg) are very effective in suppressing pseudopregnancy and there is usually a return to normal behaviour within three days. However, after the use of megestrol acetate, relapse has been observed in some bitches.

Androgens

Methyltestosterone (Orandrone, Intervet UK Ltd.), testosterone esters (Androject, Intervet UK Ltd.; Durateston, Intervet UK Ltd.) may be more useful than progestagens or oestrogens since they do not have any adverse effects on the uterus. Dose rates are 5—30mg daily for 5—7 days (Orandrone), 25—150mg monthly (Durateston) and 5—10 mg every 7 days (Androject).

Bromocriptine. The specific prolactin inhibitor bromocriptine (Parlodel, Sandoz Pharmaceuticals) administered daily (0.01mg/kg) is often successful in terminating pseudopregnancy.

PYOMETRA

Canine cystic endometrial hyperplasia-pyometra complex occurs during the progesterone-dominant phase of the oestrous cycle. Progesterone-induced cystic endometrial hyperplasia usually preceeds the development of pyometra which is associated with bacterial invasion of the uterus during oestrus.

Following the accurate diagnosis of cases of 'open' pyometra in the absence of mummified foeti, prostaglandins may be used to induce uterine emptying. Dinaprost (Lutalyse, Upjohn Ltd.) at a dose rate of 0.25mg/kg parenterally for five days and combined with antibiotics, may be successful. Repeated therapy is required in approximately one third of cases. In bitches which are extremely ill prostaglandins are not indicated since a clinical response is not observed for at least forty-eight hours. The use of prostaglandins in cases of 'closed' pyometra, or where mummified foeti are present, is contraindicated. Ovario-hysterectomy should be carried out in such cases.

METOESTRUS ACROMEGALY

As previously discussed, progestagen therapy may induce acromegaly. The elevated plasma progesterone that occurs during metoestrus may induce transient acromegaly in the bitch. The signs are similar to those recorded with progestagen therapy and there is spontaneous recovery at the end of metoestrus. Therapy should be aimed at decreasing plasma progesterone concentrations usually by ovariohysterectomy, although prostaglandin therapy has been suggested (see 'Termination of pregnancy' and 'Pyometra').

DIABETES MELLITUS

Progesterone acts as a potent insulin antagonist and some bitches may become diabetic for the duration of metoestrus. Diabetic bitches will be particularly difficult to stabilise during this period. Ovariohysterectomy is recommended as soon as diabetes is diagnosed.

CLINICAL CONDITIONS OF THE PREGNANT BITCH

FAILURE TO HOLD TO SERVICE

Bitches that repeatedly fail to conceive are sometimes given a single injection of hCG (200 – 500 I.U.) on the assumption that ovulation has not occurred or that early development of the corpora lutea is inadequate; there is no evidence of the efficacy of this treatment.

HABITUAL ABORTION

It is suggested that habitual spontaneous abortion may be due to low plasma progesterone concentrations and abortion following induced oestrus may be correlated with low plasma progesterone levels. Exogenous progestagens may have a protective value to the pregnancy by increasing uterine protein secretion and possibly due to their suppressant effect upon myometrial contractions. Daily – weekly injections of progesterone (25 – 50mg), daily oral medroxyprogesterone acetate (2.5 – 10mg) and subcutaneous progesterone implants (100 to 500mg) have all been recommended, although there is little evidence to support the theory that progesterone deficiency is an important factor in foetal loss.

TERMINATION OF PREGNANCY

Unwanted pregnancies are best treated by early (2 – 4 weeks after mating) ovariohysterectomy or left to go the term.

Canine corpora lutea are unresponsive to prostaglandin therapy for at least the first two or three weeks of pregnancy. After this time a single dose of prostaglandin (dinoprost) will produce luteolysis although the effective dose (1mg/kg) is similar to the lethal dose (5mg/kg). Prolonged therapy (for approximately one week) with lower doses (0.02mg/kg) is safer and sometimes effective.

Prostaglandin analogues have been designed to provide improved luteolytic and ecbolic actions with reduced adverse effects. Cloprostenol can effectively produce abortion after day twenty-five when given intravaginally as a twenty-four hour release plastic device. This method achieves a long luteolytic effect with reduced adverse effects, but is not commercially available at the present time.

Corticosteroids (5mg dexamethasone daily for 10 days) will produce abortion but the repeated administration and high doses required make this method impractical and inadvisable.

Non-hormonal abortifacients (e.g. L12717) have been shown to be effective in terminating pregnancy in the bitch. The way these compounds work is not clear, but they are maximally effective at 15—20 days after mating. These agents are not available commercially in the United Kingdom.

UTERINE INERTIA

Cases of primary uterine inertia may respond to parenteral oxytocin therapy. It has a short half life and repeated administration (every 15—30 mins) may be necessary. The use of a continuous low dose intravenous infusion appears not to have been evaluated in this condition in non-human females. Oxytocin is contraindicated in cases of obstructive dystocia since uterine rupture may result.

Ergometrine should not be used during parturition because it induces uterine spasm.

DYSTOCIA

Tocholytic agents e.g. hyoscine 4—10mg (Buscopan Compositum Inj, Boehringer Ing. Ltd.), monzaldon, 25—100mg (Monzaldon, Boehringer Ing, Ltd.) and proquamerzine 3mg/kg (Myspamol, RMB Animal Health Ltd.) cause uterine relaxation and may be used in cases of dystocia with relative foetal oversize to allow further dilation of the distal reproductive tract.

PLACENTAL RETENTION

The persistence of a green discharge *post partum* may indicate a retained placenta (and possibly also a puppy).

Parenteral administration of oxytocin is usually effective at producing uterine contraction and expulsion of the placenta although hysterotomy may be necessary to remove the puppy.

POST PARTUM HAEMORRHAGE

Haemorrhage due to physical injuries or placental necrosis occurs *post partum* and may be controlled by the parenteral administration of oxytocin (1—2 I.U./kg) or ergometrine (0.2—0.5mg).

POST PARTUM METRITIS

Hormones are sometimes used in conjunction with antibiotic therapy in cases of acute metritis following parturition. Oxytocin (1—2 I.U./kg) and ergometrine (0.2—0.5mg) have been used to stimulate myometrial activity and induce uterine drainage; these are the two drugs of choice. Dinaprost given twice daily in a similar regime to that for pyometra may also stimulate uterine evacuation. Oestrogens are contraindicated because of the possibility of increasing the absorption of toxins.

SUB-INVOLUTION OF PLACENTAL SITES

This condition is characterised by intermittent haemorrhagic discharge from the vulva for up to six months after parturition. Ecbolic agents and antibiotics have no effect but the condition may be prevented by the administration of oxytocin after parturition.

AGALACTIA

Lack of milk production is rare in the bitch. However, an absence of milk *letdown* is fairly common and can be treated with a single dose of oxytocin (0.2—1.0 I.U./kg). Oxytocin does not increase milk production; this would require prolactin, which is not available.

SUPPRESSION OF LACTATION

Oestrogens, androgens, progestagens and bromocriptine will suppress lactation by inhibiting prolactin production (see 'Pseudopregnancy').

CLINICAL CONDITIONS OF THE OVARIECTOMISED BITCH

URINARY INCONTINENCE

Urinary incontinence is frequently described as a complication of ovariectomy or ovariohysterectomy. The aetiology is unknown, with the onset occurring between months and many years after surgery. Some cases respond to oestrogen therapy whilst in others the response is short lived or absent. The precise role that oestrogens play is unclear, although the major action is on the urethra, probably increasing its contribution to the external sphincter mechanism.

Parenteral oestradiol benzoate is recommended at doses of 1mg/day for three days with subsequent injections every third day. The use of oral diethylstilboestrol (0.5—1mg) is also effective. Daily therapy is administered for up to three weeks with a response being observed after the first few days; the length of treatment is kept to the minimum for effect and the course is repeated as necessary.

ALOPECIA IN THE OVARIECTOMISED BITCH

The epitheliotrophic action of oestrogen may be useful in cases of alopecia following ovariectomy. The primary effects on the skin are to promote keratinisation and to suppress sebum production. The dose used must, however, be low enough to avoid stimulating sexual attractiveness. Affected bitches have blood oestrogen concentrations similar to those of normal bitches.

SIGNS OF OESTRUS AFTER OVARIECTOMY

This may be due to a piece of ovary having been left *in situ* during surgery. It may take many months for the development of follicles and signs of oestrus to occur. Oestrus can be suppressed with progestagens.

Some ovariectomised bitches are attractive to male dogs and have a swollen vulva, but are not in oestrus. They usually respond to antibiotic therapy. The two conditions can be differentiated by examining a vaginal smear.

VULVAL HYPOPLASIA

An infantile vulva has been described in some ovariectomised bitches. Oestrogen therapy may be effective but surgical removal of excess perivulvular skin is the treatment of choice.

CLINICAL CONDITIONS OF THE AGEING BITCH

OESTROGEN-DEPENDENT MAMMARY TUMOURS

Both oestrogen and progesterone receptors have been identified in maglignant and benign tumours.

Progestagens

Megestrol acetate administered for ten to fifteen days is a potential method of hormonal therapy, but this should be used with care since benign mammary nodules have been produced using progestagens.

Androgens

Androgens may also be used in the control of certain mammary tumours. Weekly to monthly parenteral therapy (Masteril, Syntex Animal Health) is recommended, whilst oral therapy is given daily.

It is not possible to differentiate these tumours except by the response to therapy.

AGEING AND DEBILITY

Various androgens (e.g. Androject (Intervet UK Ltd.), Durateston (Intervet UK Ltd.) and Testosterone Implants (Intervet UK Ltd.) are used for their anabolic effect in debilitated and aged dogs. Parenteral therapy is usually given every one to two weeks, whilst oral therapy is recommended daily.

DIAGNOSTIC USE OF HORMONES IN THE BITCH

PREDICTING THE TIME OF OVULATION

Progesterone

During pro-oestrus, progesterone concentrations in plasma are low and fluctuate between 1.59—3.18 nmol/l. There is a rapid increase (>15.9 nmol/l) during the onset of the pre-ovulatory LH surge.

This increase due to pre-ovulatory luteinisation is consistent and can be a useful indicator of ovulation time. Daily estimation is required which is expensive but this may be done rapidly and relatively simply using a plasma/serum progesterone enzyme-linked immunoassay (Ovucheck, Cambridge Life Sciences).

Luteinising hormone

During pro-oestrus there is an increase in the frequency of LH pulse release. A pre-ovulatory surge (which lasts 1—2 days on average) is observed in plasma approximately two days prior to ovulation. The diagnostic value of LH determination is limited by the expense and availability of the assay, and the requirement of serial sampling (at least 4 times daily).

Oestrogen

During proestrus, oestrogen concentrations increase and peak (50—100 pg/ml) 1 to 2 days prior to the pre-ovulatory surge of LH. The levels are thus highest in late pro-oestrus and early oestrus. However, there is considerable variation both within and between bitches and serial sampling similar to LH is required.

CONFIRMING OVULATION

Progesterone — in bitches which fail to conceive, particularly those which have a short interoestrus interval, measurement of plasma progesterone 2 to 3 weeks after the end of oestrus may be helpful in determining whether the bitch had ovulated or not. A progesterone concentration above 1ng/ml probably indicates the presence of corpora lutea although this does not exclude the possibility of follicles luteinising without ovulation.

PREGNANCY DIAGNOSIS

Progesterone — although plasma progesterone concentrations in the second half of pregnancy are higher than in non-pregnant animals, the variation is so large that progesterone estimation is of no value for confirming pregnancy.

Oestrogen — most reports suggest that there is no difference in oestrogen levels between pregnant and non-pregnant animals. However, Richkind (1983) found that three weeks after mating total oestrogens in urine increased in pregnant animals; the use of this for pregnancy diagnosis is to be evaluated.

Acute-phase proteins — at around the thirtieth day of gestation there is an increase in circulating acute-phase proteins. Measurement of these proteins can therefore be used as a potential pregnancy test.

DIAGNOSING OESTROGEN-RESPONSIVE ALOPECIA

Measurement of circulating concentrations of oestrogen, testosterone or progesterone is of no diagnostic value in cases of alopecia.

REFERENCES

CHRISTIANSEN, Ib. J. (1984). *Reproduction in the Dog and Cat.* Bailliere Tindall, London. p. 136.

REED, R. A. and THORNTON, J. R. (1982). Stilboestrol toxicity in a dog. *Aust. Vet. J.* **58** 217.

RICHKIND, M. (1983). Possible use of early morning urine for detection of pregnancy in dogs. *Vet. Med./Small Anim. Clin.* **78**, 1067.

FURTHER READING

ARNOLD, S., HUBLER, M., CASAL, M., FAIRBORN, A., BAUMANN, D., FLUECKIGER, M. and RUESCH, P. Use of low dose prostaglandin for the treatment of canine pyometra. *J. small Anim. Pract. (1988)* **29**, 303.

BURKE, T. J. (1986). *Small Animal Reproduction and Infertility, A Clinical Approach to Diagnosis and Treatment.* Lea and Febiger, Philadelphia.

CHRISTIANSEN, Ib. J. (1984). *Reproduction in the Dog and Cat.* Bailliere Tindall, London.

CHAPTER 8

REPRODUCTIVE ENDOCRINOLOGY OF THE CAT

Tim J. Gruffydd-Jones, B.Vet.Med., Ph.D., M.R.C.V.S.

The number of pet cats in this country has steadily risen over recent years and cats are becoming increasingly important to the veterinary surgeon in practice. There has been a corresponding greater interest in pedigree cats and their breeding and this is likely to lead to an increased demand for the investigation of reproductive problems in cats. However, it is only relatively recently that any data on the endocrinology of the normal reproductive process has become available for cats.

NORMAL REPRODUCTIVE PROCESS

QUEENS

Reproductive patterns in cats are very variable and are influenced both by breed and the system of management.

Puberty

In free-living cats of mixed breeding, the age of puberty is usually around seven months but is probably more closely correlated with body weight than age. The season of birth is also an important factor. Puberty usually occurs early in the spring and therefore queens born late in the previous year will mature at a younger age than those born early in the preceding breeding season.

The age of puberty is much more variable in pedigree cats and the differences are largely breed-dependent. The oriental cats (Siamese, Burmese, Abyssinians, foreign short-hairs) tend to be very precocious and may mature as young as five months of age. In contrast, pedigree long-hairs may not mature until over a year of age.

Breeding season

Free-living and feral cats are seasonally polyoestrous. The period of anoestrus usually begins around October and lasts until the end of the year. The most important factor in controlling the breeding season is daylight length; breeding activity will usually recommence soon after the shortest day of the year. However, the first oestrus cycles may be rather half-hearted and regular cyclical activity may not begin for a month or two.

Provision of 14 hours of lighting a day will abolish the anoestrous period and ensure that breeding activity continues throughout the year. Changing the photoperiod has been shown to alter the circadian pattern of melatonin production. Since most pet cats are housed and exposed to artificial lighting, they may show no period of anoestrus.

Oestrous cycle

Cats are induced ovulators and the conventional nomenclature of the oestrous cycle is not applicable. There is no metoestrous phase and pro-oestrus is not usually recognisable as a distinct phase. Full oestrous behaviour develops remarkably rapidly (within 24 hours) and there are usually no changes in the appearance of the external genitalia apart, perhaps, from an occasional slight mucoid vulval discharge. The reproductive cycle is most appropriately divided into a follicular phase corresponding to follicular growth and activity with oestrogen production and a luteal phase (corresponding to dioestrus) associated with either pregnancy or pseudopregnancy and involving progesterone dominance.

The oestrous cycle lasts around two to three weeks in cats of mixed breeding with an average duration of oestrus of around seven days. However, oestrous cycle patterns are much more variable in pedigree cats. Oriental queens tend to have a shorter oestrous cycle and longer oestrus. The interoestrual period may become progressively shorter with successive cycles if they are left unmated and they may then show a prolonged, almost permanent display of oestrous behaviour. Long-hairs and British short-hairs often cycle less frequently.

The extent of the oestrual display is also very variable. In oriental cats, there may be a marked increase in vocalisation, rubbing, rolling and general activity with frequent presentation of the oestrous posture whereas behavioural changes may be much less marked and easily overlooked in long-hairs.

Endocrine changes in the oestrous cycle have been studied mainly in cats of mixed breeding. These show a remarkably consistent picture of follicular activity as judged by oestrogen concentrations (Table 1). The follicular cycles average around ten days in duration.

Table 1
Follicular phase activity of mixed-breed queens
assessed by daily monitoring of serum oestradiol concentrations
(based on 17 follicular cycles)

Follicular phase duration	9.7 $\pm$ 3.1 days
Interval between follicular phases	5.9 $\pm$ 2.9 days
(A follicular phase was defined as the period of sustained increase in oestradiol concentrations above base line)	

The major oestrogen produced by cats is oestradiol-17β. Concentrations vary between troughs of 60 pmol/l and peaks of 300 pmol/l. These can change dramatically over a short period of time and may double within 24 hours as a new follicular cycle begins. This may explain why oestrous behaviour develops so abruptly in cats.

Follicular activity correlates well with oestrous behaviour in most cats. However, some queens will show extended periods of oestrous behaviour or no oestrous behaviour despite the presence of normal regular follicular cycles.

Mating does not appear to influence the duration of oestrus and cats are unusual in that they may continue to display oestrous behaviour even though ovulation has occurred and significant progesterone secretion has resulted.

Little information is available to indicate whether the breed variations in oestrous cycle patterns are related to differences in patterns of oestrogen secretion. In a limited survey, no significant difference in peak oestradiol concentrations was found comparing follicular cycles in Burmese and mixed breed cats (Gruffydd-Jones, 1982).

Ovulation

Cats are induced ovulators and mating is therefore normally required to trigger ovulation. Receptors within the queen's vagina are stimulated during coitus to cause release of gonadotrophin releasing hormone (GnRH) from the hypothalamus which leads to release of luteinising hormone (LH) from the pituitary. Baseline levels of LH are around 1.3 ng/ml and once a significant increase in these has occurred, ovulation will result. If ovulation fails to occur, there is no, or a hardly discernible, increase in LH concentration. The critical factor is therefore the initial release of LH and not the concentrations achieved. Ovulation is an 'all or none' phenomenon and all ripe follicles will usually ovulate simultaneously. Recent studies have provided some further information on the factors which may influence the initial release of LH. A major determinant is the number of matings and it is clear that in some cases multiple matings are required to ensure release of LH. Multiple matings may facilitate LH secretion by priming either the hypothalamus or pituitary gland. The time course of LH release is relatively short, peak concentrations of up to 40 ng/ml being achieved by about 90 minutes with levels returning to baseline within eight to 24 hours. It is therefore probably important also that the multiple matings take place in quick succession. This is the pattern that is observed in cats allowed to mate at will, with as many as six matings occurring within an hour. Successive matings cause further increments in release of LH although this response is finally exhausted, which suggests that a finite pool of LH exists.

Oestrogens are thought to be important in priming either the hypothalamus or the pituitary gland for LH release and therefore queens may be more responsive to mating later in oestrus once sustained increases in oestrogens have been achieved.

Pregnancy

Progesterone concentrations increase rapidly over baseline values after ovulation to reach a peak of 95 nmol/l after one to four weeks. These concentrations are maintained until around five weeks when a gradual decrease occurs which becomes precipitous, levels returning to baseline in the last few days of pregnancy. The magnitude of the peak of progesterone concentration does not appear to be dependent on the number of corpora lutea. The foetoplacental units take over the role of progesterone production and pregnancy maintenance during the latter stages. Ovariectomy and hence removal of the luteal source of progesterone will cause abortion if performed before day 45, but not after day 50.

Oestradiol also appears to be the major oestrogen produced during pregnancy. Concentrations fall rapidly to baseline soon after ovulation. There may be a slight preparturient increase in oestrogens with a sharp fall just before parturition. A small proportion of queens will display oestrous behaviour during pregnancy but it is not known whether this is associated with any follicular activity.

Relaxin can first be detected after around the first month of pregnancy. Levels fall during the last week and become undetectable again around the time parturition. The placentae appear to be the source of this hormone.

Pseudopregnancy

Pseudopregnancy will inevitably follow matings which successfully induce ovulation but fail to produce viable embryos. The pattern of progesterone production seen during pseudopregnancy is very simiilar to the pattern in pregnancy until around the third week when concentrations begin to fall, reaching baseline around seven weeks. This probably corresponds with the regression of the corpora lutea in a normal pregnancy. Oestrus is usually suppressed during pseudopregnancy leading to a prolonged inter-oestrual interval in comparison with anovulatory cycles, although oestrus will follow shortly after cessation of the pseudopregnancy.

Lactation

Prolactin concentrations increase in the last month of pregnancy and remain high for a further month if lactation is maintained. This will usually suppress oestrous activity which resumes shortly after the kittens are weaned. If the queen is not allowed to suckle her litter, prolactin concentrations fall rapidly to baseline after parturition and post-partum oestrus is seen after seven to ten days.

TOMS

Male cats tend to mature a little later than queens, usually around eight to nine months of age. Very little is known about the normal reproductive physiology of toms. Both serum testosterone and LH concentrations are extremely variable and may range between 0.4—25 nmol/l for testosterone and 2.2—29.2 ng/l of LH. LH release does not appear to be pulsatile in male cats in contrast to male dogs (Goodrowe, Chakraborty and Wildt, 1985).

THE USE OF ENDOCRINE ASSAYS IN THE INVESTIGATION OF REPRODUCTIVE FAILURE

QUEENS

The value of endocrine assays in investigating reproductive function is limited by the difficulty in interpreting the significance of the concentrations found in a single sample. Oestrogen concentrations change dramatically during the oestrous cycle, often more than doubling within 24 hours. Therefore, daily determinations are necessary to investigate follicular function in, for example, a case of apparent failure of oestrus. Although progesterone concentrations do not fluctuate so markedly from day to day during the luteal phase, nevertheless, serial progesterone assays are necessary to assess any possible luteal inadequacy as a cause of reproductive failure.

The one exception when a single estimation is of value is in the assay of progesterone to document whether or not ovulation has occurred. This can be useful both in differentiating between ovulation failure and either fertilisation failure or pre-implantation loss, and in assessing whether anoestrus is due to luteal phase activity. If ovulation has occurred recently, serum progesterone concentrations will be well in excess of 10 nmol/l whilst at other times baseline levels will be considerably below this.

TOMS

The response of the male pituitary-gonadal axis to stimulation with exogenous gonadotrophin releasing hormone (GnRH) has been used to investigate male reproductive function in a number of species. There are no reports of the application of this to the investigation of male cats with reproductive failure although the response of normal cats has been described (Goodowe, Chakraborty and Wildt 1985). LH concentrations peak at 42—136 ng/ml at 30 minutes and testosterone between 9—41 nmol/l at 30—60 minutes after administration of 10 ng of GnRH. The magnitude of the increment of testosterone appears to be approximately inversely proportional to the basal level resulting in less variation in post-stimulation than resting concentrations.

ENDOCRINE FACTORS AS A CAUSE OF REPRODUCTIVE FAILURE

QUEENS

Since serial hormonal estimations are necessary to adequately document endocrine imbalances as a cause of reproductive failure and these are frequently impractical, it is often difficult to verify such a diagnosis — or to disprove it. Although endocrine factors may be involved in some of the earlier stages of the reproductive process, there is little evidence that they are of any importance in pregnancy failure in queens.

Ovarian cysts and parovarian cysts are a frequent finding in cats. However, they are often found in queens with a normal reproductive history and their histological appearance suggests that they are likely to be endocrinologically inactive.

There are three main situations in which endocrine factors may contribute to reproductive failure and in which hormonal treament may be indicated -

1. Failure of oestrus
2. Failure of ovulation
3. Resorption and abortion

Failure of oestrus

Hormonal induction of oestrus using FSH or eCG can be employed in queens with apparent failure of oestrus using the regimes described below although several factors should be considered before embarking on this treatment. Firstly, it is important to ensure that pseudopregnancy-associated luteal activity is not responsible for the anoestrus. Even though the queen may have had no recent contact with an entire tom, contact with other cats may result in ovulation and pseudopregnancy. Neutered toms, even if castrated prepubertally, may mate the queen and induce ovulation. If this occurs early in oestrus it may suppress the full oestrous behavioural display. Receptors similar to those found in the vagina are found in the lumbar area and it is possible that in some particularly receptive queens, simply mounting, which may be performed by other queens maintained in the same group, may provide sufficient stimulation to induce LH release. Demonstration of high serum progesterone concentrations will confirm whether this has occurred.

It is also important to ensure that there is no normal follicular activity. Some queens, particularly if timid and stressed by environmental or social factors, may fail to display oestrous behaviour despite normal follicular activity as discussed earlier. Serial oestrogen determinations or vaginal cytology can be used to eliminate this possibility.

Finally, although the precise underlying cause of failure of oestrus is usually unclear, basic physiological defects may be responsible. Although it may be possible to successfully induce oestrus and breed from an affected queen, the possibility that such a trait may be heritable should be considered with its implications for using such a queen as breeding stock.

Failure of ovulation

Identification of failure of ovulation depends on the demonstration of low serum progesterone concentrations after mating. It is important to ensure that multiple matings have taken place, preferably throughout oestrus to ensure that every opportunity has been provided for natural ovulation to occur. Pharmacological induction of ovulation using the regimes of human chorionic gonadotrophin (hCG) or gonadtrophin releasing hormone (GnRH) described below can be used but the same considerations of the probability of a basic physiological defect and a possible inherited basis, discussed in relation to pharmacological induction for failure of oestrus, should be borne in mind.

Resorption and abortion

Progesterone deficiency is sometimes suggested as a cause for habitual resorption or abortion but no data has been reported to substantiate such a diagnosis. The proposed basis for the progesterone deficiency is premature luteal regression which would therefore be expected to occur before day 50 of pregnancy, before the foetoplacental units are able to assume the role of progesterone production and maintenance of pregnancy.

Demonstration of low progesterone concentrations in serial serum samples would be required to confirm this diagnosis. Despite using such an approach to investigate a number of queens with unexplained habitual resorption in our clinic, little evidence of progesterone deficiency has been found.

TOMS

The causes of reproductive failure in toms are not well understood and there are no reports substantiating specific endocrine factors.

USES OF REPRODUCTIVE HORMONES

INDUCTION OF OESTRUS

A number of methods have been recommended for the pharmacological induction of oestrus in cats and these have been based mainly on the use of equine chorionic gonadotrophin (eCG), follicle stimulating hormone (FSH) and gonadotrophin releasing hormone (GnRH). These drugs are not licensed for use in the United Kingdom. Suggested usage is based on clinical experience or reports from the U.S.A. Oestrogens can be used to induce behavioural oestrus in both entire and oraviectomised queens. This may be useful to check libido in a tom.

Equine chorionic gonadotrophin (eCG). A variety of different regimes employing dosages of 50–1000 I.U. given as single injections — or multiple injections of the lower dosages for up to seven days — have been used to induce oestrus (Wildt, Kinney and Seager, 1978; Cline, Jennings and Sojka, 1980). The dosage regime employed in our clinic is 100 I.U. for two days followed by 50 I.U. for a further three days. The main disadvantage of eCG is that it does not have pure FSH activity. It also has some LH action and this may lead to premature luteinisation of follicles. Another potential disadvantage of eCG is possible immunogenicity in cats.

Follicle stimulating hormone (FSH). Pure FSH (Sigma Chemicals Co.) is preferred to eCG but is less readily available in this country. The recommended dosage of this gonadotrophin is 2.0 mg daily until signs of oestrus are observed but for not more than five days (Wildt *et al.,* 1978). Single, higher dosages of up to 15 mg will induce follicular growth but are less effective in inducing oestrous behaviour.

Gonadotrophin releasing hormone (GnRH). Limited data are available on the efficacy of GnRH administration for inducing oestrus in queens. A regime of twice daily injections of 5 μg for six days and four injections of 10 μg on alternate days induced follicular growth and behavioural oestrus in a proportion of treated cats. Synthetic GnRH is available in the United Kingdom as 'Fertagyl' (Intervet) and 'Receptal' (Hoechst) but is not licensed for use in cats.

There are a number of drawbacks with all these pharmacological strategies for inducing oestrus. Most require multiple injections which may not be practical. However, the major problem is the variability of response. Most treatment regimes will cause overstimulation in a proportion of cases and this may result in cystic follicle development and superovulation. There is clearly considerable variability in response which may partly reflect different stages of the oestrous cycle at the initiation of treatment and partly inherent individual variability. This last factor may be particularly relevant in practice situations as induction of oestrus is most likely to be required in pedigree cats coming from a variety of different environmental backgrounds and managemental regimes whilst the reported dosage schedules have been developed using cats of mixed breeding maintained under controlled laboratory conditions.

Induction of ovulation

In most circumstances, ovulation is induced by natural matings although the need for multiple matings has already been stressed. Exogenous hormones to induce ovulation may be used to facilitate ovulation in queens with a history of ovulation failure and human chorionic gonadotrophin (hCG) and GnRH can be used for this purpose.

hCG. Although lower dosages may be effective in some queens, 500 I.U. is recommended to ensure that ovulation occurs. This can be given i/v or i/m as close to a natural mating as possible. hCG, like eCG, may be immunogenic in cats and may possibly induce antibody formation.

GnRH. GnRH is not as readily available as hCG. A dosage of 25 μg is recommended to ensure that ovulation occurs (Chakraborty, Wildt and Seager, 1979). A lower dosage of 5μg will sometimes induce ovulation but the response is variable and unpredictable.

Oestrus suppression

There are three main indications for the use of pharmacological agents to suppress oestrus in cats:

1. **To delay breeding in queens having precocious puberty**
   Some queens of the oriental breeds such as Siamese and Burmese mature at a very early age, as young as four months and long before they are considered physically mature enough to breed. Oestrus suppression is useful in such queens until they are mature enough to be bred.

2. **Suppression of oestrus *post partum* and during lactation**

   As discussed earlier, lactation will usually suppress oestrus if a queen is suckling a litter of average size and oestrous activity will not normally resume until a short while after weaning. However, oestrus is often seen during lactation in queens suckling only one or two kittens and occasionally in queens suckling larger litters. Lactation places considerable demands on a queen and it is inadvisable to allow her to breed again until she has regained some bodily condition. Oestrus suppression is therefore useful in this situation.

3. **For planned litters**

   There are many reasons of convenience why owners may elect to postpone oestrus in a queen — for example, to stagger litters from queens in a breeding colony throughout the year, or to fit in with exhibiting the queen at shows and around holiday times.

Some queens, especially of the oriental breeds, may have a particularly prominent display of oestrous behaviour. Not only may the resulting constant vocalisation and attempts to solicit the attention of a tom be socially unacceptable but the queen may also become inappetent during oestrus, rapidly losing bodily condition. Queens with particularly prominent oestrual display frequently show longer periods of oestrus with an interoestrual interval which becomes progressively shorter with successive oestrous cycles until an extended continual oestrual display results. Breeders occasionally experience difficulties in breeding from such individuals, probably because of the difficulty in coordinating mating with periods of follicular activity when the follicles are capable of ovulation, and therefore it may be preferable to avoid leaving such queens unmated for more than one or two oestrous cycles.

Progestagens are not suitable for indefinite, long-term oestrus suppression in queens that are not intended for future breeding. They do not represent an acceptable alternative to surgical ovario-hysterectomy.

A variety of pharmacological agents may be used to suppress oestrus, most of which are progestagenic drugs. These are available as depot injectable forms with a prolonged duration of activity which avoids the need for frequent tablet administration, and oral preparations which have the advantage of greater flexibility of usage should the need to withdraw the drug arise.

Any progestagenic drug carries a slight risk of predisposing to chronic endometritis since the uterus is more susceptible to infection by opportunist organisms when under progesterone dominance. Although this risk is small, their use should be avoided in queens with any history suggestive of endometritis, such as the presence of a vaginal discharge or unexplained reproductive failure. These drugs may also induce a variety of progesterone-dependent changes such as an increased appetite; weight gain with fat redistribution and fluid retention; behavioural changes, usually shown as reduced activity. These side-effects may be considered unacceptable by some owners. Other more serious complications may arise with long-term usage and these are described below.

Megestrol acetate. This oral preparation is the most widely used preparation in the United Kingdom. The manufacturers recommend two dosage regimes: 2.5 mg given twice weekly will prevent oestrus indefinitely or 2.5 mg can be given on three consecutive days as soon as signs of oestrus are observed to postpone a single oestrous period. The latter regime is seldom employed since postponement of a single oestrus is rarely required and oestrous behaviour usually develops very abruptly without any distinctive prooestrous phase. In practice, breeders frequently find that prolonged prevention can be achieved using considerably lower dosages than those recommended. The minimum effective dose can be determined by experimentation in individual queens and this may be as low as 0.6 mg once or twice weekly. The lowest possible dose is preferable as it minimises the risk of side effects.

Proligesterone. Proligesterone is available as a depot injection of aqueous suspension. It is given at a dosage of 100 mg and this will have a duration of action of around six to seven months. Repeated injections every five months will prevent oestrus indefinitely. Discolouration of the overlying fur may occasionally occur at the site of injection and for this reason it is recommended that show queens should be injected in the groin area.

Medroxyprogesterone acetate. Medroxyprogesterone acetate is available both in tablet form (Perlutex, Leo) and as a depot injection in oil (Perlutex, Leo; Promone E, Upjohn). This preparation is not licensed for use in cats in the United Kingdom but is sometimes used.

Other agents. Some other drugs have been used for suppressing oestrus in cats but are not widely used in the United Kingdom. For example, mibolerone, an androgenic steroid, has been used in the U.S.A.

Misalliance

There is no treatment that has been adequately assessed both for efficacy and safety in treating misalliance in cats. If the queen is not required for future breeding, ovariohysterectomy early in pregnancy is, therefore, the preferred course of action.

Oestrogens will interfere with oviductal transport of the eggs and oestradiol cyprionate given as a single intramuscular dose of 0.25 mg, 40 hours after mating will block oviductal transport (Herron & Sis, 1974). However, this may prolong the period of oestrus and in some cases may predispose to subsequent development of endometritis. Oestradiol benzoate is the only readily available injectable oestrogen in the United Kingdom but it is not licensed for this purpose in cats.

Progestagens There is limited evidence that megestrol acetate given at a dosage of 2.5 mg/kg up to 12 hours after mating will prevent pregnancy (Skerritt, 1978) but its use for this purpose has not been satisfactorily evaluated.

Prostaglandins can be used as abortifacient agents. However, this is mediated through an ecbolic effect and prostaglandins are not effective until the later stages of pregnancy.

In view of inadequate evaluation, it is advisable to avoid the use of hormones for treating misalliance in queens required for future breeding.

Induction of abortion

Prostaglandins produce only a short lived suppression of progesterone production and appear to have either no effect on luteal life span or possibly cause slight prolongation (Shille & Stabenfeldt, 1979). Administration late in pregnancy will induce abortion and this action is potentiated by corticosteroids. This results from stimulation of uterine contractions rather than from any luteolytic action.

Treatment of endometritis

Prostaglandin $F_2\alpha$ has also been used as an adjunct in the treatment of the endometritis-pyometritis complex given at a dosage of 0.2—1.0 mg/kg (Arnbjerg & Flagstad, 1985; Henderson, 1984; Johnson & Wasserfall, 1982). This ecbolic effect is particularly beneficial in acute cases in expelling the uterine exudate. Some treated cats may breed again but if the endometrial changes are severe, these are likely to be irreversible. Synthetic forms of prostaglandin $F_2\alpha$ ('Estrumate', Coopers; 'Lutalyse', Upjohn; 'Prosolvin', Intervet) are available in the U.K. but are not licensed for this purpose in cats.

TOMS

There are no reports of the use of reproductive hormones for the treatment of infertility in toms.

Testosterone has been used for treatment of so-called 'feline symmetric alopecia' but there are no conditions in cats in which a deficiency of this hormone has been demonstrated nor has any beneficial effect of testosterone been documented in controlled trials. A side effect of testosterone administration may be the development of spraying behaviour together with other male secondary sex characteristics. Since spraying is such a socially unacceptable behaviour which may persist as a learned behaviour despite cessation of testosterone treatment, sometimes leading to a request for euthanasia, it is questionable whether it should ever be used in cats.

MISCELLANEOUS USES OF PROGESTAGENS

In addition to their use for oestrus suppression, progestagens are now employed for a wide range of conditions in cats. These conditions include behavioural problems such as spraying and aggression, chronic gingivitis, idiopathic epilepsy, eosinophilic granulomas and skin conditions, most notably miliary eczema. Their usage is based on clinical experience although, for many of these conditions, no controlled trials have been conducted to confirm any beneficial effect. The mode of action of progestagens in these conditions is not known. They can clearly have potent behaviour modifying effects and it is suggested that this may be due to a direct central action (Middleton, 1986). An anti-inflammatory effect may also be important in some conditions and megestrol acetate has been shown to cause adrenocortical suppression in cats (Chastain, Graham & Nichols, 1981).

Adverse effects of progestagens

Recently, a greater appreciation has arisen of some of the potential side effects of progestagens, summarised in Table 2, which has led to caution in their usage. There is evidence of some variation depending on the individual progestagen used (Watson et al., 1989). The behavioural effects of increased appetite, weight gain and lethargy may be particularly marked in some individuals and may be unacceptable to the owner. In extreme cases the cat may develop a pot bellied, almost Cushingoid, appearance with truncal hair loss. Some cats may also show a heavy moult leading to alopecia following withdrawal of progestagens after long-term usage. There is also evidence of prolonged adrenocortical suppression which may lead to inability to respond to stress.

Table 2
Some side effects reported with the use of progestagens in cats

Weight gain

Lethargy

Alopoecia

Uterine infections

Adrenal suppression

Diabetes mellitus

Mammary hyperplasia

A small proportion of cats receiving long-term treatment develop mammary hypertrophy (Hinton & Gaskell, 1977). This condition may affect all or just one or two of the mammary glands which appear grossly enlarged due to fibrous hyperplasia and glandular proliferation. Affected cats are usually otherwise well although in extreme cases there may be marked oedema of the mammae and the overlying skin may become ulcerated. The condition will usually regress if the progestagen is withdrawn.

The most serious effect which has been reported is development of diabetes mellitus (Moise & Reimers, 1983). Induction of growth hormone secretion and development of insulin resistance due to a direct effect of the progestagens or an indirect insulin insensitivity resulting from obesity induced by the progestagens are possible mechanisms in the development of impaired glucose homeostasis. This problem can develop after only a short course of progestagens and in some cases may persist despite withdrawal of the drug. In view of these side effects, progestagens should be used with care and alternative drugs should be considered where appropriate.

REFERENCES

ARNBJERG, J. and FLAGSTAD, A. (1985). Protaglandin $F_2\alpha$ treatment of feline open pyometra. *Nor. Vet. Med.* **37**, 286.

CHAKRABORTY, P. K., WILDT, D. E. and SEAGER, S. W. J. (1979). Serum luteinizing hormone and ovulatory response to luteinizing hormone-releasing hormone in the estrous and anestrous domestic cat. *Lab. Anim. Sci.* **29**, 338.

CHASTAIN, C. B., GRAHAM, C. L. and NICHOLS, C. E. (1981). Adrenocortical suppression in cats given megestrol acetate. *Am. J. vet. Res.* **42**, 2029.

CLINE, E. M., JENNINGS, L. L. and SOJKA, N. J. (1980). Breeding laboratory cats during artificially induced oestrus. *Lab Anim. Sci.* **30**, 1003.

GOODROWE, K. L., CHAKRABORTY, P. K. and WILDT, D. E. (1985). Pituitary and gonadal response to exogenous LH-releasing hormone in the male domestic cat. *J. Endocr.* **105**, 175.

GRUFFYDD-JONES, T. J. (1982). Ph.D. Thesis, University of Bristol.

HENDERSON, R. T. (1984). Prostaglandin therapeutics in the bitch and queen. *Aust. Vet. J.* **61**, 317.

HERRON, M. A. and SIS, R. F. (1974). Ovum transport in the cat and the effect of estrogen administration. *Am. J. vet. Res.* **35**, 1277.

HINTON, M. and GASKELL, C. J. (1977). Non-neoplastic mammary hypertrophy in the cat associated either with pregnancy or with oral progestagen therapy. *Vet. Rec.* **100**, 277.

JOHNSON, C. A. and WASSERFALL, J. L. (1983). Prostaglandin therapy in feline pyometra. *J. Am. Anim. Hosp. Ass.* **20**, 247.

MIDDLETON, D. J. (1986). Megestrol acetate and the cat. *Vet. Annual* **26**, 341.

MOISE, N. S. and REIMERS, T. J. (1973). Insulin therapy in cats with diabetes mellitus. *J. Am. vet. med. Ass.* **182**, 158.

SHILLE, V. M. and STABENFELDT, G. H. (1979). Luteal function in the domestic cat during pseudopregnancy and after treatment with prostaglandin F_2. *Biol. Reprod.* **21**, 1217.

SKERRITT, G. C. (1978). Treatment of feline misalliance. *Vet. Rec.* **103**, 543.

WATSON, A. D. J., CHURCH, D. B., EMSLIE, D. R. and MIDDLETON, D. J. (1989). Comparative effects of proligesterone and megestrol acetate on basal plasma glucose concentrations and cortisol responses to exogenous adrenocorticotrophic hormone in cats. *Res. Vet. Sci.* **47**, 374.

WILDT, D. E., KINNEY, G. M. and SEAGER, S. W. J. (1978). Gonadotrophin induced reproductive cyclicity in the domestic cat. *Lab. Anim. Sci.* **28**, 301.

Part Two

DIFFERENTIAL DIAGNOSIS OF PRESENTING SYMPTOMS

CHAPTER 9

DIFFERENTIAL DIAGNOSIS OF POLYURIA AND POLYDIPSIA

John K. Dunn, B.V.M.& S., M.A., M.Vet.Sci., M.R.C.V.S.

Polyuria signifies the formation and excretion of large volumes of urine, usually of low specific gravity. In dogs, volumes in excess of 50 mls/kg/24 hrs constitute polyuria. *Polydipsia* can be defined as increased thirst which is manifested as an increased fluid intake (greater than 100mls/kg/24 hrs in the dog). Compensatory polydipsia is caused by an obligatory polyuria; less frequently the polydipsia is primary and compensatory polyuria occurs in response to the excess water load.

Two mechanisms are responsible for balancing water loss with water intake:

1. the thirst mechanism
2. renal concentrating mechanisms

Under normal circumstances renal concentrating defects which result in polyuria initiate compensatory changes in the thirst mechanism (polydipsia) and vice versa. Hence, polyuria is usually accompanied by compensatory polydipsia which effectively maintains the volume of total body fluids within normal limits. Simultaneous defects in both the thirst and renal concentrating mechanisms may result in two possible outcomes:

1. Polyuria without a compensatory polydipsia i.e. volume depletion of both extracellular and intracellular fluid compartments resulting in hypernatraemia, hypovolaemia and cellular dehydration.

2. Polydipsia without a compensatory polyuria i.e. cellular overhydration with resultant severe consequences on cerebral and pulmonary function.

Water balance is closely related to the osmolality of the extracellular fluid (ECF) and therefore also to sodium regulation since the osmolality of the ECF is almost entirely determined by the concentration of sodium ions (see Figure 1, page 166).

The term polyuria should not be confused with *pollakiuria* (increased frequency of urination) or *nocturia* (a desire to urinate at night). Although polyuria is frequently accompanied by pollakiuria and nocturia the converse is not always the case i.e. pollakiuria and nocturia are not necessarily indicative of polyuria and may be caused by numerous inflammatory, neoplastic or functional disorders of the lower urinary tract which compromise the normal function or filling capacity of the bladder (e.g. cystitis, cystic or urethral calculi, or bladder neoplasia).

Normal water balance

Water may be taken into the body by drinking or in food. It is also produced in the body during the oxidation of carbohydrate, fat and protein.

Water is lost from the body in faeces, urine and by evaporation from the skin and respiratory tract. The balance between water input and output is so precise that daily fluctuations in body weight are less than 1% (O'Connor and Potts, 1988).

The amount of water lost in faeces in the normal animal is unimportant compared to the volumes lost in the urine and by evaporation. An obligatory loss of urine is necessary for the excretion of the end products of dietary protein metabolism. Adjustments to the rate of release of antidiuretic hormone (ADH) from the neurohypophysis ensure that the urine is not only maximally concentrated but that the volume is the minimum required for solute excretion (urea, sulphate and phosphate ions). Post-prandial drinking together with the water contained in food provides sufficient fluid to match the obligatory urine loss. Water derived from food is particularly important in cats.

Evaporative losses occur at a basal rate in the resting animal but increase significantly during periods of activity associated with panting and barking. The volume of water drunk during periods of high activity immediately matches the evaporative losses and prevents dehydration.

A healthy dog drinks an average of 50—60 mls/kg/24 hrs depending on the water content of the diet. Normal urine output varies between 20—40 mls/kg/24 hrs.

Thirst mechanism

Thirst is the conscious desire for water and is regulated by centres in the hypothalamus.. The neurones of the thirst centre respond to increases in ECF osmolality and decreases in effective blood volume. A 2% increase in ECF osmolality is sufficient to stimulate thirst via osmoreceptors in the hypothalamus. An 8—10% reduction in blood volume also stimulates the thirst centre via input from volume and pressure receptors in the left atrium and major vessels (carotid sinus and aortic arch).

Renal concentrating mechanisms

1. Secretion of ADH

ADH or vasopressin is synthesised by the supraoptic and paraventricular nuclei of the hypothalamus, which are located near the neurones of the thirst centre, and is stored in nerve endings in the neurohypophysis (posterior pituitary). ADH acts on the cells of the distal tubules and collecting ducts via a specific receptor mechanism. The major stimuli for ADH release are:
a.   plasma hypertonicity
b.   hypovolaemia
In response to ADH, water is reabsorbed along concentration gradients established in the renal medulla by the countercurrent multiplier system involving the loop of Henle and vasa recta. High levels of sodium chloride and urea within the medullary interstitium preserve this concentration gradient thereby maximising the antidiuretic effect of the hormone.

In summary, the ability of the kidney to concentrate urine depends on three factors:
a.   The amount of circulating ADH
b.   The responsiveness of the distal tubules and collecting ducts to ADH
c.   The degree of hypertonicity of the renal medulla

2. Renal tubular function

Glomerular filtrate is isosthenuric i.e. it has a specific gravity equal to that of plasma (1.008—1.012). Approximately 70% of the filtered sodium load is actively reabsorbed in the proximal tubule by a process which is dependent on the activity of the sodium/potassium ATPase pump in the tubular epithelial cells. The continuous reabsorption of sodium and other solutes such as glucose, amino acids, potassium, chloride and bicarbonate, sets up osmotic gradients for the passive reabsorption of water.

As much as 25% of sodium is reabsorbed with chloride from the thick ascending limb of the loop of Henle which contributes significantly to the maintenance of renal medullary hypertonicity. Since this part of the nephron is impermeable to water, the glomerular filtrate is actively diluted and on entering the distal tubule is hypotonic to plasma. The reabsorption of sodium from the loop of Henle can be blocked by 'loop' diuretics such as frusemide.

In the distal tubule, sodium (less than 10% of the filtered load) and water are reabsorbed while potassium is actively secreted into the tubular lumen, a process which is enhanced by aldosterone (see below). In the presence of ADH, water is reabsorbed with urea from some distal tubule segments and the collecting ducts which results in the production of a concentrated urine.

Table 1
Polyuria and polydipsia

History check list

Consider breed, age and sex; sexually intact or neutered?

Quantify water intake (mls/kg/24 hours)

Urination:
　Abnormal volume, colour and smell of urine?
　Nocturia?
　Incontinent?
　Frequency?
　Dysuria?

Diet:
　Dry or moist?
　Recent changes?

Appetite:

Normal or polyphagic?	— psychogenic polydipsia
	— diabetes insipidus
	— diabetes mellitus
	— hyperadrenocorticism
	— hyperthyroidism
Inappetent or anorexic?	— pyometra
	— chronic renal insufficiency
	— liver disease
	— diabetes mellitus (ketoacidosis)
	— hypoadrenocorticism
	— hypercalcaemia

General Health
　Weight loss?
　Lethargic or depressed?
　Vomiting or diarrhoea?
　　　　— toxaemia eg
　　　　　endotoxaemia (pyometra)
　　　　　uraemia (chronic renal failure)
　　　　　ketoacidosis (diabetes mellitus)
　　　　— liver disease
　　　　— hypoadrenocorticism
　　　　— hypercalcaemia

Behavioural abnormalities or CNS signs?
　　　　— hepatic encephalopathy
　　　　— expanding pituitary neoplasm

Exercise intolerance
　　　　— hyperadrenocorticism

Reproductive history
　Recent oestrus?
　Vaginal discharge?
　Recent administration of oestrogens?
　Loss of libido?

Environmental changes?
　　　　— psychogenic polydipsia

Trauma?
　　　　— acquired diabetes mellitus

Recent or current drug administration?
　Frusemide
　Mannitol
　Dextrose
　Intravenous fluids
　Anticonvulsant drugs
　　(phenytoin, primidone or phenobartitol)
　Glucocorticoids

Clinical examination check list

Weigh

Assess hydration status

Abdomen:

Kidneys enlarged and/or painful?	— glomerulonephritis
	— renal lymphosarcoma
	— pyelonephritis
Kidneys small and mis-shapen?	— chronic interstitial nephritis
	-- congenital renal hypoplasia
Liver enlarged?	— diabetes mellitus
	— hyperadrenocorticism
	— chronic active hepatitis
	— feline lymphocytic cholangiohepatitis
	— hepatic neoplasia
Uterus distended?	— pyometra (closed-cervix)
Pendulous abdomen?	— hyperadrenocorticism

Peripheral lymphadenopathy?
　　　　— multicentric lymphosarcoma
　　　　　(check for hypercalcaemia)

Palpable thyroid mass?
　　　　— hyperthyroidism
　　　　　(functional benign thyroid
　　　　　adenoma or less frequently
　　　　　thyroid carcinoma)

External genitalia

Vaginal discharge?	— open-cervix pyometra
Testicular atrophy?	— hyperadrenocorticism
Cataract formation?	— diabetes mellitus

Skin

Endocrine alopecia?	
Thin, non-elastic skin?	— hyperadrenocorticism
Comedone formation?	
Pendulous abdomen?	

Heart

Bradycardia?	— hypoadrenocorticism
	— hypercalcaemia

3. Aldosterone

Aldosterone is a steroid hormone produced by the zona glomerulosa of the adrenal cortex. Aldosterone acts on the cells of the distal convoluted tubule where it promotes the reabsorption of sodium and excretion of potassium and hydrogen ions. The secretion of aldosterone is influenced by the circulating levels of potassium and sodium. Increased potassium concentrations increase aldosterone secretion via a direct effect of potassium on the adrenal cortex. Alterations in serum sodium concentration affect aldosterone release via the renin-angiotensin system which can be summarised as follows:

a.　Sodium depletion causes a reduction in circulating blood volume which diminishes renal perfusion. Reduced renal perfusion is detected by specialised myoepithelial cells of the juxtaglomerular apparatus which secrete the proteolytic enzyme renin. Conditions which decrease ECF volume and/or decrease arterial blood pressure such as dehydration, shock, haemorrhage or congestive heart failure, also stimulate the release of renin into the systemic circulation.

b.　Renin cleaves angiotensin I from angiotensinogen, a plasma alpha-2 globulin produced in the liver.

c.　Angiotensin converting enzyme (ACE) converts angiotensin I to angiotensin II. The latter is a powerful vasoconstrictor which increases peripheral vascular resistance. Angiotensin II has a direct negative feedback effect on renin and stimulates the release of aldosterone from the adrenal cortex thereby restoring the ECF volume deficit and increasing arterial blood pressure (Figure 1). Interestingly, in dogs with congestive heart failure, the renin-angiotensin system is activated as a compensatory mechanism. However, the high levels of aldosterone that are present in many dogs with congestive heart failure are detrimental since they exacerbate the clinical signs associated with congestion and oedema by causing further retention of sodium and water. Activation of the renin-angiotensin system may also explain why many dogs with congestive heart failure, particularly those in the early stages of decompensation, are polydipsic since angiotensin has a direct dipsogenic effect on the thirst centre. Aldosterone antagonists such as spironolactone especially if used in conjunction with the more conventional thiazide or loop diuretics may prove beneficial in such cases.

4. Natiuretic factors (factors which promote the urinary excretion of sodium).

Natiuretic factors or hormones have recently been discovered which may influence sodium balance in the short term. In particular an atrial natiuretic hormone produced in response to volume overload has been identified, which, in addition to promoting the urinary excretion of sodium, also has hypotensive effects.

DIAGNOSTIC APPROACH TO POLYURIA AND POLYDIPSIA

HISTORY

An accurate history is essential if unnecessary laboratory tests and expense are to be avoided. Polydipsia should be quantified at an early stage of the diagnostic investigation and consideration should be given to the general health of the patient, diet, environmental factors, reproductive history and recent or current drug administration. These aspects are summarised in Table 1.

Primary versus secondary polydipsia

Primary polydipsia is a relatively uncommon disorder but has been reported in the dog. It is characterised by a marked increase in water intake which cannot be explained as a compensatory mechanism for excessive fluid loss. Water consumption exceeds the body's demand and results in a compensatory polyuria. Specific causes of primary polydipsia include psychogenic polydipsia (compulsive water drinking) and central nervous system lesions.

More frequently polydipsia is a secondary compensatory response to an obligatory polyuria. Although an observant owner may notice an increase in drinking, it is often the polyuria that provides the initial stimulus for veterinary consultation, particularly if the animal is unable to retain large volumes of urine overnight (see next section).

A more variable increase in water intake occurs in response to dehydration or hypovolaemia i.e. high environmental temperatures, excessive exercise, acute haemorrhage, lactation, vomiting or diarrhoea, dyspnoea or prolonged hyperventilation, and severe or extensive burns.

Urinary incontinence versus nocturia

Nocturia must, in the first instance, be differentiated from urinary incontinence. Typically, oestrogen-responsive incontinence or incontinence associated with sphincter mechanism incompetence is characterised by the leakage of urine when the dog is either lying down resting or sleeping ('bed-wetting'). The problem is most frequently observed in overweight, middle-aged spayed bitches. A higher incidence has been reported in medium and large breed dogs (Holt, 1985). It is also worth noting that nocturia and urinary incontinence may be initiated or exacerbated in any dog that is concomitantly polyuric.

Breed, age and sex

Some polyuric/polydipsic disorders are more common in certain breeds of dog. Poodles are predisposed to hyperadrenocorticism (Cushing's disease) and diabetes mellitus; Dobermann pinschers to hepatic disease and Lhasa apsos and shih tzus to familial renal dysplasia. Pyometra is more common in middle-aged (8—10 year old) bitches and *the three major differential diagnoses for polydipsia and polyuria in the elderly cat are chronic renal insufficiency, diabetes mellitus and hyperthyroidism.* Psychogenic polydipsia, although a relatively rare condition, is more common in large breed dogs. Affected animals are often highly excitable or nervous but appear otherwise healthy.

Verify and quantify the polydipsia

In most cases this can be performed simply by the owner measuring the daily water intake at home. However, an *accurate* estimate may be difficult, if not impossible, to obtain in the severely polydipsic animal which persists in drinking from puddles, toilets, or which drinks its own urine. Similar difficulties may be encountered in multipet households and in many cases hospitalisation is necessary to obtain a more accurate assessment of the animal's water intake.

Animals with diabetes insipidus or psychogenic polydipsia are usually *severely* polydipsic i.e. there may be a four to sixfold increase in water consumption. Not infrequently hospitalisation alone may significantly reduce the water intake in dogs with psychogenic polydipsia, presumably by removing or altering the precipitating emotional or stress factor.

Appetite and diet

The nature and composition of the diet should be taken into account when assessing water intake. Animals fed a complete dry diet invariably drink more water than do those fed a semi-moist or moist diet.

Many systemic disease conditions which are associated with polydipsia also affect appetite. Disease states which increase or diminish appetite are summarised in Table 1.

General health

Many of the diseases associated with polydipsia produce other systemic clinical signs. Some of these signs such as anorexia, lethargy, depression and weight loss are non-specific and are of limited diagnostic value. Other signs which are more informative relate directly to the underlying disease process responsible for the polydipsia and polyuria.

Vomiting, with or without diarrhoea, is a feature of pyometra (endotoxaemia), chronic renal insufficiency (uraemia), hepatic failure, hypoadrenocorticism, hypercalcaemia and diabetes mellitus (ketoacidosis).

Hepatic encephalopathy (congenital portosystemic shunts or acquired chronic liver disease) and expanding pituitary neoplasms (pituitary-mediated Cushing's disease) may result in a variety of behavioural abnormalities and CNS signs (ataxia, apparent blindness, seizures, stupor and aimless wandering).

Dogs with hyperadrenocorticism become exercise intolerant due to progressive muscle weakness.

Reproductive history

Although pyometra is typically a disorder of middle-aged bitches, open or closed-cervix pyometra may occur in younger animals following the administration of oestrogens for misalliance. The clinical signs appear during or immediately after the dioestrous phase of the oestrus cycle. Open-cervix pyometra is characterised by a purulent and/or sanguinous, vaginal discharge which is usually first noted 4—8 weeks post-oestrus.

Hyperadrenocorticism is frequently associated with prolonged anoestrus and, in the male, the excessive secretion of cortisol results in testicular atrophy which, in the stud dog, may be manifested as a loss of libido.

Environmental changes/trauma

Occasionally, in dogs with psychogenic polydipsia, it is possible to identify a precipitating stress factor in the form of a sudden change in the animal's environment (e.g. moving house, new baby etc.) which precedes the onset of the polydipsia. Secondary central diabetes insipidus has been reported in dogs and cats following trauma to the head and disruption of the pituitary stalk.

Recent or current drug administration

Numerous drugs are capable of causing marked polyuria and polydipsia and can therefore influence and modify urine specific gravity and urine output. Polydipsia can occur secondary to an obligatory solute diuresis (e.g. following the administration of frusemide, dextrose, mannitol or intravenous crystalloid solutions) or as a result of interference either with the release of ADH from the pituitary or the action of ADH on the renal tubules (glucocorticoids and anticonvulsant drugs such as phenytoin, primidone and phenobarbitol).

CLINICAL EXAMINATION

The nature of any clinical abnormalities is dependent on the underlying aetiology for the polydipsia or polyuria. Very few, if any, clinical abnormalities will be detected in dogs with *diabetes insipidus* or *psychogenic polydipsia*.

A thorough clinical examination should include a careful and systematic palpation of the abdomen, peripheral lymph nodes and external genitalia. Skin elasticity ('tenting') provides only a rough assessment of an animal's hydration status and is unreliable in the very obese or emaciated patient or those suffering from hyperadrenocorticism. *Canine hyperadrenocorticism* is characterised by bilaterally symmetrical alopecia, thin, non-elastic skin, comedone formation and a pendulous abdomen.

During abdominal palpation particular attention should be paid to the size and shape of the kidneys and the size of the liver. If closed-cervix *pyometra* is suspected, palpation of the abdomen should be performed with care to avoid perforating the distended uterine wall.

The neck should be palpated for evidence of a thyroid mass *(hyperthyroidism)* and the eyes should be examined for cataract formation *(diabetes mellitus)*. These aspects are summarised in Table 1.

LABORATORY TESTS

Routine haematology, biochemical screening and urine analysis are essential components of the initial diagnostic plan. A complete biochemical profile should include glucose, urea, creatinine, sodium, potassium, chloride, calcium, phosphate, alanine aminotransferase (ALT), alkaline phosphatase (ALP), and gamma-glutamyl transferase (γ-GT) determinations. Such a profile provides a cost effective means of identifying or ruling out some of the more obscure electrolyte abnormalities associated with polydipsia and polyuria e.g. the hyponatraemia and hyperkalaemia typical of Addison's disease.

Urine analysis

Urine specific gravity (S.G.) depends on molecular size and weight as well as the total number of solute molecules. An approximate relationship exists between S.G. and the total concentration of urinary solute. Typical values for urine S.G. range from 1.015—1.045 in the dog and 1.035—1.060 in the cat.

Osmolality represents the concentration of osmotically active particles in solution and is expressed in mOsm/kg. Osmolality is directly related to osmotic pressure and is not influenced by molecular weights or particle size. Normal values for urine S.G. and plasma and urine osmolality are given in Table 2.

Table 2
Urine specific gravity (S.G.), urine and plasma osmolality : normal values* in the dog and cat.

	Urine S.G. (typical)	Urine S.G. (extremes)	Urine Osmolality (mOsm/kg)	Plasma Osmolality (mOsm/kg)
Dog	1.015—1.045	1.001—1.065	500—1400	275—305
Cat	1.035—1.060	1.001—1.080	1250—2100	275—305

*normal values vary with the state of hydration

A patient can be classified into one of four categories on the basis of urine S.G.:

1. Hyposthenuric (S.G. 1.001—1.007) urine more dilute than plasma
2. Isosthenuric (S.G. 1.008—1.012) urine with a similar concentration to plasma i.e. 'fixed range' urine typical of end-stage renal failure.
3. Range of minimal urine concentration (S.G. 1.013—1.029)
4. Hypersthenuric (S.G. >1.030) urine more concentrated than plasma.

The production of persistently dilute solute-free urine with a S.G. less than 1.007, although suggestive of a deficiency of, or a lack of responsiveness to ADH, does not indicate abnormal tubular function since urine is *actively* diluted in the ascending limb (diluting segment) of the loop of Henle.

In addition to S.G., urine should be routinely examined for protein, blood, bilirubin and urobilinogen; spun sediment should be examined for the presence of white and red blood cells, bacteria, casts and crystals.

Pathophysiological classification of polyuric/polydipsic conditions

Water diuresis may be associated with:

1. Impaired secretion of ADH
2. Impaired action of ADH
3. Excessive water intake e.g. primary or psychogenic polydipsia

The net result is the production of a large volume of dilute solute-free urine.

Solute diuresis

A large amount of solute, e.g. glucose, urea or sodium, in the glomerular filtrate overwhelms the reabsorptive capacity of the proximal tubular epithelial cells and results in the obligatory excretion of water.

Medullary washout

Renal medullary hypertonicity is required for ADH to exert its maximal antidiuretic action. The cortical medullary osmotic gradient is maintained by the efflux of high levels of sodium chloride and urea from the loop of Henle and collecting ducts. Loss of this osmotic gradient results in submaximal concentration of urine even in the presence of adequate amounts of ADH.

Certain diseases produce polyuria by decreasing these renal medullary osmotic gradients:

1. Hypoadrenocorticism (sodium depletion)
2. Liver disorders (reduced hepatic conversion of ammonia to urea)
3. Low protein diet (decreased production of urea)

4. Pyelonephritis (decreased reabsorption of urea and water from the collecting ducts)
5. Primary or psychogenic polydipsia (prolonged ingestion of large volumes of water may result in sodium and urea depletion of the medullary interstitium and hence an inability to concentrate urine despite maximal levels of ADH).

In many cases the cause of the polyuria and polydipsia is multifactorial. For example, the polyuria/polydipsia associated with liver disease may be partly due to medullary washout and partly to other mechanisms (decreased renin catabolism, reduced metabolism of glucocorticoids or interference with the action of ADH). The polyuria associated with primary polydipsia may be due partly to medullary washout and partly to overhydration resulting in a relative lack of ADH. In some disorders the mechanism for polyuria/polydipsia has not been established. The proposed pathophysiological mechanisms for the numerous endocrine and non-endocrine disorders which cause polyuria and polydipsia are summarised in Tables 3 and 4.

INVESTIGATION OF PERSISTENT HYPOSTHENURIA (DILUTE URINE)

Persistent hyposthenuria may be caused by:
1. A partial or complete lack of ADH (central diabetes insipidus). Partial deficiency may result in the production of urine in the isosthenuric range.
2. Disease affecting the distal tubules or collecting ducts resulting in an interference in the action of ADH (nephrogenic diabetes insipidus)
3. Excessive water intake e.g. primary or psychogenic polydipsia.

DIAGNOSTIC INVESTIGATIONS
1. A water deprivation test
2. A modified or partial water deprivation test
3. Response to exogenous ADH test (vasopressin)
4. Intravenous administration of hypertonic saline (the Hickey-Hare test).

A. Water deprivation test
1. 12 hour fast
2. Catheterise and empty bladder
3. Check urine specific gravity
4. Record body weight
5. ± Record urine and plasma osmolalities, packed cell volume, total plasma protein, blood urea
6. Withold all water
7. Catheterise bladder every one or two hours and record parameters 3, 4 and 5

The test is discontinued when the animal has lost 5% of its body weight or the urine specific gravity exceeds 1.030. Values between 1.020 and 1.030 indicate submaximal concentration and should be regarded as equivocal. Failure to concentrate above 1.010 is highly suggestive of diabetes insipidus. Equivocal results may be obtained in animals with a partial deficiency of ADH or when primary polydipsia is complicated by a loss of the renal medullary concentration gradients.

B. A modified or partial water deprivation test

A modified or partial water deprivation test is indicated when medullary washout is suspected i.e. when equivocal results are obtained using the standard water deprivation test or following the injection of ADH (see below). The modified test involves a gradual reduction (5—10% per day) in daily water intake over a three day period. Daily water intake should not exceed 100mls/kg. Hydration status and urine S.G. are monitored daily. Failure to concentrate urine during the procedure suggests that medullary washout was not the cause of polyuria. The test is, therefore, useful in differentiating nephrogenic diabetes insipidus from primary polydipsia associated with renal medullary washout. *Both forms of water deprivation are contraindicated in animals which are azotaemic, hypercalcaemic, or dehydrated.*

C. ADH (Vasopressin) response test

An ADH response test is indicated in all animals which fail to concentrate urine in response to water deprivation. *A positive response to ADH is not significant unless it has been demonstrated that the animal cannot concentrate its urine in response to water deprivation.* ADH can be administered immediately following the standard water deprivation test as follows:

1. Catheterise and empty bladder; check urine S.G.

2. Inject desmopressin (DDAVP, Ferring)
    $2.0\mu g$ intramuscularly for dogs <15kg (and cats)
    $4.0\mu g$ intramuscularly for dogs >15kg

3. Catheterise and check urine S.G. at thirty minute intervals for two hours.

    The animal may be fed and offered *small* amounts of water before starting the test. Large amounts of water given either during or immediately after the test may result in water intoxication.

    A positive response to ADH (urine S.G. >1.025 or in most cases a S.G. >1.030) is consistent with a diagnosis of central diabetes insipidus. Failure to concentrate urine in response to ADH suggests nephrogenic diabetes insipidus or medullary washout. Equivocal cases may show a positive response if ADH is administered on two or three consecutive days.

D. The Hickey-Hare test

The Hickey-Hare test involves the administration of an intravenous bolus of hypertonic saline. The protocol is as follows:

1. 20mls/kg of water is given by stomach tube

2. Catheterise and empty bladder

3. 2.5% sodium chloride is infused intravenously at a rate of 2.5mls/kg/min over 45 minutes.

4. Measure urine volume and S.G. ($\pm$ urine osmolality) every 15 minutes after the start of the infusion. In normal dogs urine volume progressively decreases with an increase in urine S.G. and osmolality. Failure to do so is suggestive of central or nephrogenic diabetes insipidus. *The development of central nervous system signs due to sodium overload is a potential hazard which has restricted extensive use of this test.*

Diagnosis of diabetes insipidus is discussed more fully in Chapter 1. The clinicopathological features of the numerous endocrine and non-endocrine disorders which cause polyuria and polydipsia in the dog and cat are summarised in Tables 3 and 4.

Table 3. Non-endocrine causes of polydipsia/polyuria

Condition	Clinical signs other than polyuria and polydipsia*	Haematology	Biochemistry	Urine analysis	Radiology	Special diagnostic tests	Mechanism of polyuria/polydipsia*
Chronic renal failure:							
1. Chronic interstitial nephritis (CIN)	weight loss, anorexia, depression, vomiting, 'rubber jaw', ±melaena	non-regenerative anaemia, lymphopenia	↑BUN, ↑creatinine, ↑phosphate, ↓urine:plasma ratios of urea and creatinine	isosthenuria, ±casts, ±protein	kidneys small, ±signs of renal secondary hyperparathyroidism		decrease in number of functional nephrons, osmotic diuresis
2. Glomerulonephropathy/nephrotic syndrome – renal amyloidosis – renal lymphoma – glomerulonephritis	as for CIN + peripheral oedema ± ascites (rare)	as for CIN	as for CIN ± ↑cholesterol, hypoproteinaemia (decreased albumin)	significant proteinuria	enlarged kidneys?, ± signs of renal secondary hyperparathyroidism	single urine protein: creatinine ratio, 24 hr urinary protein excretion, renal biopsy	As for CIN
3. Pyelonephritis	as for CIN + pyrexia, sublumbar pain	as for CIN + neutrophilic leucocytosis	as for CIN	WBCs, protein, bacteria	kidney size variable	intravenous urography, urine culture	as for CIN
Chronic liver disease – chronic active hepatitis – fibrosis/cirrhosis – cholangiohepatitis (cats) – portosystemic shunts – neoplasia	vomiting, diarrhoea, weight loss, ± jaundice, ± ascites, ± CNS signs	mild non-regenerative anaemia, variable thrombocytopenia	hypoproteinaemia(↓albumin), ↓BUN, ↑ALT, ↑ALP, ↑γGT, ±↑bile salts, ±↓↑glucose, ±↑bilirubin	variable urine S.G., biurate crystals (portosystemic shunts), ±↑bilirubin	↓liver size (portosystemic shunts, cirrhosis), ↑liver size (CAH, neoplasia)	prolonged retention of BSP. ↑blood clotting parameters (OSPT/APTT), ↑blood ammonia, ammonia tolerance test, liver biopsy	↓medullary hypertonicity, ↓catabolism of renin, hypokalaemia, ↓degradation of glucocorticoids, impaired action of ADH
Pyometra and other toxaemic states	anorexia, depression, weight loss, vomiting, abdominal distension, vaginal discharge (if open)	neutrophilia/left shift, may be normal if open	non-specific, ± prerenal azotaemia	WBCs, protein	coiled soft tissue dense viscus in mid-caudal abdomen		renal tubular insensitivity to ADH induced by E. coli endotoxins, immune-complex glomerulonephritis
Primary or psychogenic polydipsia	severe polyuria/polydipsia		plasma osmolality low normal e.g. 280 mOsm/kg	hyposthenuria		equivocal response to water deprivation and exogenous ADH indicating sub-maximal concentration of urine	failure of collecting ducts to respond to ADH, medullary washout
Primary renal glycosuria	inherited in Norwegian elk-hounds		normal blood glucose	glycosuria			osmotic diuresis
Fanconi's syndrome	inherited in Basenjis		normal blood glucose	glycosuria, ↑urinary excretion of aminoacids, phosphate, sodium and bicarbonate			osmotic diuresis
Hypercalcaemia – hypercalcaemia of malignancy – metastatic bone tumours – renal dysplasia	weakness, depression, anorexia, muscle tremors, bradycardia, vomiting, constipation plus signs associated with neoplasia (enlarged lymph nodes etc.)	± non-regenerative anaemia	initially ↑calcium with decreased phosphate, ↑BUN, creatinine and phosphate in later stages (nephrocalcinosis)	frequently isosthenuria, ± casts		identify underlying cause e.g. lymph node or bone marrow aspirate to rule out neoplasia	nephrocalcinosis resulting in chronic renal failure, impaired action of ADH on renal receptors
Hypokalaemia – excessive gastrointestinal losses – excessive urinary loss e.g. diabetes mellitus, diuretic therapy	muscle weakness (hypokalaemic myopathy), gastric atony, paralytic ileus, cardiac arrhythmias		↓potassium	non-specific		response to potassium supplementation	intracellular dehydration resulting in stimulation of thirst centre, failure of collecting duct to respond to ADH, medullary washout
Hyperviscosity syndromes – polycythaemia vera – hypergammaglobulinaemia e.g. plasma cell myeloma	bleeding diathesis, CNS signs or CHF	↑haemoglobin, PCV and total RBCs				serum protein electrophoresis, bone marrow aspiration	uncertain

*The mechanisms responsible for the polyuria/polydipsia associated with many of the non-endocrine disorders listed above involve an endocrine component, for example, hypercalcaemia interferes with the action of ADH on renal receptor sites (acquired or secondary nephrogenic diabetes insipidus).

Table 4. Endocrine causes of polydipsia/polyuria

Condition	Clinical signs other than polyuria/polydipsia	Haematology/Biochemistry	Urine analysis	Radiology	Special diagnostic tests	Mechanism of polyuria/polydipsia
Diabetes insipidus (DI) 1. Central or pituitary DI	*Severe* polyuria/polydipsia ± marginal dehydration, ± CNS signs, ± weight loss (restlessness), ± vomiting following excessive water intake	± slight increase in PCV, plasma proteins and plasma osmolality, ±↑ BUN, creatinine, sodium and chloride (mild dehydration)	hyposthenuria, urine osmolality 40-200 mOsm/kg		negative response to water deprivation with a positive response to exogenous ADH	decreased secretion of ADH
2. Nephrogenic DI	as for central DI	as for central DI	as for central DI		negative response to water deprivation and to exogenous ADH	distal tubules/collecting ducts unresponsive to ADH
Diabetes mellitus — may be associated with Cushing's disease	obese or progressive weight loss, polyphagia, lethargy, vomiting/anorexic if ketoacidotic, hepatomegaly, dry scurfy hair coat, cataract formation	± leucocytosis or stress haemogram, ↑ glucose, ↑ ALT/ALP, ±↑ cholesterol, lipaemic plasma, low or normal potassium, ± prerenal azotaemia, ↑ amylase/lipase if concurrent pancreatitis	glycosuria, ± ketonuria, urine S.G. typically > 1.030	enlarged liver	insulin assays to establish aetiology	osmotic diuresis
Hyperadrenocorticism — may be associated with diabetes mellitus	alopecia, hyperpigmentation, loss of skin elasticity, calcinosis cutis, muscle weakness/atrophy, exercise intolerance, polyphagia, hepatomegaly, pendulous abdomen, testicular atrophy	stress haemogram i.e. neutrophilia, eosinopenia, lymphopenia ± monocytosis, increased ALP and ALT, ± increased glucose, ± increased cholesterol	variable urine specific gravity (frequently hyposthenuric or isosthenuric), urinary tract infections common, ± glycosuria	hepatomegaly, bronchial/tracheal calcification, calcification along fascial planes, calcinosis cutis, osteoporosis, mineralisation of adrenal gland (neoplasia)	ACTH response test Dexamethasone suppression test	excessive production of cortisol interferes with the action of ADH, inhibition of ADH release
Hypoadrenocorticism Acute	hypovolaemia, shock (collapse), dehydration, bradycardia, ± gastrointestinal haemorrhage, abdominal pain	variable eosinophilia/lymphocytosis, mild non-regenerative anaemia (regenerative if GI haemorrhage), pre-renal azotaemia, ↓ sodium, ↑ potassium	variable urine S.G. (1.016 – 1.028)	microcardia, hyperlucent lung fields (decreased pulmonary perfusion), narrow PVC	ECG: peaked T waves, absent P waves and bradycardia consistent with hyperkalaemia, negative response to ACTH stimulation	medullary washout, hypovolaemia
Chronic	polyuria/polydipsia in 15% of cases, weight loss, depression, muscle weakness, tremors, anorexia, intermittent vomiting/diarrhoea	sodium potassium :ratio <25:1, ± mild hypercalcaemia, ± ↓ glucose				
Hyperthyroidism — benign thyroid adenoma (cats) — thyroid carcinoma (cats & dogs)	palpable thyroid mass, weight loss, polyphagia, poor hair coat, restlessness/aggressiveness, voluminous stools, vomiting/diarrhoea, cardiac arrhythmias (cardiomyopathy), ± CHF (dyspnoea etc)	↑ ALT and ALP, ↑ glucose (stress), ± prerenal azotaemia	non-specific, ± glycosuria (cat)	cardiomegaly (cat) ± signs of CHF, occasionally ectopic thyroid mass	T3/T4 assays, ECG	multifactorial, ? impaired action of ADH, increased total renal blood flow resulting in medullary washout ? compulsive polydipsia
Acromegaly Dog: — iatrogenic administration of progestagens — spontaneous during dioestrus phase of oestrus cycle Cat: — functional pituitary adenoma	excessive skin folds around head, neck and limbs (myxoedema), inspiratory stridor, general increase in body size, protruding mandible, increased interdental spaces, polyarthropathy, ± CNS signs	± ↑ glucose, ↑ ALP/ALT, ↑ phosphate (mild)	± glycosuria	hyperostosis of the skull, soft tissue swelling head, neck, limbs and oropharyngeal region	skin biopsy (increased dermal collagen deposition), growth hormone assays not routinely available	excessive production of growth hormone resulting in insulin-resistant diabetes mellitus
Hypocalcaemia — idiopathic hypoparathyroidism — thyroid carcinoma (hypercalcitonism)	CNS signs predominate (seizures, ataxia, muscle tremors, tetany) ± vomiting and diarrhoea, cataract formation	↓ calcium, ↑ phosphate			PTH assays not routinely available	uncertain
Hypercalcaemia — functional parathyroid adenoma — hypervitaminosis D	see non-endocrine causes of hypercalcaemia	see non-endocrine causes of hypercalcaemia	see non-endocrine causes of hypercalcaemia	skeletal osteoporosis	exploratory surgery, PTH assays not routinely available	see non-endocrine causes of hypercalcaemia

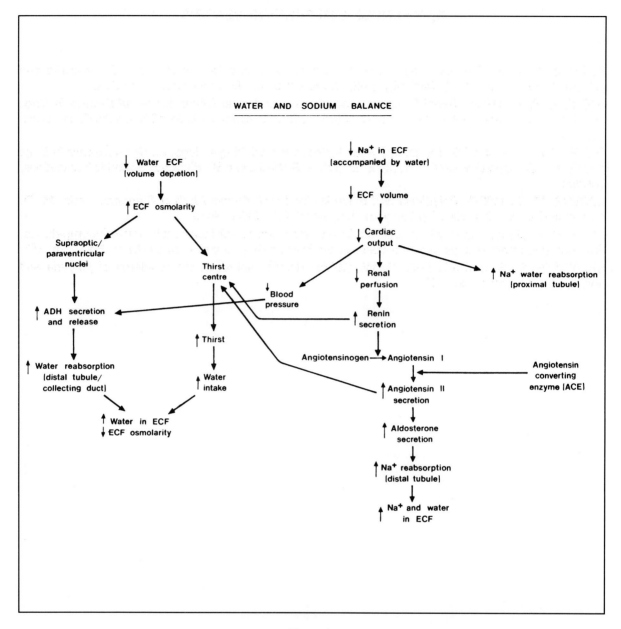

Figure 1
Water and sodium balance
(ECF = extra cellular fluid)

REFERENCES AND FURTHER READING

BUSH, B.M. (1988). Polyuria and polydipsia. In: *Renal Disease in Dogs and Cats — Comparative and Clinical Aspects.* (ed. A. R. Michell.) p 48. Blackwell Scientific Publications, London.

MICHELL, A. R. (1988). Renal function, renal damage and renal failure. In: *Renal Disease in Dogs and Cats — Comparative and Clinical Aspects.* (ed. A. R. Michell.) p 5. Blackwell Scientific Publications, London.

O'CONNOR W. J. and POTTS, D. J. (1988). Kidneys and drinking in dogs. In: *Renal Disease in Dogs and Cats — Comparative and Clinical Aspects.* (ed. A. R. Michell.) p 30. Blackwell Scientific Publications, London.

LORENZ, M. D. (1987). Polydipsia and polyuria. In: *Small Animal Medical Diagnosis.* (eds. M. D. Lorenz and L. M. Cornelius.) p 39. J. B. Lippincott Co., Philadelphia.

HOLT, P. E. (1985). Urinary incontinence in the bitch due to sphincter mechanism incompetence: prevalence in referred dogs and retrospective analysis of sixty cases. *J. small Anim. Pract,* **26,** 181.

BRUYETTE, D. S. and NELSON, R. W. (1986). How to approach the problems of polyuria and polydipsia. *Vet. Med.,* **81,** 112.

CHAPTER 10

DIFFERENTIAL DIAGNOSIS OF ALOPECIA

David I. Grant, B.Vet.Med., F.R.C.V.S., Cert S.A.D.

Hair loss is a common presenting sign in small animal practice. Although the major cause is ectoparasitism, and this must always be eliminated first, a number of other conditions, including endocrine disorders, may also be causative.

Most endocrinopathies present with bilaterally symmetrical alopecia. Pruritus is never a feature initially, although the condition may later become pruritic as a result of secondary infection. Hyperpigmentation is a feature of many chronic skin disorders, including most endocrinopathies, although this may be seen in other chronic dermatoses such as demodicosis and hypersensitivity disorders. In order to make a diagnosis when confronted with non-specific bilaterally symmetrical alopecia, a logical step by step approach is necessary, for example, that suggested by Lloyd (1985) for skin disease in general and given in Table 1.

Table 1
Sequence of diagnostic procedures

1.	Take the history
2.	Make a physical examination
3.	Evaluate the differential diagnosis
4.	Do initial diagnostic tests
5.	Narrow the differential diagnosis
6.	Do definitive tests for probable endocrine disorders
7.	Arrive at a diagnosis

Much information is derived from the history, and care should be taken to obtain as much detail as possible. A careful physical examination follows, after which the diagnosis is frequently suggested. Initial diagnostic tests will then make the diagnosis — or narrow it to a few possibilities.

In this chapter emphasis will be placed on important aspects of the history and physical examination in order to assist the practitioner to evaluate the differential diagnosis when confronted with a possible endocrine dermatosis. Flow charts will aid in a logical approach and are outlined in Tables 3 and 4.

HISTORY TAKING

Careful questioning of the owner may reveal many significant abnormalities. It is commonly stated that 70% of diagnostic information is supplied by the history.

Background information

1. Breed

Some conditions are seen far more commonly in certain breeds. Growth hormone responsive dermatosis has been described in poodles, pomeranians, chow chows, keeshonds, samoyeds and Lhasa apsos. Hyperadrenocorticism occurs most commonly in Boston terriers, poodles, boxers and dachshunds.

Congenital and hereditary disorders occur in various breeds. For example, colour mutant alopecia is seen in the blue (occasionally red and fawn) Dobermann, great dane, standard poodle, whippet, chow chow and the fawn Irish setter.

Pituitary dwarfism is seen predominantly in the German shepherd dog and the Carnelian bear dog.

2. Age

In the conditions listed above young adults are most commonly affected, but other endocrinopathies are more usually found in middle-aged or older animals.

3. Sex

Consider whether the animal is male or female, entire or neuter.

If male — is there loss of libido, attractiveness to other male dogs, squatting to urinate? These signs are suggestive of oestrogen-secreting Sertoli's cell tumour.

If female — are the oestrous cycles abnormal or absent? This occurs in hypothyroidism, ovarian imbalance type 1 and hyperadrenocorticism.

4. Previous or current illness

Hepatopathy, maldigestion/malabsorption, food hypersensitivity and nephropathy may induce dermatoses and hair loss.

5. Previous or concurrent treatment

Long-term administration of glucocorticoids may produce iatrogenic hyperadrenocorticism.

Key questions

1. Is the animal pruritic?
2. Over what period of time has the hair loss developed?
   Endocrinopathies are usually slowly developing.
3. Are the lesions constant or intermittent?
   Hypersensitivity disorders and ectoparasitic dermatoses may be seasonal.
4. Has there been any change in body weight?
   Hepatopathy and maldigestion/malabsorption may induce loss in weight.

5. Is the animal drinking or urinating more frequently?
    Polydipsia is an important sign in hyperadrenocorticism.

6. Behavioural changes — is the animal lethargic?
    Lethargy is a frequent finding in hyperadrenocorticism and hypothyroidism.

7. Is the animal intolerant to cold, spending much of its time near a source of heat?
    Thermophilia is often noted in hypothyroidism.

8. Does there appear to be any muscle stiffness or weakness?
    Muscle weakness is commonly seen in the later stages of hyperadrenocorticism.

9. Are any other animals in the household affected?
    Evidence of contagion to other animals or the owners suggests parasitic or fungal conditions.

10. Have any ectoparasites, particularly fleas, been seen and have anti-parasitic measures been effectively carried out?
    Flea control is frequently inefficiently done.

CLINICAL FINDINGS

Examination of the hair

Hair growth and replacement is a cyclic phenomenon initiated via the hypothalamus and anterior pituitary gland. It is useful to pluck several hairs and examine the roots and tips under a microscope.

In most endocrinopathies the majority of the hairs will be in the resting (telogen) phase, with only a small number in the growing (anagen) phase. Anagen hairs are pigmented, and square at the root end and surrounded by a root sheath. Telogen hairs show a club root with no root sheath and no pigmentation.

When examining the hair a careful examination is made for evidence of parasites and associated lesions and the skin is examined for pyoderma lesions.

Having taken a careful history, performed a physical and dermatological examination, an endocrinopathy may be suggested. Table 2 lists the endocrine disorders which may present as bilaterally symmetrical alopecia.

In order to differentiate these conditions it is necessary to evaluate key aspects of the history and physical examination, perform non-specific laboratory investigations and finally apply specific tests for each condition. This is summarised in Tables 3 and 4 at the end of the chapter. Important specific aspects of the history and physical examination of endocrine disorders are discussed below.

CANINE			FELINE
MALES ONLY	**BOTH SEXES**	**FEMALES ONLY**	
Sertoli cell tumour	Hypothyroidism	Ovarian imbalance Types I and II	Hyperthyroidism
Testosterone-responsive dermatosis	Hyperadrenocorticism		Iatrogenic feline symmetric alopecia (IFSA)
Castration-responsive dermatosis	Growth-hormone responsive dermatosis		
	Pituitary dwarfism		

Table 2
Possible causes of non-pruritic bilaterally symmetrical alopecia

CANINE CONDITIONS

HYPOTHYROIDISM

History

Careful questioning of the owner may reveal some of the following abnormalities:-

1. Lethargy. This is a common sign, and usually one of the first to improve following correct therapy
2. Obesity
3. Intolerance to cold
4. Abnormal oestrous cycles — oestrous cycles that are almost inapparent or completely absent or which recur after variable periods of time.
5. Lack of libido in the male
6. Variable appetite and gastro-intestinal disorders
7. Muscle weakness and stiffness
8. Hair loss, which may be patchy or unilateral in the early stages, but eventually becomes bilaterally symmetrical
9. Pruritus is only present if there is secondary pyoderma. Some cases present initially as recurrent pyodermas.

Physical examination

1. Dermatological abnormalities. These are usually the most obvious.
   They include: —
   > Bilaterally symmetrical alopecia (occasionally unilateral in the early stages)
   > Cool skin
   > Thickened skin (compare hyperadrenocorticism)
   > Hyperpigmentation
   > Seborrhoea
   > Comedones
   > Pyoderma

2. Cardiovascular abnormalities.

   There may be a bradycardia, or more commonly a low normal heart rate. Cardiac arrhythmias are also possible.

3. Ocular abnormalities.

   These include corneal lipid deposits, corneal ulceration and keratoconjunctivitis sicca.

HYPERADRENOCORTICISM

Hyperadrenocorticism (Cushing's disease) is seen in older dogs of either sex. It is seen more commonly in Boston terriers, poodles, boxers and dachshunds, (Peterson 1984), although any breed may be affected.

History

Key features of the history include: — polydipsia, polyuria, polyphagia, lethargy, muscle weakness, exercise intolerance and panting at rest, anoestrus in the bitch and decrease in libido in the male.

Physical examination

Bilaterally symmetrical alopecia is a frequent finding, with the head and extremities usually spared.

In dark coloured breeds there is often a lightening of the coat colour. The skin is very thin, inelastic and easily bruised. Subcutaneous vessels become visible, particularly on the ventral abdomen. Any skin wounds heal poorly as a result of the excessive thinness.

Hyperpigmentation is seen later in the course of the disease.

Comedones, particularly along the ventral abdominal and inguinal areas, are other features commonly noted. In advanced cases there may be calcinosis cutis.

Most dogs develop a pendulous abdomen and are obese. Hepatomegaly is a frequent finding and accentuates the pendulous abdomen. Generalised muscle atrophy also contributes to the appearance of the abdomen, and is an important factor in the lethargy and poor exercise tolerance reported by the owners. The muscle atrophy is often marked, particularly over the temporal area.

GROWTH HORMONE RESPONSIVE DERMATOSIS

History

This rare condition has been described in adult poodles, pomeranians, chow chows and keeshonds (Parker and Scott, 1980, Eigenmann and Patterson, 1984).

Growth hormone responsive dermatosis has also been reported in the samoyed and Lhasa apso. Most of the cases have been in males, but the number of cases is too small to be sure of a sex predilection. Signs usually, but not always develop in young animals.

The animals are usually presented because of the development of alopecia. Apart from the reported breed incidence, there is nothing in the history of help to the clinician.

Physical examination

The dogs are normal except for alopecia. Hair in affected areas is easily epilated. The alopecia affects the trunk, neck, pinnae, tail and thighs. Hyperpigmentation develops in affected areas, and in chronic cases the skin becomes thin and hypotonic. A curious feature of this condition is that hair tends to grow back at biospy sites, and at injection sites or areas of skin trauma.

CASTRATION-RESPONSIVE DERMATOSIS OF MALE DOGS

This is a rare dermatosis in which the Siberian huskie, malamute and keeshond may be predisposed.

Adult male dogs are affected.

Physical examination

The dogs are normal apart from dermatological abnormalities. These consist of initially a fluffy woolly coat, with the subsequent development of bilaterally symmetrical alopecia over the gluteal region, caudomedial thighs, ventral abdomen, thorax and collar region of the neck. The testicles are usually macroscopically normal.

PITUITARY DWARFISM

This condition has been described principally in the German shepherd dog, and Carnelian bear dog with other breeds being affected only rarely.

Affected animals fail to grow beyond 3 months of age. Initially, the hair coat is soft and puppy-like, and is not replaced by the adult coat. A bilaterally symmetrical alopecia develops, with only the face and extremities spared.

Hyperpigmentation, excessive scale, comedones and secondary pyoderma are frequent complications.

SERTOLI CELL TUMOUR

Sertoli cell tumour is seen in older dogs. The tumour is more common in undescended testicles, especially in abdominally located testes. Feminisation is a frequent sign. The owner may note that the dog has become sexually attractive to other male dogs, and adopts a squatting posture to urinate. Libido decreases and occasionally the dog becomes more aggressive.

Physical examination

If the tumour is in the inguinal canal it is easily palpable, and the other testicle may be atrophied. If the tumour is in the abdomen, it may be possible to palpate it. This will depend on the temperament of the dog, the size of the tumour and the degree of obesity.

Alopecia is a consistent finding, with easily epilated hair, especially of the genital area, medial thighs, and ventral abdomen. In the early stages, the skin may be soft, but in advanced cases there is thickening of the skin and secondary seborrhoea. In these cases hyperpigmentation, gynecomastia and pendulous prepuce are commonly seen.

Rectal examination may reveal an enlarged prostate gland. In addition, as approximately 10% of Sertoli cell tumours are malignant (Crow, 1980), careful palpation of the abdomen and regional lymph nodes should form part of the physical examination.

A few dogs develop severe bone marrow depression, believed to be due to the effects of persistently elevated plasma oestrogen concentrations. This complication is suggested by pallor of mucous membranes, and petechial haemorrhages.

TESTOSTERONE RESPONSIVE DERMATOSIS

Testosterone responsive dermatosis is a rare poorly documented condition of older male dogs. The alopecia begins in the perineal and genital area and spreads to the flanks and legs. The skin is thin, but other pathological changes do not occur. The condition has been described in intact male dogs with normal or diseased testicles, and also in dogs that have been castrated. Diagnosis is usually made on clinical grounds, and response to testosterone administration.

OVARIAN IMBALANCE TYPE 1 (Hyperoestrogenism)

The ovarian imbalances are clinical terms only, for conditions which are recognised by clinicians. The precise endocrinology, however, is not understood, and therefore reliable diagnostic tests do not exist. Ovarian imbalance type1 is seen in middle aged entire bitches. There is a bilaterally symmetrical alopecia beginning in the perineal and genital areas. Later, hyperpigmentation of these areas may occur, with enlargement of the teats. A secondary seborrhoea with pruritus may occur later in the course of the disease. A frequent finding noted in the history is irregular or abnormal oestrus cycles, often with persistent oestrus. The condition is often associated with ovarian tumours or cystic ovaries.

OVARIAN IMBALANCE TYPE 2 (Oestrogen-responsive dermatosis of the bitch)

Ovarian imbalance type 2 is a rare disorder that is usually seen in female dogs that have been prematurely neutered (Muller et al, 1983). There is alopecia which begins in the perineal and genital regions, spreading to the flanks and upper legs. The teats and vulva are often small and infantile. There is usually no abnormality of the skin. In some animals there may be urinary incontinence.

FELINE CONDITIONS

FELINE HYPERTHYROIDISM

Feline hyperthyroidism is a common entity in cats and is the most common endocrinopathy affecting cats above 8 years of age (Feldman and Nelson, 1987).

Typical features noted in the history include weight loss (in spite of a good appetite), polydipsia, diarrhoea and hyperactivity.

Physical examination

These cats are invariably thin and, in advanced cases, emaciated. In a series of 94 cases (Feldman and Nelson), 52% had hair loss and an unkempt coat. Thoday (1986), reporting on 74 cats, found skin lesions in 32% of the cats. These lesions consisted of matting, seborrhoea sicca or oleosa, patchy or regional alopecia and hyperaemia of the pinnae.

FELINE SYMMETRIC ALOPECIA

This is a poorly documented condition in the cat, of unknown aetiology. The term 'endocrine alopecia' was previously used because of empirical response to various hormonal therapies. Most cases are said to occur in neutered animals, and there is no breed predilection reported. Apart from dermatological abnormalities, these animals are normal, though some may have low functional thyroid reserve (Thoday, 1986 a and b).

Physical examination

In early cases a bilaterally symmetrical alopecia develops in the perineum and genital areas, base of the tail and medial thighs. In some cats alopecia also develops on the forelegs, below the elbow and above the carpus. Later this alopecia spreads ventrally to involve the ventral two thirds of the flanks.

The dorsum is invariably spared. In affected areas the skin is macroscopically normal and there is usually no pruritus.

DIFFERENTIAL DIAGNOSIS

Following a detailed history, physical examination and preliminary laboratory tests such as skin scrapings and fungal culture, a list of differential endocrine diagnoses may be made.

Routine haematological, biochemical and urine screening tests are often of great value in assisting the clinician in the selection of specific diagnostic laboratory investigations.

FURTHER INVESTIGATIONS

A. HAEMATOLOGY

Hypothyroidism

Hypothyroid dogs classically exhibit a normocytic, normochromic non-regenerative anaemia. In such cases the PCV is frequently less than 25. In those cases where there is a secondary pyoderma, there may be a leucocytosis.

Hyperadrenocorticism

Excessive production of cortisol usually results in neutrophilia, monocytosis, lymphopenia and eosinopenia.

Growth hormone responsive alopecia

Routine haematological and biochemical investigations are usually normal. This is of use, however, in differentiating this condition from hypothyroidism and hyperadrenocorticism.

Sertoli cell tumour

Some cases may develop bone marrow depression. Haematology in these cases will reveal non-regenerative anaemia with leucopenia, lymphocytosis and thrombocytopenia.

Feline hyperthyroidism

There are no marked haematological abnormalities in feline hyperthyroidism, but in one series (Peterson et al, 1983), 47% of cats with hyperthyroidism had an elevated PCV, and there was a tendency for leucocytosis, neutrophilia, lymphopenia and eosinopenia.

Iatrogenic feline symmetric alopecia

The eosinophil count is normal in this condition. The vast majority (92%) of cats with bilaterally symmetrical alopecia and a *raised* (>1.5 x 10⁹/l) eosinophil count are infested with fleas (Thoday, 1986).

B. BIOCHEMISTRY

Hypothyroidism

Hypercholesterolaemia is the most common abnormality and is seen in more than 75% of dogs with hypothyroidism, (Feldman and Nelson, 1987). This abnormality may also be associated with hyperadrenocorticism, diabetes mellitus, protein-losing enteropathy, protein-losing nephropathy, pancreatitis, hepatopathies or starvation. In spite of being non-specific, hypercholesterolaemia is a useful indicator when taken along with clinical signs.

In a few cases, there is an increase in serum alkaline phosphatase, alanine aminotransferase, aspartate aminotransferase and lactate dehydrogenase (Muller *et al,* 1983). Such increases are non-specific, however.

Hyperadrenocorticism

Dogs with hyperadrenocorticism frequently show increased alkaline phosphatase, ALT, cholesterol, fasting blood glucose and plasma lipids.

Feline hyperthyroidism

In cases of feline hyperthyroidism there are commonly elevations in serum alkaline phosphatase (SAP), alanine aminotransferase (ALT) and aspartate aminotransferase (AST). In one series (Feldman and Nelson), 91% had an elevation in the SAP, 75% had an elevation in the ALT, and 63% had an elevation in the AST. 92 out of the 94 cats in this series had an elevation in at least one of the enzymes.

C. URINALYSIS

Examination of the urine is a useful procedure particularly in hyperadrenocorticism cases. The majority of such cases have dilute urine, (specific gravity <1.007). These dogs are able, however, to concentrate the urine to an osmolarity above that of the plasma although less than that of normal dogs, (Joles and Mulnix, 1977).

Urine should be tested for glucose, since in 10% of cases (Meijer 1980) there is a concurrent diabetes mellitus.

D. BIOPSY

Skin biopsy is a very useful but frequently neglected procedure. Endocrine diseases are suggested by hyperkeratosis, follicular keratosis and/or atrophy, follicular dilatation and plugging, predominance of telogen hair follicles, hair follicles devoid of hair, epidermal hyperpigmentation and sebaceous gland atrophy. Samples should be sent to a veterinary histopathologist with experience in skin histopathology. Close liaison between the clinician and pathologist is essential in order to achieve the best results from biopsy specimens.

Having completed the history, physical examination and screening tests, the physician should be able to make a tentative diagnosis or limit the diagnosis to a few possibilities. Definitive diagnosis may then be made by specific tests. Detail of these is described in the appropriate chapters.

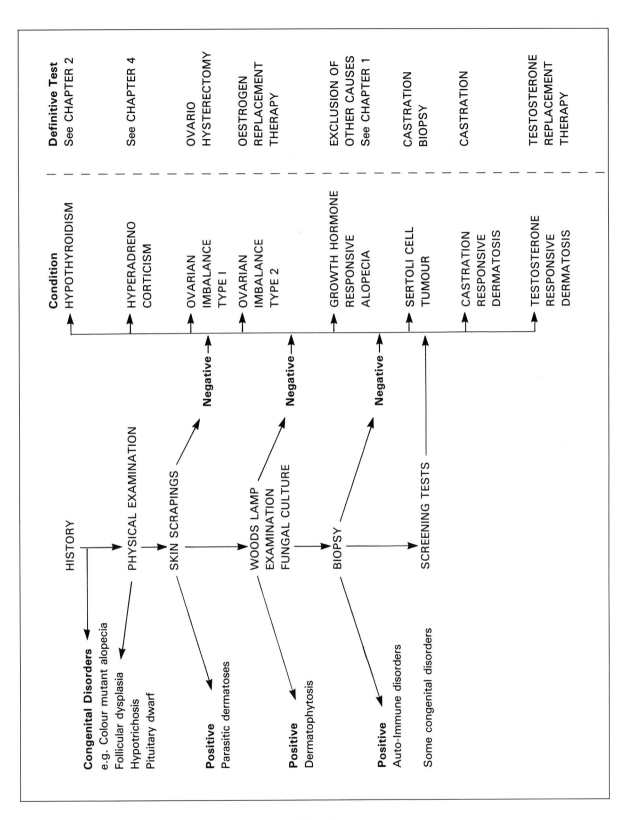

The flowchart describes the investigation of non-pruritic alopecia of the dog.

Investigation pathway:

HISTORY → PHYSICAL EXAMINATION → SKIN SCRAPINGS → WOODS LAMP EXAMINATION FUNGAL CULTURE → BIOPSY → SCREENING TESTS

Congenital Disorders
e.g. Colour mutant alopecia
Follicular dysplasia
Hypotrichosis
Pituitary dwarf

Positive
Parasitic dermatoses (SKIN SCRAPINGS)

Positive
Dermatophytosis (WOODS LAMP EXAMINATION FUNGAL CULTURE)

Positive
Auto-Immune disorders (BIOPSY)
Some congenital disorders

Condition	Definitive Test
HYPOTHYROIDISM	See CHAPTER 2
HYPERADRENO CORTICISM	See CHAPTER 4
OVARIAN IMBALANCE TYPE I	OVARIO HYSTERECTOMY
OVARIAN IMBALANCE TYPE 2	OESTROGEN REPLACEMENT THERAPY
GROWTH HORMONE RESPONSIVE ALOPECIA	EXCLUSION OF OTHER CAUSES See CHAPTER 1
SERTOLI CELL TUMOUR	CASTRATION BIOPSY
CASTRATION RESPONSIVE DERMATOSIS	CASTRATION
TESTOSTERONE RESPONSIVE DERMATOSIS	TESTOSTERONE REPLACEMENT THERAPY

Table 3
Investigation of non-pruritic alopecia of the dog

177

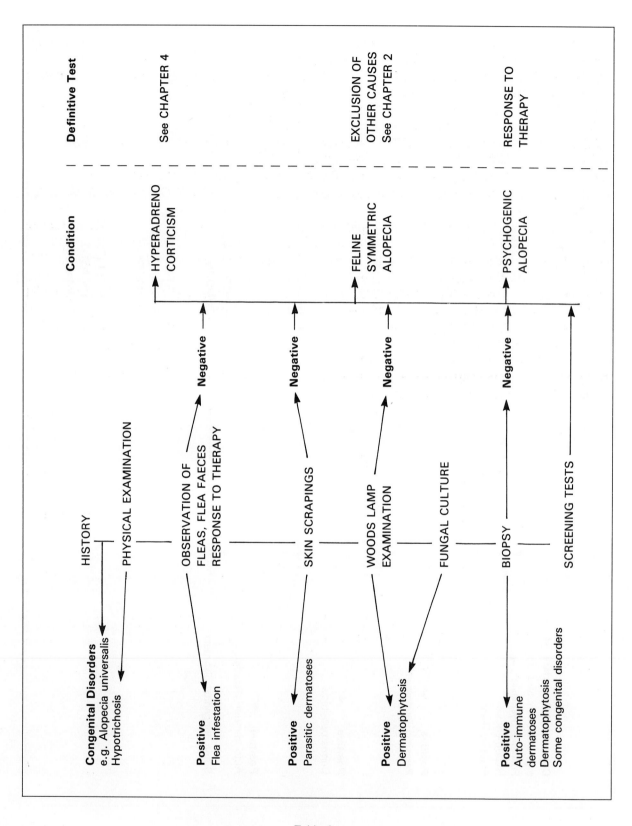

Table 4

Investigation of non-pruritic alopecia of the cat

REFERENCES

CROW, S. E. (1980) Neoplasms of the reproductive organs and mammary glands of the dog. In: *Current Therapy in Theriogenology* (ed. D. A. Morrow.) p. 640. W. B. Saunders, Philadelphia.

EIGENMANN, J. E. and PATTERSON, D. F. (1980) Growth hormone responsive alopecia in the mature dog — a discussion of thirteen cases. *J. Am. Anim. Hosp. Ass.* **16**, 824.

FELDMAN, E. C. and NELSON, R. W. (1987) In: *Canine and Feline Endocrinology and Reproduction.* p. 92. W. B. Saunders, Philadelphia.

JOLES, J. A. and Mulnix, J. A. (1977) Polyuria and polydipsia. In: *Current Veterinary Therapy* (ed. R. W. Kirk.) p. 1050 W. B. Saunders, Philadelphia.

LLOYD, D. H. (1985) Diagnostic Methods in Dermatology. *Br. Vet. J.* **141**, 463.

MEIJER, J. C. (1980) Canine hyperadrenocorticism. In: *Current Veterinary Therapy* (ed. R. W. Kirk.) p. 975.

MILNE, K. L. and HAYES H. M. (1981) Epidemiological features of canine hypothyroidism. *Cornell Vet.* **71**, 3.

MULLER, G. H., KIRK, R. V. and SCOTT, D. W. (1983) *Small Animal Dermatology* (3rd edn) p. 537. W. B. Saunders, Philadelphia.

PARKER, W. M. and SCOTT, D. W. (1980) Growth hormone responsive alopecia in the mature dog — a discussion of thirteen cases. *J. Am. Anim. Hosp. Ass.* **16**, 824.

PETERSON, M. E. (1984) Hyperadrenocorticism. *Vet. Clins. N. Am.: Small Anim. Pract.* **14**, 731.

REIF, J. S. and BRODEY, R. S. (1969) The relationship between cryptorchidism and canine testicular neoplasia. *J. Am. vet. med. Ass.* **155**, 2005.

THODAY, K. L. (1986) Differential diagnosis of symmetrical alopecia in the cat. In: *Current Veterinary Therapy* (ed. R. W. Kirk.) p. 545. W. B. Saunders, Philadelphia.

DIFFERENTIAL DIAGNOSIS OF OBESITY AND ABDOMINAL ENLARGEMENT

Barry M. Bush, B.V.Sc., Ph.D., F.R.C.V.S.

An animal is considered obese when its body weight has increased by 15% or more above the optimum for its breed, age and sex. Most cases of obesity in small animals are the result of an excessive intake of calories relative to the amount of exercise taken, i.e. simple over-eating. Approximately a third of dogs in the United Kingdom are overtly obese, though rather less that 10% of cats. The disorder is twice as common in neutered animals, demonstrating the influence of sex hormones and the need to reduce calorific intake following castration and spaying if obesity is to be avoided.

Apart from this association with neutering, obesity or apparent obesity, is a possible feature of six endocrine disorders. In addition, there are a number of other causes of abdominal enlargement that may be confused with obesity. These are listed in Table 1.

DIAGNOSIS

The history and clinical manifestations of a case of abdominal enlargement play a major role in its diagnosis, especially in eliminating non-endocrine causes, most of which are unlikely to be confused with obesity by an experienced clinician. Diagnosis is aided by radiography and non-specific laboratory tests. The flow chart in Figure 1 may prove helpful in eliminating possibilities. Specific tests will be required to establish conclusively the presence of an endocrine cause of abdominal enlargement.

HISTORY TAKING

1. **Background details**

    a. **Genetic predisposition** to simple obesity exists in certain breeds of dog i.e. Scottish terriers, Labrador retrievers, cairns, west highland whites, cocker spaniels.

    b. **Age.** Older dogs have a tendency to simple obesity due to a reduction in metabolic rate and physical activity.

    c. **Sex.** Pregnancy and pyometra must be considered in cases of abdominal enlargement in the entire bitch or queen.

    d. **Breeding history.** Pyometra typically, though not invariably, occurs in the older bitch some 9 weeks post-oestrus. It may also be associated with the use of progestagens to suppress oestrus or oestrogens for misalliance.

e.   **Previous illness**

f.   **Concurrent treatment.** Certain drugs (e.g. glucocorticoids) may stimulate appetite and long-term cause changes that produce or resemble obesity.

g.   **Exercise.** Modern lifestyles of pet-owners may result in dogs having little exercise and cats being confined permanently to the house, thus enhancing the likelihood of obesity.

h.   **Feeding management.** It is a popular misconception that cats should be fed or given milk *ad lib,* with the result that they may consume far in excess of their energy requirements. It is important to establish how much food the animal is offered and whether it is given table-scraps or 'tit-bits' which may not be regarded as food.

i.   **Thirst.** Is the animal drinking an increased amount? (See Chapter 9)

2.   Consider whether the animal is genuinely overweight. Older cats and dogs should weigh no more than they did in the first year of maturity: a record of the weight at that ages is a useful parameter. If it is not overweight, then abdominal enlargement is due to other causes than simple obesity. (See Table 1)

3.   Is the onset of abdominal enlargement gradual or rapid? Rapid abdominal enlargement is invariably due to emergency situations of non-endocrine origin. (See Table 1)

CLINICAL FINDINGS

The most practical and useful technique for assessing obesity is observation and palpation of the rib cage. The ribs should be easily felt but not seen in a dog or cat of normal weight.

A complete physical examination should be carried out, which may reveal signs of a pathological condition causing obesity or abdominal enlargement. Particular attention should be paid to abdominal palpation in order to detect hepatomegaly, enlargement of other abdominal organs or accumulation of gas or fluid. For details see Figure 1.

Skin should be examined for changes which may be endocrine in origin (i.e. bilateral alopecia, follicular plugging, hyperpigmentation, prominence of superficial blood vessels, thinning of the skin).

Our present knowledge indicates that in both dogs and cats obesity *predisposes* to Type II (insulin-resistant) diabetes mellitus, *accompanies* hypothyroidism (including hypothyroidism associated with pituitary dwarfism) and is a *consequence* of hyperinsulinism and sometimes hyperadrenocorticism. *Abdominal enlargement not due to obesity* is a common feature of hyperadrenocorticism and acromegaly.

Obesity due to overeating and unassociated with any of these endocrine conditions may be strongly suspected if there is a history of excessive food consumption but can only be established after eliminating other possibilities. An association with hypothyroidism is usually the most difficult to rule out, only being definitely eliminated after performing a T_4 estimation, which in the dog is preferably in the form of a TSH test.

Confusion can arise when obesity occurs at the same time as, though unconnected with, signs that are due to, or suggestive of, endocrine disease. In particular the combination of obesity and the male feminisation syndrome (producing endocrine alopecia and hyperpigmentation of the skin) strongly resembles hyperadrenocorticism, although the typical haematological and biochemical changes are absent. Usually this syndrome is due to a Sertoli cell tumour in a retained testis, though sometimes a seminoma or interstitial cell tumour is responsible for the feminisation; exceptionally in a small dog, massive enlargement of the retained neoplastic testicle can itself be the cause of abdominal distention.

In considering the inter-relationship between endocrine diseases it is appropriate to observe that both acromegaly and hyperadrenocorticism are potential (and often actual) causes of insulin-resistant diabetes mellitus, in one case due to the effect of growth hormone and in the other of cortisol.

Phaechromocytomas [tumours which occur in the adrenal medulla of the dog but which are seldom recorded in the cat (Carpenter *et al*, 1987)] can have a similar effect due to their secretion of catecholamines — adrenaline and noradrenaline (epinephrine and norepinephrine). Any abdominal enlargement is confined to occasional cases with ascites

A. Endocrine causes of obesity/abdominal enlargement

These causes are discussed in more detail in the text.

1. Diabetes mellitus.
2. Hypothyroidism.
3. Pituitary dwarfism.
4. Hyperadrenocorticism
5. Hyperinsulinism.
6. Acromegaly.

B. Non-endocrine causes of obesity/abdominal enlargement

True obesity, due to over-eating (predisposes to Type II diabetes mellitus).

Slow enlargement of one or more abdominal organs.

Neoplasia of one or more abdominal organs; principally the liver and spleen (including vascular tumours that intermittently become engorged with blood), less often the kidney(s), prostate gland, retained testicle, ovary, lymph nodes or gut.

Pregnancy.

Pyometra.

Liver enlargement due to right-sided or congestive heart failure.

Myeloproliferative disorders resulting in hepatomegaly and/or splenomegaly.

Hydronephrosis due to a post-renal obstructive lesion; unilateral or, if partial, bilateral.

Gross distension of the bladder due to atony or urethral obstruction.

Faecal accumulation due to atony of the gut.

Prostatic abscessation.

Slow accumulation of fluid.

Ascites arising from right-sided or congestive heart failure, hypoproteinaemia and/or obstruction of the posterior vena cava.

Peritonitis, due to infection (e.g. from a perforated gut) or irritation (e.g. leakage of bile, chyle or urine); 'wet' i.e. effusive, form of feline infectious peritonitis.

Rapid distension of the abdomen.

Traumatic haemoperitoneum (i.e. extensive bleeding into the peritoneal cavity following trauma) e.g. following rupture of the spleen or liver or abdominal penetration. Haemoperitoneum can also occur more slowly due to anticoagulant poisoning, perforation of a gastric or duodenal ulcer or bleeding from an abdominal tumour.

Bladder rupture and the accumulation of urine in the peritoneal cavity.

Gastric dilatation and torsion associated with the accumulation of gas.

Splenic torsion.

Pneumoperitoneum.

Rarely, air may enter the abdomen following penetration by a foreign body or during abdominal surgery and produce abdominal distension. At times, the abdomen may be deliberately distended, but only for short periods, with fluid injected to perform intermittent peritoneal dialysis, or carbon-dioxide for endoscopic examination.

Table 1
Differential diagnosis of obesity/abdominal enlargement

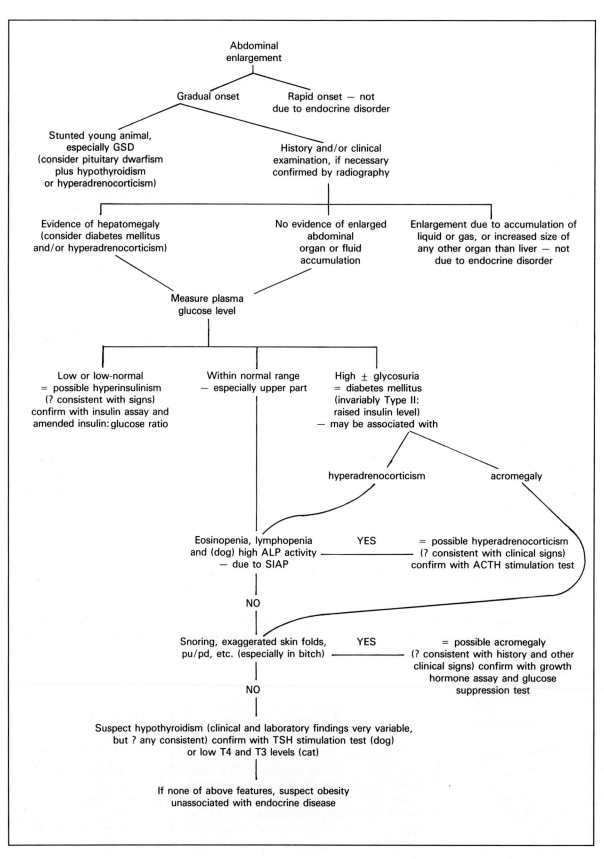

Figure 1
Diagnosis of the cause of abdominal enlargement

FURTHER INVESTIGATIONS INTO ENDOCRINE CAUSES OF OBESITY/ABDOMINAL ENLARGEMENT

Diabetes mellitus

Obesity is not a *consequence* of diabetes mellitus, rather it is a factor which *predisposes* to it, both obesity and diabetes mellitus being consequences of over-eating. In human medicine this fact is well recognised. Obese, non-insulin-dependent diabetics have fewer insulin receptor sites than normal, as a consequence of hyperinsulinism induced by overeating. As a result, such individuals are unable to respond fully to the effects of insulin, i.e. they become insulin resistant, the level of blood glucose rises and, if the hyperglycaemia is sufficient, glucose will appear in the urine.

Type I diabetes mellitus is *not* linked with obesity in either man or the dog. Obesity is, however, seen in many, possibly 50%, of the cases of Type II diabetes mellitus in the dog, as well as in Type III cases (impaired glucose tolerance). Unlike the situation in man, canine Type II diabetes is not ketosis-resistant and roughly half the dogs in all the groups, Type I, non-obese Type II and obese Type II are found to have ketonuria at the time of initial diagnosis (Mattheeuws *et al,* 1984b). Although there is little difference in their elevated plasma glucose levels these three groups can readily be distinguished by their insulin levels which are abnormally low in Type I, normal or slightly elevated in non-obese Type II and significantly elevated in obese Type II.

Mattheeuws *et al,* (1984a) showed that with increasing age and degree of obesity, dogs demonstrated progressive increases in the plasma level of insulin and insulin resistance. Eventually post-receptor defects also develop, adversely affecting the transport and metabolism of glucose. The final phase in the sequence of events is the onset of Type II diabetes mellitus.

Consequently the correction of obesity should be one aim in the treatment of diabetes mellitus.

Hypothyroidism

Obesity is a classical sign of hypothyroidism, along with lethargy and endocrine alopecia. However, it is now recognised that the importance of obesity has been over-estimated in the past and that many dogs of normal weight, and even thin, active animals may be hypothyroid. (Indeed, some veterinary consultants have stated that frankly obese dogs are probably *not* hypothyroid; Muller *et al,* 1983). The obesity appears to be attributable to relative over-eating by an animal that has become considerably less active, rather than to the hypothyroidism *per se.*

The signs of hypothyroidism have been re-appraised in recent years and it is clear that they are very diverse and may be present in any combination, a fact which can cause hypothyroidism to mimic several other diseases. In addition to obesity it may have many features in common with Cushing's syndrome, including:

1. Endocrine alopecia affecting the same areas (including a 'rat-tail'), plus follicular plugging and hyperpigmentation, although the skin is thicker than usual and not thinner, and there is no calcinosis cutis,

2. depression

3. muscle weakness

4. an elevated cholesterol level in up to 50% of cases (although the higher the value the more likely it is that the condition is hypothyroidism rather than anything else)

5. elevated alkaline phosphatase and ALT activities due to secondary liver damage (though usually *not* the enormous increases in alkaline phosphatase that can occur in canine Cushing's syndrome; i.e. 3—4 times the upper limit of normal or more)

6. low resting T_4 (thyroxine) and T_3 (tri-iodothyronine levels) in plasma are particularly confusing. In Cushing's syndrome, and in a number of other illnesses or following drug therapy, the levels of T_4 and T_3 can also fall below the lower level of the normal range but are seldom markedly depressed. Such individuals have been termed 'euthyroid sick' e.g. 50% of dogs with generalised demodicosis have low baseline levels of T_3 and T_4.

Findings in up to half of hypothyroid cases in the dog which are generally not present in Cushing's syndrome include an increase in creatinine phosphokinase activity and a *mild,* non-regenerative anaemia due to depression of bone marrow activity and therefore not accompanied by such regenerative signs as reticulocytosis.

Obesity is also a feature of feline hypothyroidism, as are anaemia and hypercholesterolaemia, though alopecia and other skin changes are rare. It seldom arises spontaneously but may follow therapy (involving surgery or drug treatment) for hyperthyroidism.

The performance of a TSH stimulation test usually clarifies the diagnosis in the dog, although it is easier and more certain to make the distinction between hypothyroidism and Cushing's syndrome using the ACTH stimulation test (see pages 90 and 211).

The diagnosis of hypothyroidism in the cat is best established by the finding of low levels of T_3 and T_4; there is currently some doubt about the value of the TSH stimulation test in this species.

Pituitary dwarfism

As well as a lack of growth and dermatological abnormalities, pituitary dwarfs may occasionally develop obesity due to concurrent secondary hypothyroidism. Exceptionally, abdominal enlargement may be the result of hyperadrenocorticism (Feldman and Nelson, 1987).

Hyperadrenocorticism

Excessive levels of cortisol in the circulation cause a redistribution of fat deposits. This is not true obesity because often the total body weight is not increased, but rather a transference of fat to the trunk from other storage areas. In dogs it produces a very broad back, and in some individuals there may also be an accumulation of fat in the mediastinum, causing it to appear abnormally wide on radiographs (Ticer, 1979). The distension of the abdomen, seen in 95% of dogs, is only in part due to the redistribution of fat. Other factors which contribute are enlargement of the liver, and, in particular, weakness of the abdominal muscles due to a loss of tone and atrophy which permits them to sag. In combination, these changes produce the typical pot-belly or barrel-shaped abdomen, that in extreme cases appears to be supported on stick-like legs which are also the result of severe muscle atrophy.

Cats, in which the disorder appears much less commonly and in which it is difficult to induce by the administration of corticosteroids, also have a pot-bellied appearance in 95% of cases although actual weight gain is seen in only 50%.

Diagnosis, especially in the dog, is clarified by the plethora of other clinical signs, many of which are present in any one case. Prominent amongst them are polyuria and polydipsia, polyphagia, panting at rest, and a variety of skin changes (endocrine alopecia, thinning of the skin, loss of elasticity, prominence of superficial blood vessels, follicular plugging, hyperpigmentation, easy bruising, delayed healing and calcinosis cutis). There *may* at times be signs attributable to neoplasia, i.e. pituitary enlargement (giving rise to blindness, confusion, circling, head pressing, etc.), or adrenal malignancy (with an absence of skin changes in the early stages, because these take longer to develop, and later metastasis, with the possible development of coughing or chronic renal failure).

Affected animals show typical steroidal changes on haematological examination, especially eosinopenia (often the complete absence of eosinophils), lymphopenia, neutrophilia, and in the dog monocytosis. (Monocytosis *can* occur in cats but much less frequently). Although total leucocyte counts are often in the upper part of the normal range, this is not necessarily the case and the recognition of the typical steroidal pattern demonstrated by the differential white cell count can be more valuable than the absolute counts of each cell type.

Alkaline phosphatase activity is increased in 95% of canine cases due to a specific isoenzyme (steroid-induced alkaline phosphatase, SIAP) produced by the liver, and which can now be measured independently (Eckersall and Douglas, 1988). However, dramatic increases in ALP activity are not seen in cats, and where there are mild increases they are more likely to result from the development of diabetes mellitus. Overt diabetes mellitus develops in approximately 80% of cats though only 10% of dogs. Secondary liver damage results in increased ALT activity and hypercholesterolaemia in approximately 50% of affected dogs, though 85% of cats show an increased cholesterol value.

Resting cortisol levels are often not diagnostic unless either markedly raised (> 330 nmol/l) or very low (< 55 nmol/l, indicating an iatrogenic case).

Confirmatory tests for hyperadrenocorticism include:

the ACTH stimulation test (the time of peak action varies — in the dog it is two hours after ACTH injection but in the cat half an hour; estimating cortisol levels after only half an hour in the dog would cause several cases to remain unrecognised),

the dexamethasone low dose (screening) test, or

the urinary corticoid-creatinine ratio (Rijnberk et al, 1988).

To distinguish cases of adrenal neoplasia from those that are pituitary-dependent requires either the dexamethasone high dose (suppression) test, based on the assumption that cases of adrenal neoplasia will not show suppression, (although unfortunately some pituitary cases are also incompletely suppressed and exploratory laparotomy may be required to provide absolute confirmation), or estimation of the ACTH level (which is low in cases of adrenal neoplasia and high/high-normal with pituitary dependency). The use of a combined dexamethasone suppression and ACTH stimulation test (Eiler and Oliver, 1980) is not now recommended. For further details see Chapter 4, page 92 and Chapter 14, page 211)

Hyperinsulinism

Obesity has been reported in up to 20% of dogs with functional tumours (primarily, or solely, malignant) of the β cells in the pancreatic islets. These tumours are responsible for the intermittent and usually short-lived appearance of signs of hypoglycaemia, principally seizures, weakness, ataxia, collapse and depression. Generally they arise following periods of exercise or excitement, or 2-6 hours after feeding.

The weight gain has been attributed to inhibition of the hypothalamic satiety centre and the unchecked activity of the feeding centre in the hypothalamus which provoke polyphagia, and to the potent anabolic effects of insulin which promote the storage of nutrients in adipose tissue and muscle.

Hyperinsulinism is extremely rare in the cat.

Acromegaly

Although true obesity does not occur, abdominal enlargement is a prominent sign of canine acromegaly. The condition is usually associated with bitches in which the excessive output of growth hormone is stimulated by the progesterone produced in the dioestrus phase of the oestrus cycle or by the use of progestagens to control oestrus. There may also be an increased production of growth hormone by pituitary and hypothalamic tumours, and possibly by neoplasms elsewhere. The overgrowth of soft tissues and/or bony structures results in exaggerated skin folds on the head, neck and legs, a snoring respiration and a broad face with enlarged interdental spaces. In addition, polyuria/polydipsia and reduced exercise tolerance are shown.

In the cat, agromegaly is most often caused by a growth hormone-secreting tumour of the pituitary gland (Peterson and Randolph, 1989) and weight gain has been a feature of 50% of cases.

Most affected bitches (90%) show hyperglycaemia and in about a third of cases glycosuria develops, i.e. there is an overt Type II diabetes mellitus, as can be demonstrated by their normal or raised insulin levels. Hyperphosphataemia is a feature and two thirds show increased ALP activity. All affected cats (the majority of which are males) have shown hyperglycaemia.

All cases have increased plasma levels of growth hormone which are not suppressed following the oral or intravenous administration of glucose, but unfortunately in the United Kingdom. growth hormone assay has yet to become routinely available.

REFERENCES

CARPENTER, J. L., ANDREWS, L. K. and HOLZWORTH, J. (1987). Tumours and tumour-like lesions. In: *Diseases of the Cat: Medicine and Surgery* (ed. J. Holzworth) pp 544 and 554. W. B. Saunders, Philadelphia.

ECKERSALL, P. D. and DOUGLAS, T. A. (1988). New biochemistry tests. *Vet. Rec.* **122**, 240.

EILER, H. and OLIVER, J. (1980). Combined dexamethasone suppression and cosyntropin (synthetic ACTH) stimulation test in the dog: a new approach to testing of adrenal gland function. *Am. J. Vet. Res.* **41**, 1243.

FELDMAN, E. C. and NELSON, R. W. (1987). *Canine and Feline Endocrinology and Reproduction,* p 36, W. B. Saunders, Philadelphia.

MATTHEEUWS, D., ROTTIERS, R., BAEYENS, D. and VERMEULEN, A. (1984a). Glucose tolerance and insulin response in obese dogs. *J. Am. Anim. Hosp. Ass.* **20**, 287.

MATTHEEUWS, D., ROTTIERS, R., KANEKO, J. J. and VERMEULEN, A. (1984b). Diabetes mellitus in dogs: relationship of obesity to glucose tolerance and insulin response. *Am. J. vet. Res.* **45**, 98.

MULLER, G. H., KIRK, R. W. and SCOTT, D. W. (1983). *Small Animal Dermatology,* 3rd edn, p. 551. W.B. Saunders, Philadelphia.

PETERSON, M. E. and RANDOLPH, J. F. (1989). Endocrine diseases. In: *The Cat: Diseases and Clinical Management* (ed. R. G. Sherding) p 1097 and 1098, ed. R.G. Sherding. Churchill Livingstone, New York.

RIJNBERK, A., VAN WEES, A. and MOL, J. A. (1988). Assessment of two tests for the diagnosis of canine hyperadrenocorticism. *Vet. Rec.* **122**, 178.

TICER, J. W. (1979). Roentgen signs of endocrine disease. *Vet. Clinics N. Am.* **7**, 465.

CHAPTER 12

DIFFERENTIAL DIAGNOSIS
OF WEAKNESS
AND COLLAPSE

Peter G. G. Darke, B.V.Sc., Ph.D., D.V.R., D.V.C., M.R.C.V.S.

Episodes of weakness or collapse are commonly encountered in practice, particularly in dogs. As with fainting (syncope) in man, the aetiologies are manifold and may be elusive or obscure. Although it is often assumed that the cause of most episodes of collapse is cardiovascular, detailed investigations suggest that these may represent a minority of cases. In many animals the cause may be metabolic, often associated with endocrine disturbances. Animals may also be presented in a continuous state of collapse or weakness.

The range of clinical signs exhibited by cases of episodic weakness or collapse is very variable and they overlap those of epileptiform convulsions. Indeed, convulsions can also be caused by metabolic disturbances.

One problem commonly encountered in trying to establish a diagnosis can be the very episodic nature of the seizures. As they occur infrequently they are not likely to be witnessed by the clinician, who must rely on an indirect history that has been absorbed in many cases by a client under stress. Careful history-taking is therefore essential to establish a full mental image of the nature of attacks and thus help to establish the type of cause.

Although many diagnostic tests may be applied to these cases (e.g. radiology, ECG and bio-chemistry), the results of investigations may be normal between episodes. This is less likely in most endocrine diseases than in some cardiovascular or biochemical disturbances. Metabolic disturbances may be provoked particularly by exercise, excitement or activity or by feeding.

In some metabolic disturbances and in most endocrine diseases that can cause weakness or collapse, there will be signs of disease at times without episodes of collapse. These are likely to include depression, lethargy, ataxia, trembling and/or other neurological disturbances. Continuous weakness, ataxia or trembling can indicate spinal, neuromuscular or muscular disorders.

Most causes of episodic weakness or collapse are finally mediated through neurological dysfunction, whether due to cardiovascular, metabolic or primary neurological disease.

SOME TERMS DEFINED (Stedman, 1982)

1. **Seizure:**   'an attack; the sudden onset of a disease, or of certain symptoms, such as convulsions'.

2. **Convulsion:** 'a violent spasm or series of jerkings of the face, trunk or extremities'.

3. **Syncope:**   'a fainting or swooning'.

CLASSIC CAUSES OF SEIZURES

1. Cardiac output failure
2. Conditions affecting the central nervous system e.g.
    — infections (encephalitis, meningitis)
    — hypoxia
    — functional disorders (e.g. primary epilepsy, narcolepsy)
    — metabolic disturbances
3. Psychogenic/idiopathic syncope
    — fainting with no apparent cause
4. Neuromuscular disorders
5. Metabolic disorders e.g.
    — hyperkalaemia
    — hypocalcaemia
6. Hypoxia due to airway obstruction, severe coughing or severe pulmonary disease

ENDOCRINE DISTURBANCES CAUSING SEIZURES OR COLLAPSE

1. Hyperinsulinism:
    — islet cell tumour (insulinoma)
    — iatrogenic
    — ectopic production by neoplasms?
2. Hypoadrenocorticalism:
    — adrenal atrophy — immune-mediated
                       — iatrogenic
    — adrenal neoplasia
3. Hyperparathyroidism:
    — idiopathic
    — parathyroid neoplasia
    — ectopic production of parathyroid-like product
4. Hypoparathyroidism
    — immune-mediated atrophy
    — surgical removal
    — neoplasia
5. Hyperthyroidism (thyroid adenoma) occasionally causes seizures in cats.

ENDOCRINE CONDITIONS CAUSING WEAKNESS:

1. Hypothyroidism (dogs)
2. Hyperadrenocorticalism
3. Diabetes mellitus (especially if ketoacidotic)

LIKELY AETIOLOGIES FOR VARIOUS PRESENTING SIGNS

1. PERSISTENT WEAKNESS (ASTHENIA) OR ATAXIA (WITHOUT BEHAVIOURAL SIGNS INDICATING UPPER CNS DISTURBANCES OR GENERALISED ILLNESS)

This usually indicates a spinal disorder e.g.

    a. Canine 'Wobbler' Syndrome

    b. Prolapsed intervertebral discs

    c. Spinal neoplasia, CDRM

Muscle weakness or tremors can also be found with myopathies e.g.

    a. Rhabdomyolysis
    b. Polymyositis
    c. Myotonia
    d. Neuromuscular disease (e.g. myasthenia gravis)
    e. Circulatory disturbances (e.g. iliac thrombosis in cats)

In these cases there may be evidence of disturbance to muscles other than just those associated with locomotion e.g.

    Changes in facial expression
    Temporal muscle wasting
    Inability to swallow or regurgitation
    Dysphonia

Episodes of collapse are uncommon with these diseases.

2. EPISODES OF WEAKNESS OR COLLAPSE IN ANIMALS SHOWING BEHAVIOURAL SIGNS INDICATIVE OF UPPER CNS DISTURBANCES OR OTHER SIGNS OF NEUROLOGICAL DISTURBANCE

These may indicate primary neurological disease e.g.

    Trauma
    Encephalitis
    Hydrocephalus
    Neoplasia
    Metabolic disturbances (see 5 below)

3. EPISODIC CONVULSIONS

Isolated convulsions in animals with no other signs of illness very often suggest epilepsy. Epilepsy usually causes seizures in which there is *activity* with tonic-clonic spasm, and the animal shakes or paddles, salivates and has dyspnoea (and therefore froths at the mouth). The animal is usually unconscious and prolonged post-ictal bewilderment (or confusion) is common. Seizures are often seen when the animal is at rest or waking, rather than being provoked by activity, and idiopathic epilepsy is often first seen in young mature animals, particularly German shepherd dogs and miniature poodles. The post-ictal bewilderment can last for an hour or more and in these cases epilepsy may require differentiation from metabolic disturbances (see 5 below). Most cases of epilepsy, especially when developing in young mature animals, are idiopathic.

CNS disorders that can give rise to seizures include encephalitis (e.g. distemper, toxoplasma, FeLV), hydrocephalus, trauma, neoplasia, lead poisoning and storage diseases and (in cats) thiamine deficiency or benzoic acid poisoning.

Status epilepticus can be induced by:

Metabolic disturbances (e.g. hypoglycaemia or hepatic encephalopathy)

Poisoning (e.g. heavy metals, metaldehyde, strychnine, chlorinated hydrocarbons or organophosphates and benzoic acid or alphachloralose in cats) even in the absence of other clear-cut clinical signs.

4. EPISODES OF SYNCOPE OR WEAKNESS

Episodes of weakness or flaccid syncope (fainting) are typically caused by *cardiovascular insufficiency*, especially if they develop with excitement or exercise. In such circumstances the animal is usually flaccid during the seizure (although tonic spasm is not unknown) and recovery may be very rapid, with few further signs of distress. The aetiology is typically transient cardiac dysrhythmia (e.g. sinus arrest which is quite common in brachycephalic dogs), although syncope can also occur with:

    Congenital cardiac deformities (e.g. aortic stenosis) in young dogs
    Mitral regurgitation (common in ageing, small breeds of dog)
    Cardiomyopathy (especially large dogs).
    Cardiac dysrhythmias (bradycardias and tachycardias)

The mucous membranes are usually pale, rather than cyanosed, in these circumstances. Cyanosis is more likely to be a feature of respiratory embarrassment, as in airway obstruction or epilepsy.

There may be further episodes of weakness, exercise intolerance or dyspnoea in cardiac insufficiency, especially with cardiac dysrhythmias. Other signs of congestive cardiac failure (e.g. weight loss, ascites, coughing) may also be encountered.

Certain bradydysrhythmias (e.g. sinus bradycardia, sinus arrest) can be caused by endocrine disturbances, and animals with significant bradycardias when showing signs of cardiac insufficiency should be checked for hypothyroidism, hypoadrenocorticalism and calcium disturbances.

Episodes of weakness can occur with recurrent haemorrhage (e.g. with haemangiosarcoma or coagulopathy).

Syncopal attacks can also occur with the functional neurological disturbance known as narcolepsy and many cases have no obvious aetilogy, despite intensive investigation.

5. EPISODIC COLLAPSE IN ANIMALS WITH OTHER SIGNS OF SYSTEMIC DISEASE

Episodes of weakness or collapse and seizures that occur in animals with other signs of illness may particularly indicate metabolic or endocrine disease. In many of these cases other disturbances will include restlessness or depression, tremors or ataxia and behavioural signs such as vagueness, head pressing, apparent blindness, lack of response to commands and temperament changes at times separate from the seizures. Metabolic disorders that can cause these signs include:

hypoglycaemia	<3.0 mmol/l (dog)	3.3 mmol/l (cat)
hyperkalaemia	>5.6 mmol/l (dog)	5.0 mmol/l (cat)
hypokalaemia	<3.6 mmol/l (dog)	4.0 mmol/l (cat)
hypercalcaemia	>3.0 mmol/l (dog)	2.9 mmol/l (cat)
hypocalcaemia	<2.3 mmol/l (dog)	2.1 mmol/l (cat)
hyponatraemia(?)	<139 mmol/l (dog)	145 mmol/l (cat)

Other metabolic disturbances include:

hepatic encephalopathy
hyperlipidaemia
azotaemia
poisonings

Hypoglycaemia can be associated with hyperinsulinism, hypoadrenocorticalism, hepatic failure, malignancies and storage diseases.

Hyperkalaemia can be found with hypoadrenocorticalism, hepatic or renal failure or diabetes mellitus.

Hypokalaemia can be a feature of severe enteric loss of potassium in diarrhoea or vomiting.

Hypercalcaemia is caused by hyperparathyroidism, hypervitaminosis D and malignancy.

Hypocalcaemia is found in lactation tetany and in hypoparathyroidism (including surgical removal), and rarely, in dietary deficiency, malabsorption or renal failure.

Hyponatraemia can be associated with hypoadrenocorticalism, diarrhoea, haemorrhage, neoplasia, renal failure or excessive diuresis or isotonic intravenous fluid administration. Thus, hypoadrenocorticalism, hyperinsulinism, diabetes mellitus and parathyroid disturbances can each cause episodic collapse.

Anaemias and polycythaemia are further disturbances to be considered in animals with these signs.

6. CONTINUOUS COLLAPSE OR COMA

A state of continuous weakness, collapse or in extremis, coma, can be due to circulatory shock, central nervous system disturbances, severe anaemia, myopathies or metabolic or endocrine diseases such as those quoted in (5) above. Sudden onset can indicate crises such as trauma, poisoning (e.g metaldehyde, organophosphates), acute haemorrhage, heat stroke or hypothermia.

Circulatory shock may be primary due to hypovolaemia or acute cardiac failure (cardiac output failure), but it can also be induced by endocrine disease: the presence of bradydysrhythmia should stimulate investigation for hypothyroidism, hypoadrenocorticalism and hyperparathyroidism, for example. In dogs, debilitating tachydysrhythmia has been reported with the catecholamine-secreting phaeochromocytoma of the adrenal cortex, while in cats, tachydysrhythmias are commonly found in hyperthyroidism.

DIAGNOSTIC PROCEDURE

I. HISTORY

It is very important to establish the pattern and secure clear details of the episodes of weakness or collapse in any attempt to identify the cause.

1. **Circumstance at the collapse:** does it occur :
   — at exercise or with excitement (e.g. circulatory insufficiency)?
   — when the animal is resting (e.g. idiopathic epilepsy)?
   — in association with feeding or starvation (e.g. hypoglycaemia, hepatic encephalopathy)?
   — are there prodromal signs (epilepsy)?
   — is the animal conscious or unconscious?
   — how long does the episode last?

2. **Is the animal otherwise well?** Usually it is not in central nervous system, metabolic or endocrine diseases - there may be depression, weight loss, muscle tremors, polydipsia or inappetance. In episodic seizures due to functional central nervous system disturbances (e.g. epilepsy or narcolepsy) and with episodic cardiac dysrhythmias, the animal is likely to be normal between attacks.

3. **Seizures**

   Are there prodromal signs?
   Is there clonic-tonic spasm during the seizure?
   Is there postictal bewilderment (as typical of epilepsy)?
   Is the attack syncopal, with the animal flaccid, with an undramatic recovery (cardiac insufficiency, narcolepsy)?

4. **Continuous collapse: what preceded the collapse?**
   a. was the animal unwell? (poisoning, metabolic disturbance, cardiovascular, central nervous system)
   b. was the animal under observation, or does it roam free?
      Was there access to trauma, poisons, etc.?

II. CLINICAL EXAMINATION

While clinical examination may give clues as to the cause of weakness or collapse, it is often frustratingly unrewarding. The most obvious abnormalities are likely to be cardiological. A thorough examination is very likely to yield abnormalities if the disease is spinal or neurological. However, some cardiac abnormalities, notably dysrhythmias, are transient and may only be evident at the time of collapse.

Neurological or cardiac disturbances are most likely to be found in animals with continuous weakness or collapse, rather than with intermittent seizures.

Body temperature may be *raised* by activity in a seizure due to;
   meningitis
   heat stroke
   hyperthyroidism
It may be *depressed* by;
   hypothermia   hypothyroidism
   hyperventilation   chloralose poisoning
   circulatory shock

Non-specific signs of depression, weight loss or muscle weakness (or tremors) may be seen in endocrine disturbances.

Cardiac dysrhythmias may be found with electrolyte disturbances (e.g. hypoadrenocorticism).

Any animal with weakness or recurrent collapse with bradycardia or dysrhythmia muscle weakness or tremors should be screened for:-

Serum potassium
Serum calcium
Thyroid function
Adrenal function
Plasma glucose

Endocrine disturbance (diabetes mellitus, hyperadrenocorticalism, hypothyroidism) should be suspected in animals presenting with;

weakness and lethargy
polydipsia
skin changes (alopecia, melanosis, keratinisation, comedones)
hepatomegaly

III FURTHER INVESTIGATIONS

1. Episodic collapse

In episodic collapse, metabolic screening is probably well justified, given the paucity of clear-cut clinical signs in many of theses cases.

However, some disturbances, notably in hypoadrenocorticalism, hyperparathyroidism and hyperinsulinism, are very variable from day to day and hour to hour. There may only be serious abnormalities at the time of collapse. Therefore, marginal biochemical abnormalities should be pursued with repeat sampling and/or provocative testing by sampling before and after feeding or exercise, as indicated by the history.

Similarly, unless a dysrhythmia has already been detected by clinical examination, or there is evidence of neurological disturbance present at clinical examination, electrophysiology such as ECG or EEG is unlikely to be rewarding between attacks.

Routine screening might include the following:
i. routine haematology (background information, mainly)
ii. urea (elevated in renal insufficiency, circulatory disturbances and hypoadrenocorticalism, depressed in hepatic encephalopathy)
iii. glucose (elevated in diabetes mellitus, depressed in hyperinsulinism)
iv. sodium, potassium, calcium

Secondary testing might include:
i. glucose tolerance test, insulin/glucose ratios (for hyperinsulinism)
ii. ACTH stimulation of cortisol levels (for adrenal dysfunction)
iii. liver enzyme levels, bile acids, ammonia, BSP retention (hepatic dysfunction)
iv. inorganic phosphate, creatinine (for renal failure)
v. EMG, CPK levels, CSF tap; (for CNS disturbances)
vi. Blood gas analysis (cardiovascular/respiratory hypoxia)
vii. X-ray (liver size, cardiac size, spinal lesion?)
viii. Ultrasonic examinations (heart, liver)

If ECG is unrewarding, 24 hour tape recording of ECGs can be carried out.

2. Weakness or depression

In animals with weakness and/or depression, a similar range of tests is indicated, with thyroid screening and TSH stimulation being added if other signs suggest thyroid dysfunction.

3. Coma

In comatose animals ECG or EEG may be more appropriate. A routine screen is again indicated.

REFERENCES AND FURTHER READING

CHRISMAN, C. L. (1982). Seizures. In: *Problems in Small Animal Neurology.* Lea and Febiger, Philadelphia.

ETTINGER, S. J. (1983). Weakness and Syncope. In: *Textbook of Veterinary Internal Medicine, Diseases of the Dog and Cat,* 2nd ed. (ed. S. J. Ettinger). W. B. Saunders, Philadelphia.

FARROW, B. R. H. (1980). Episodic Weakness. In: *Current Veterinary Therapy VII* (ed. R. W. Kirk), W. B. Saunders, Philadelphia.

HERRTAGE, M. E. and McKERRELL, R. E. (1989). Episodic Weakness. In: *Manual of Small Animal Neurology (ed. S. L. Wheeler)* p. 223, BSAVA, Cheltenham.

HOLLIDAY, T. A. (1980). Seizure disorders. *Vet. Clin. N. Amer.* **10**, 3.

OLIVER, J. E. (1987). Seizure disorders and narcolepsy. In: *Veterinary Neurology.* (Eds. J. E. Oliver, B. F. Hoerlein and I. G. Mayhew), W. B. Saunders, Philadelphia.

STEDMAN, T. L. (1982). In: *The Medical Dictionary,* 24th ed. Williams and Wilkins, Baltimore.

CHAPTER 13

PARANEOPLASTIC SYNDROMES

Neil T. Gorman, B.V.Sc., Ph.D., F.R.C.V.S., D.A.C.V.I.M.
and Jane Dobson, B.Vet.Med., M.R.C.V.S.

There are a number of systemic metabolic and haematologic derangements that can be associated with tumours. The major recognised ones are listed along with the clinical signs and the associated tumours in Tables 1 and 2. In those cases where the metabolic effects in some way mimic an endocrinopathy, the systemic effects are referred to as a *paraneoplastic syndrome.*

TOPIC PARANEOPLASTIC SYNDROME

Tumours that originate from endocrine glands can be functional in that they continue to produce hormones that act upon the target organ(s). The endocrine gland tumour can be benign (e.g. feline thyroid gland adenoma) or malignant (e.g. canine pancreatic islet-cell carcinoma, insulinoma). *The systemic effects of endocrine tumours are commonly known as topic paraneoplastic syndromes.* The serum hormone levels are elevated, but are often independent of the normal control mechanisms, as exemplified by the abnormal dexamethasone suppression test seen in patients with adrenal tumours. The elevated hormone levels exceed the capacity of the compensatory mechanisms, for instance, the many counter-regulatory hormones of insulin (glucagon, epinephrine growth hormone, and glucocorticosteroids) are insufficient to block the hypoglycaemia associated with insulinoma.

There are no specific topic paraneoplastic syndromes unique to the dog. Hyperadrenocorticism may be associated with either pituitary or adrenal tumours. Hypergastrinaemia, hyperhistaminaemia and hyperinsulinaemia are also worthy of note.

Hypergastrinaemia

The secretion of gastrin by pancreatic tumours, known as Zollinger-Ellison syndrome, and the release of histamine by mast cell tumour degranulation promote gastric acid secretion and can lead to gastroduodenal ulcers. Vomiting, acute intraluminal bleeding and gastric perforations can all ensue.

Hyperhistaminaemia

Hyperhistaminaemia associated with mast cell tumours is more common than is generally appreciated. In those animals with cutaneous mast cell tumours that have a history of fluctuating in size, pruritus at the tumour site and a tendency to bleed there are often vomiting episodes and melaena due to gastroduodenal intraluminal bleeding. In addition, mast cell degranulation may precipitate an anaphylactic reaction and anaphylactic shock which requires emergency treatment with fluids, corticosteroids and antihistamines.

Cimetidine blocks the gastric histamine H_2 receptors and thereby reduces the secretion of gastric acid and the related complications. The use of cimetidine is strongly recommended in the management of these cases. The drugs ranitidine (Zantac, Glaxo) and omeprazole (Losec, Astra) can also be used to control hyperacidity.

Pancreatic islet cell tumours

Hyperinsulinaemia is associated classically with functional tumours of the pancreatic islet-cells. Unfortunately, the majority of these tumours prove to be malignant rather than benign. The clinical signs in these cases are directly associated with hypoglycaemia, but are not necessarily related to the absolute severity of the hypoglycaemia; rather, they reflect the rapidity of the decline in blood glucose level. Because of the limited carbohydrate reserve in the brain, hypoglycaemia primarily effects central nervous system functions. Thus, commonly observed signs with glucose levels < 2mmol/l are intermittent weakness and muscle tremor, abnormal behaviour, syncope, seizure and coma. If an extrapancreatic tumour cannot be localised, diagnostic laboratory tests include immediate blood glucose measurement, with concomitant serum insulin determination.

In hypoglycaemia due to physiological fasting, serum insulin levels are suppressed. In contrast, hypoglycaemia caused by a pancreatic ß cell tumour is associated with inappropriately *elevated* serum levels of insulin. Thus, a high (>30) amended insulin:glucose ratio has proved to be most reliable for the diagnosis of an insulin-secreting pancreatic tumour in the dog.

Complications	Clinical Signs	Associated Tumours
Dehydration	Decreased skin turgor. Increased PCV and electrolyte imbalances	Any tumour and associated metabolic and endocrine disturbances
Hypercalcaemia	Polydipsia/polyuria, nephropathy, anorexia vomiting, diarrhoea, cardiac arrhythmias and neuropathy	Lymphoma, multiple myeloma Tumours (metastasis) infiltrating bone Apocrine gland adenocarcinoma of the anal sac Parathyroid gland adenoma/carcinoma
Hypoglycaemia	Weakness, coma, seizures	Insulinoma, hepatic tumours, Large intra-abdominal tumours, Lymphoma/leukaemia
Hyperthyroidism	Polyphagia, polydipsia, polyuria, cachexia, tachycardia, dyspnoea, hypertrophic cardiomyopathy	Thyroid gland adenoma (cat) Thyroid gland carcinoma (dog, rat)
Syndrome of inappropriate antidiuretic hormone (SIADH) secretion	Oedema, hyponatremia, hypo-osmolality, urinary osmolality greater than plasma	Small cell carcinoma (man)
Hypergastrinaemia Zollinger-Ellison syndrome	Gastroduodenal ulcer, bleeding gastro-enteritis, gastric perforations	Gastrinoma (Pancreatic and islet cells)
Hyperhistaminaemia Mast cell degranulation	Gastroduodenal ulcer as above Anaphylactoid reaction	Mast cell tumour
Myasthenia gravis	Intermittent weakness and collapse	Thymoma
Hypertension	Renal and cardiac failure Blindness	Phaeochromocytoma

Table 1
Metabolic and endocrine complications caused by systemic effects of tumours

Treatment. The treatment of choice for insulinomas is surgical removal. This is generally not totally successful as the majority of pancreatic islet-cell adenocarcinomas have metastasised by the time the diagnosis is made. In some cases emergency treatment is required to control the hypoglycaemic seizures and establish a normal blood glucose level. Emergency treatment entails an intravenous bolus of 2—10 ml of 40—50% dextrose (0.5ml/kg) followed by a 5 to 10% dextrose infusion. Blood glucose levels should thereby be maintained within a normoglycaemic range as determined by serial blood glucose samples. If appropriate glucose administration fails to control the neurologic signs, more severe nerve damage with brain oedema has to be suspected requiring additional therapy with diazepam (2—10mg intravenously), dexamethasone (1—2mg/kg intravenously), and/or mannitol (1—2g/kg administered slowly intravenously). For further details see 'Insulinomas', Chapter 5.

Adenoma of the thyroid gland in the cat

In the cat probably the most important topic paraneoplastic syndrome is associated with a functional thyroid gland adenoma. Hyperthyroid cats typically have a history of hyperactivity, weight loss, polyphagia, and increased defecation and urination. Some animals may present in an advanced hypermetabolic state, which causes hyperthermia, tachypnoea, tachyarrhythmia, and signs of congestive heart failure (including pulmonary oedema, pleural effusion and shock). This fulminant presentation is called thyrotoxic storm in humans. Unilateral or bilateral thyroid gland enlargement, elevated serum T3/T4 levels, or the presence of both are diagnostic.

Complications	Clinical Signs	Associated Tumours
Anaemia (acute/chronic)	Hypovolaemia, bleeding, lethargy, pale mucous membranes	Haematopoietic and any other tumour ($\pm$ FeLV infection)
Leukopenia (neutrophil count $<3 \times 10^9$/l)	Infection at various sites, fever	Myelophthistic tumours ($\pm$ FeLV) infection, oestrogen-producing tumours
Thrombocytopenia (platelet count $<50 \times 10^9$/l)	Mucosal surface bleeding and petechia/ecchymosis, anaemia, seizures due to CNS bleeding	Myelophthistic and oestrogen-producing tumours. Haematopoietic and certain solid tumours (immune-mediated, Ehrlichia canis, FeLV)
Pancytopenia	Any or all of the above	Haematopoietic tumours, myelophthistic tumours ($\pm$ FeLV infection), oestrogen-producing tumours
Bleeding disorders and disseminated intravascular coagulation	Bleeding and thromboembolism microangiopathic anaemia, thrombocytopenia, abnormal coagulation, positive fibrin split products	Any tumour, particularly haematopoietic tumours, haemangiosarcoma, and inflammatory mammary carcinoma
Monoclonal gammopathy	Hyperviscosity: neuropathy (seizures), bleeding disorders, nephropathy (Bence-Jones protein)	Multiple myeloma lymphoma, lymphocytic leukemia
Leukocytosis ($>100 \times 10^9$/l)	Hyperviscosity leukostasis	Lympho- and myeloproliferative disorders
Erythrocytosis (PCV>0.6l/l)	Hyperviscosity	Polycythemia vera, Renal carcinoma and lymphoma, hepatic tumour

Table 2
Haematologic complications caused by the systemic effect of tumours

The functional thyroid gland tumour is usually benign and surgical removal is probably the treatment of choice in most cases.

Initial management must address the cardiac and other related abnormalities in order to stabilise the cat prior to surgery. Treatment may involve administration of propranolol (to counter the cardiac effects of excessive thyroid hormone) and prednisolone, methimazole and sodium iodide to temporarily suppress further release and production of thyroid hormones. In certain cases, thoracocentesis, diuretics and oxygen may be required. An alternative to surgery is treatment with radioactive iodine [131]. However, this requires specialised handling lasting for up to 32 days. For further details see 'Thyroid' chapter.

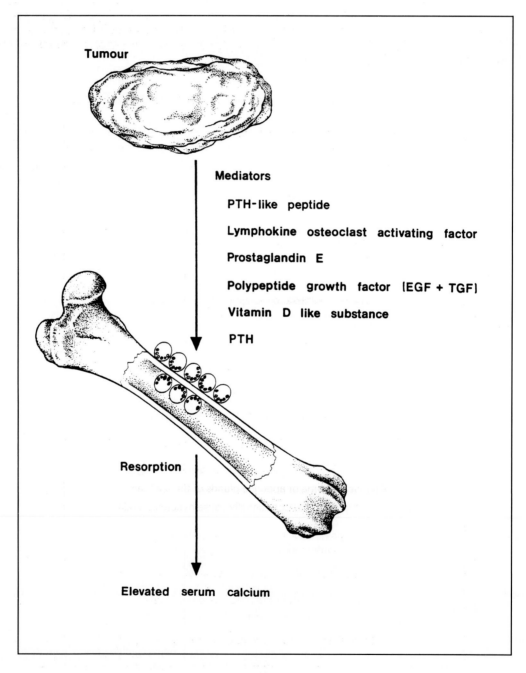

Tumour

Mediators

PTH-like peptide

Lymphokine osteoclast activating factor

Prostaglandin E

Polypeptide growth factor (EGF + TGF)

Vitamin D like substance

PTH

Resorption

Elevated serum calcium

Figure 1
Pathogenesis of cancer associated hypercalcaemia

ECTOPIC PARANEOPLASTIC SYNDROMES

Various *non-endocrine tumours* produce and release active substances into the circulation. These include peptide hormones and their precursors; prostaglandins and enzymes. Although the active tumour products have in many instances not been identified, the action of these 'ectopic hormones' can induce serious metabolic derangements mimicking primary endocrine disorders. Thus, these systemic effects are well known as *ectopic* paraneoplastic syndromes. Examples of ectopic paraneoplastic syndromes are: hypercalcaemia associated with apocrine gland adenocarcinoma of the anal sac and lymphoma, and the syndrome of inappropriate antidiuretic hormone (SIADH) secretion.

Hypercalcaemia

Hypercalcaemia is the most common ectopic paraneoplastic syndrome in the dog and cat and is frequently associated with malignant disease although other causes do exist (Table 3). Hypercalcaemia is due to an increase in bone resorption and calcium absorption, but the pathogenesis of the processes remains unknown in many cases (Figure 1). Five major groups of patients with hypercalcaemia can be identified, depending on the type of malignancy. (See Table 4).

Malignant neoplasms (see Table 4)
Hypoadrenocorticism
Primary renal failure
Hypervitaminosis D
Primary hyperparathyroidism
Bone lesions

    metastatic bone tumours
    septic osteomyelitis
    disuse osteoporosis

Others

    severe hypothermia
    miscellaneous inflammatory disorders
    haemoconcentration
    young animals
    lipaemia

Table 3
Causes of hypercalcaemia

---

1. Lymphosarcoma and other haematogemous malignancies

2. Adenocarcinoma of apocrine glands of the anal sac

3. Solid tumours that occasionally cause hypercalcaemia

        e.g.testicular interstitial cell tumour, seminoma, fibrosarcoma, thymoma

4. Solid tumours with primary or metastatic bone invasion

        e.g. carcinoma of mammary gland, prostate, exocrine pancreas, lung

5. Primary adenoma/adenocarcinoma of the parathyroid

Table 4
Malignant neoplasms which cause hypercalcaemia

Lymphoproliferative diseases

In contrast to humans, small animals develop hypercalcaemia most frequently in association with haematogenous malignancies like lymphoma and multiple myeloma. In one report, 15% of canine patients with lymphoma were shown to have hypercalcaemia at the first presentation. In these lymphocyte and plasma cell neoplasms, increased osteoclastic activity causes accelerated bone resorption.

Solid tumours with bone metastases

Patients with solid tumours that have disseminated to bone frequently develop hypercalcaemia. Carcinomata of the mammary glands, exocrine pancreas, lungs and nasal cavities are more frequently associated with either local or metastatic bone involvement and hypercalcaemia than are sarcomata.

Solid tumours without bone metastases e.g. adeno carcinoma of the apocrine glands of the anal sac of the dog.

Solid tumours (renal carcinoma and pulmonary squamous cell carcinoma in humans), and the apocrine adenocarcinoma of the anal sac in the dog *without* clinically demonstrable skeletal metastases have until recently been thought either to produce a metabolically active substance (ectopic parathormone) or to stimulate normal cells to produce and release parathormone-like substances, resulting in bone resorption (pseudohyperparathyroidism). Hypercalcaemia is a common finding in association with apocrine gland adenocarcinoma of the anal sac and may be present in >90% of such cases.

Parathyroid gland adenoma or adenocarcinoma

Primary hyperparathyroidism caused by parathyroid gland adenoma or adenocarcinoma and secondary hyperparathyroidism with renal disease can precipitate hypercalcaemia in cancer patients.

Normally, serum calcium is maintained within narrow and constant limits, with equal proportions of ionised and protein-bound calcium (mostly albumin). The regulatory mechanisms are summarised in Figure 2. Acid-base balance influences the level of ionised calcium, in that acidic conditions tend to increase the ionised calcium fraction, while alkaline status tends to decrease ionised serum calcium. The total serum calcium is usually measured in clinical laboratories, although it is the ionised calcium that is biologically active. Total calcium must be assessed in relation to serum protein, particularly albumin, in determining a patient's calcium status. Cancer patients with a low serum albumin due to malnutrition or liver dysfunction may have fatal complications of hypercalcaemia with seemingly slight elelvations of serum calcium. Rarely, severe hypercalcaemia may occur in dogs with multiple myeloma without producing clinical signs due to the fact that the paraproteins bind the excessive calcium.

The clinical manifestations of hypercalcaemia reflect the important role of calcium in maintaining the stability and excitability of cellular membranes. The effects of hypercalcaemia become particularly evident in the gastrointestinal, neuromuscular, renal and cardiovascular systems (Table 5). The early and nonspecific gastrointestinal signs include anorexia, vomiting and constipation. Pancreatitis and peptic

Gastrointestinal:	anorexia, vomiting, constipation
Neuromuscular:	muscle weakness, sluggish reflexes
CNS:	depression, stupor, coma
Renal:	polyuria, polydipsia
Cardiovascular:	bradycardia, arrhythmias, cardiac arrest

Table 5
Clinical signs of hypercalcaemia

ulcers are the most serious gastrointestinal complications. The neuromuscular effects lead to depression, lethargy, muscle weakness and finally coma. Hypercalcaemia may be associated with cardiac arrhythmias. In man the commonest cause of death in hypercalcaemic patients is cardiac arrest. A poorly understood but important adverse effect of hypercalcaemia occurs in the kidneys, resulting in polyuria with secondary polydipsia. Renal tubular defects occur, markedly exacerbating dehydration that may have already been present as a result of vomiting and reduced fluid intake. Volume depletion causes a further increase in serum calcium and decrease in glomerular filtration rate. Finally, this vicious cycle leads to further renal impairment with subsequent azotaemia, acidosis and eventual renal failure.

Hypercalcaemia, even with accompanying mild renal failure, can be reversed, but if it is not treated, it will cause fatal complications. Thus, any hypercalcaemia (>3.2 mmol/l) in a cancer patient, with or without symptoms, should be treated immediately. The management of hypercalcaemia requires

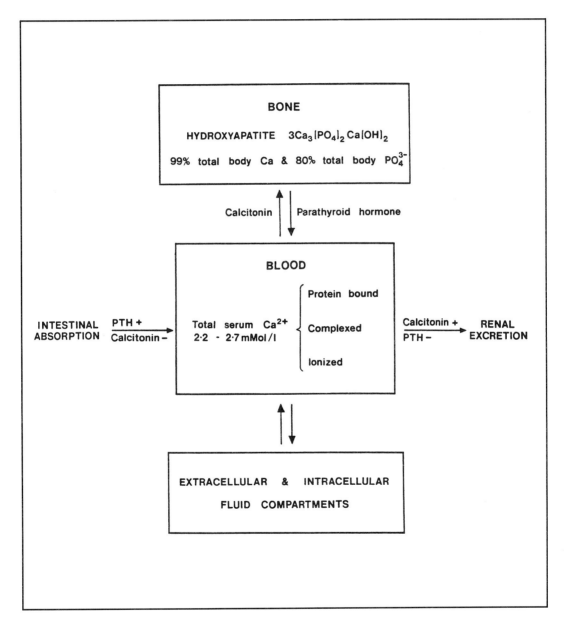

Figure 2
Distribution of calcium

restoration of the circulating volume, promotion of calciuresis and treatment of the primary cause (see Table 6). Fluid therapy is central in the treatment of hypercalcaemia, since most patients are dehydrated. Intravenous normal saline restores vascular volume and increases the glomerular filtration rate, thereby promoting the excretion of calcium. Since large volumes of saline are often required over a few hours, renal and cardiovascular statuses must be carefully monitored. As soon as adequate hydration is restored, certain diuretics like frusemide (2 mg/kg twice daily) can be used to enhance calciuresis by decreasing renal tubular resorption of sodium and calcium.

Since hypercalcaemia is most often caused by such haematologic malignancies as lymphoma and myeloma, corticosteroids are indicated. Pharmacological doses of glucocorticoids act on haematogenous malignant cells to decrease the production and release of bone resorbing factors. The efficacy of steroids in other malignant diseases, however, appears unpredictable.

The above described therapy is usually effective in normalising serum calcium levels within several hours to days and has no serious complications. In nonresponsive hypercalcaemia, a single intravenous dose of mithramycin (Mithracin, Pfizer Ltd. at a dose rate of 25 μg/kg) will usually reverse the electrolyte imbalance within days, presumably by direct inhibition of bone resorption or by alteration of vitamin D metabolism. Other methods for reversing hypercalcaemia have been described (see Table 6) but these alternatives are not generally advocated being either too toxic or ineffective. Therapy directed toward the malignancy itself follows once the hypercalcaemia is medically treated.

OTHER SYSTEMIC METABOLIC COMPLICATIONS

Alteration in the amount of hormone production and metabolism through indirect stimulatory or inhibitory mechanisms.

A renal tumour mass may cause local kidney hypoxia that can induce excess erythropoetin production and/or activation, thereby leading to a secondary and inappropriate erythrocytosis.

Alteration in the substrate level of a hormone-regulated metabolism can also mimic an endocrinopathy.

Hyperglycaemia may arise as a result of a functional islet cell tumour as previously described but may also be associated with large intra-abdominal tumours and hepatic tumours.

Table 6a. Aims of management of hypercalcaemia

1. Restore circulatory volume	0.9% NaCl
2. Promote calciuresis	Frusemide-2mg/kg bid
3. Treat primary cause	Surgery, radiation, chemotherapy

Table 6b. Clinical management of hypercalcaemia

Glucocorticoids — useful in lymphoma associated hypercalcaemia

    limit bone resorption
    decrease intestinal calcium absorption
    enhance renal excretion of calcium
    cytolytic to haematogemous malignancies

Mithramycin — 25μg/kg, single i/v injection
Calcitonin
I/V infusion of phosphate solutions
Sodium EDTA
Peritoneal dialysis

It has been postulated that the hypoglycaemia associated with large intra-abdominal tumours, particularly fibrosarcoma, results from over-utilisation of glucose, whereas, the hypoglycaemia associated with extensive primary hepatic tumours or metastasis may be due to increased gluconeogenesis. An artifactual hypoglycaemia may be seen as a test result in patients with high numbers of circulating leukaemia cells. This is, however, the result of plasma glucose metabolism by the cells while standing in the collection tube.

There is conflicting data regarding the production and secretion by extrapancreatic tumour tissue of insulin-like growth factors (IGF) that might cause hypoglycaemia.

The product of some tumours may change the capacity of a target organ or cell to respond to the hormone.

Oestrogens secreted from a Sertoli cell or granulosa cell tumour may drastically and often irreversibly reduce canine blood cell precursors in the bone marrow resulting in pancytopenia. Myasthenia gravis associated with human and canine thymoma is probably mediated by an antibody produced against acetycholine receptors.

Dehydration

Dehydration is the most common systemic metabolic effect of tumour growth. Volume depletion can be due to decreased fluid intake, prolonged vomiting and diarrhoea, kidney disease, and many other metabolic and endocrine complications that are associated with malignant diseases. Fluid replacement and correction of electrolyte and blood-gas imbalances can dramatically improve the patient's condition. Half of the fluid deficit should be replaced intravenously over the first two hours; the rest of the replacement fluid, as well as maintenance fluid, should be given over the remainder of the first 24-hour period. The patient's heart and respiratory rates, lung sounds, total serum protein, electrolytes and central venous pressure should be carefully monitored during fluid administration.

FURTHER READING

BRESLAU, N. A., McGUIRE, J. L. and ZERWEKH, J. E., et al: (1984). Hypercalcaemia associated with increased serum calcitriol levels in three patients with lymphoma. *Ann. Intern. Med.* **100**, 1.

BUNN, P. A. and MINNA, J. D. (1985). Paraneoplastic syndromes. In: *Cancer, Principles and Practice of Oncology,* 2nd ed. (Eds. V. T. DeVita, S. Hellmann and S. A. Rosenburg) p. 1797. J. B. Lippincott, Philadelphia.

CHEW, D. J. and MEUTEN, D. J. (1983). Primary hyperparathyroidism. In: *Current Veterinary Therapy VIII.* (Ed. R. W. Kirk), p. 880. W. B. Saunders Co., Philadelphia.

DRAZNER, F. H. (1981). Hypercalcaemia in the dog and cat. J. Am. vet. med. Ass. **178**, 1251.

FIELDS, A. L. A., JOSSE, R. G. and BERGSAGEL, D. E. (1985). Metabolic emergencies. In: *Cancer, Principles and Practices of Oncology,* 2nd ed. (Eds. V. T. DeVita, S. Hellmann and S. A. Rosenburg) p 1866. J. B. Lippincott, Philadelphia. p 1866.

FINCO, D. R. (1983). Interpretation of serum calcium concentrations in the dog. *Compend. Contin. Educ. Pract. Vet.* **5 (9)**, 778.

GIGER, U. and GORMAN, N. T. (1984a). Oncologic emergencies in small animals. Part I. Chemotherapy-related and hematologic emergencies. *Comp. Cont. Ed. Pract. Vet.* **6**, 689.

GIGER, U. and GORMAN, N. T. (1984b). Oncologic emergencies in small animals. Part II. Metabolic and endocrine emergencies. *Comp. Cont. Ed. Pract. Vet.* **6**, 805.

GIGER, U. and GORMAN, N. T. (1984c). Oncologic emergencies in small animals. Part III. Emergencies related to organ systems. *Comp. Cont. Ed. Pract. Vet.* **6**, 873.

GIGER, U. and GORMAN, N. T. (1986). Oncologic emergencies. In: *Current Veterinary Therapy IX: Small Animal Practice.* (Ed. R. W. Kirk) p 452. W. B. Saunders, Philadelphia.

GIGER, U. and GORMAN, N. T. (1986). Acute complications of cancer. In: *Contemporary Issues in Small Animal Practice. Volume 6, Oncology.* (Ed. N. T. Gorman). p 147. Churchill Livingstone, New York.

GRAIN, J. and WALDER, E. J. (1982). Hypercalcaemia associated with squamous cell carcinoma in a dog. *J. Am. vet. med. Ass.* **181**, 165.

JOHNSON, R. K. (1977). Insulinoma in the dog. *Vet. Clin. North Am.: Small Anim Pract.* **7**, 629.

KRUTH, S. A., FELDMAN, E. C. and KENNEDY, P. C. (1982). Insulin-secreting islet cell tumours: Establishing a diagnosis and the clinical course for 25 dogs. *J. Am. vet. med. Ass.* **181**, 54.

MacEWEN, E. G. and SIEGEL, S. D. (1977). Hypercalcaemia: A paraneoplastic disease. *Vet. Clin. North Am.: Small Anim Pract.* **7**, 187.

MacEWEN, E. G. and HURVITZ, A. I. (1977). Diagnosis and management of monoclonal gammopathies. *Vet. Clin. North Am.: Small Anim Pract.* **7**, 119.

MEUTEN, D. J. (1984). Hypercalcaemia. *Vet. Clin. North Am.* **14**, 891.

MEUTEN, D. J., CAPEN, C. C. and KOCIBA, G. J. *et al* (1982). Hypercalcaemia associated with an adenocarcinoma of the apocrine glands of the anal sac. *Am. J. Pathol.* **108**, 366.

MORGAN, R. V. (1982). Endocrine and metabolic emergencies — Parts I and II. *Compend. Contin. Educ. Pract. Vet.* **4**, **9**, 755; **10**, 814.

MUNDY, G. R., IBBOTSON, K. J. and D'SOUZA, S. M. (1985). Tumour products and the hypercalcaemia of malignancy. *J. Clin. Invest.* **76**, 391.

OSBORNE, C. A. and STEVENS, J. B. (1983). Hypercalcaemia Nephropathy. In: *Current Veterinary Therapy VI.* (Ed. R. W. Kirk) p 1080. W. B. Saunders Co., Philadelphia.

PETERSEN, M. E. and TURREL, J. M. (1986). Feline Hyperthyroidism. In: *Current Veterinary Therapy IX.* (Ed. R. W. Kirk). p 1026. W. B. Saunders, Philadelphia.

SCHAER, M. and BRIGHT, J. (1985). Endocrine emergencies. In: *Medical Emergencies.* (Ed. W. G. Sherding) p 183. Churchill Livingstone, New York.

SIMPSON, E. L., MUNDY, G. R. and D'SOUZA S. M. *et al* (1983). Absence of parathyroid hormone messenger RNA in nonparathyroid tumours associated with hypercalcaemia. *N. Engl. J. Med.* **309**, 325.

WEIR, E. C. (1986). Malignancy associated hypercalcaemia. Proc ACVIM Forum Washington. **13**, 65.

WEIR, E. C. (1988). Malignancy associated hypercalcaemia. Proc ACVIM Forum Washington. 103.

WELLER, R. E. (1982). Paraneoplastic disorders in companion animals. *Comp. Contin. Ed. Pract. Vet.* **4**, 423.

WELLER, R. E., THEILEN, G. H. and MADEWELL, B. R. (1982). Chemotherapeutic responses in dogs with lymphosarcoma and hypercalcaemia. *J. Am. vet. med. Ass.* **181**, 891.

WELLER, R. E., HOLMBERG, C. A. and THEILEN G. H. *et al* (1982). Canine lymphosarcoma and hypercalcaemia: Clinical, laboratory and pathologic evaluation of twenty four cases. *J. small Anim. Pract.* **23**, 649.

WILSON, J. W. and CAYWOOD, D. D. (1981). Functional tumours of the pancreatic β-cells. *Compend. Contin. Educ. Pract. Vet.* **3** **(5)**, 458.

WILSON, R. B. and BRONSTAD, D. C. (1983). Hypercalcaemia associated with nasal adenocarcinoma in a dog. *J. Am. vet. med. Ass.* 1982:1246.

ZENOBLE, R. D. and ROWLAND, G. N. (1979). Hypercalcaemia and proliferative, myelosclerotic bone reaction associated with feline leukovirus infection in a cat. *J. Am. vet. med. Ass.* **175**, 591.

CHAPTER 14 # LABORATORY ASSESSMENT OF ENDOCRINE FUNCTION

P. David Eckersall, B.Sc., Ph.D.

INTRODUCTION

Over the last twenty years, the laboratory assessment of endocrine function has been revolutionised by the introduction of radioimmunoassay (RIA) and associated techniques. These provide highly sensitive and specific means of measuring hormones in serum or plasma.

The hormones, commonly assayed in small animal medicine are those which have the same chemical structure in each species. Therefore, thyroxine, cortisol and progesterone which are chemically identical in human, dog and cats can be measured by assays developed for use in humans. However, differences between species in the reference ranges and in the composition of the serum, means that an assay must be validated for use in a particular species. Veterinary practitioners should ensure that the laboratory to which samples are sent has validated its assays for the species to be tested.

Radioimmunoassay is a complicated method to employ for measuring blood components and this leads to the possibility that differing results can be obtained when assays are performed on the same sample by different laboratories. For this reason it is imperative that results from one laboratory be interpreted by comparison to a reference range determined by that laboratory. However, interpretation of the result should be the same from all laboratories. The table of reference values (page 217) is included as a guide and should not be used for comparison against reported results.

Quality control, which is particularly important with radioimmunoassays, is maintained by inclusion in each assay of identical control samples to assess interassay variability. Analysis of replicate samples provides a measure of intra-assay variability. Recovery studies should also have been performed to ensure that the radioimmunoassays are accurate. Data from these quality control systems should be available from laboratories performing assays and it might be instructive to ask for details from the laboratory to which samples are sent.

In the following endocrine assays, in general, serum or heparinised plasma may be used. In some of the tests, particularly when endocrine levels are monitored in response to stimulation, it is important to follow the procedure of the laboratory which is to carry out the analysis. Interpretation will depend on consistent procedures having been followed.

For all blood samples, and this applies to those for general biochemistry as well, it is good practice to separate the serum or plasma from the blood as soon as possible after collection. This minimises the risk of haemolysis. It is particularly important to remove red blood cells if progesterone is to be assayed as progesterone is metabolised by these cells. If an unseparated blood sample was in transit for a few days the progesterone result would be meaningless. Serum or plasma should always be in an unbreakable and leak proof container, inside a reinforced package which should also contain sufficient packing material to absorb all the sample should any leakage occur. The sample must be clearly labelled and be accompanied with a covering letter or completed request form. The package should be clearly addressed to the laboratory and should also be marked as 'PATHOLOGICAL SPECIMEN'.

PITUITARY FUNCTION

Laboratory diagnosis of pituitary function is seldom concerned with the pituitary in isolation. The majority of investigations into the pathophysiology of the pituitary gland are associated with either thyroid or adrenal gland functions. The adenohypophysis is the source of trophic (i.e. stimulating) hormones for the thyroid gland and adrenal cortex, and laboratory investigations of pituitary function are valuable in determining whether malfunctions in the thyroid or adrenal glands are due to primary lesions in the respective glands or a result of a secondary lesion in the pituitary. Tests of pituitary function related to thyroid or adrenal function will be found in the sections dealing with these glands in detail.

Radioimmunoassays have been described for canine growth hormone, which record a normal range of 0—4 ng/ml. As this is at the limit of sensitivity of the assay a stimulation test with xylazine (100 μg/kg) or clonidine (10—30 μg/kg) has been recommended. Growth hormone concentration should rise to 50—70 ng/ml in the serum of a normal dog 15 minutes after intravenous injection of the stimulant, returning to normal within an hour. However, radioimmunoassay for canine (or feline) growth hormone is not available in the United Kingdom in any commercial diagnostic laboratory and should only be used after exhaustive validation of the assay if it were offered by a hospital or research laboratory.

THYROID FUNCTION

The laboratory diagnosis of thyroid gland disease in small animals is usually concerned with hypothyroidism in the dog and with hyperthyroidism in the cat. Both diagnoses use as the primary test an estimate of serum (or plasma) total thyroxine (TT4). For feline hyperthyroidism a single TT4 test is usually sufficient, but for canine hypothyroidism there is an overlap as hypothyroid dogs can have a circulating TT4 level which is at the low end of the normal range. To overcome this problem, a number of additional tests should be performed to establish the correct diagnosis.

THYROXINE ASSAY

The TT4 level in cat or dog serum is about one-fifth that in human serum so it is especially important to ensure the assay has been validated for these species as an assay designed for human use will be unreliable. In the determination of thyroid function, it is important to ensure that the dog has not been on replacement therapy at the time of the test, since both thyroid extract as well as thyroxine as the medication, are measured by the TT4 assay. Treatment should have ceased at least 3—4 weeks before the sample was taken, to allow for the clearance of the exogenous TT4.

Interpretation

Canine Hypothyroidism is confirmed if the TT4 level is below the normal range (13—50 nmol/l), but since hypothyroid dogs can have a TT4 level of up to 20nmol/l, only those dogs with a TT4 of <13 nmol/l can be confirmed as hypothyroid using results from a single test.

Interpretation can be clarified if a serum cholesterol estimate is performed on the same sample. Up to 60% of hypothyroid dogs exhibit hypercholesterolaemia due to a reduction in the rate of clearance of cholesterol. Therefore, a low TT4 in the normal range but with a raised cholesterol, would be indicative of hypothyroidism.

Certain drugs are known to affect the serum TT4 concentration either by displacing it from the serum proteins (e.g. thyroxine binding protein) to which most serum TT4 is bound, or by affecting the levels of the proteins. Salicylate, diphenylhydantoin, halofenate, chlorpropamide, tolbutamide, o,p'DDD, penicillin and diazepam displace TT4 from the plasma proteins with the result that the total TT4 level is reduced (Gershengorn et al 1980). Oestrogens increase the binding proteins in plasma, with a corresponding increase in TT4, while androgens and glucocorticoids have the opposite effect.

As the TT4 result may give equivocal results in the diagnosis of hypothyroidism, a number of secondary tests have been proposed. These are tests for triiodothyronine, T3 uptake, free TT4 and stimulation tests with TSH or TRH and are described below.

Feline Hyperthyroidism is confirmed if the TT4 level is higher than the normal range in the cat (20—60 nmol/l). In hyperthyroidism, the TT4 level is substantially greater than the top of the normal range so that there is no problem of an overlap between the low abnormal and the high normal result.

TRIIODOTHYRONINE

Triiodothyronine (T3) is a similar hormone to TT4, containing 3 iodine atoms instead of the 4 in thyroxine, but it is present in canine serum at a lower concentration (0.7—1.8 nmol/l), even though it is more active metabolically. The circulating T3 is derived largely by the post-secretory deiodination of TT4 and therefore, there is a close relation between the levels of the two hormones. Assay of the T3 level may be useful in the clarification of an equivocal TT4 result.

Interpretation

A T3 level below the normal range would confirm that a low TT4 is from a hypothyroid animal. This is another approach to differentiating the low euthyroid animal from a hypothyroid animal with a TT4 level within the normal range.

T3 UPTAKE

T3 uptake is a measure of the vacant binding capacity of serum proteins for T3. In the circulation the thyroid hormones are bound to thyroxine binding globulin (TBG), thyroxine binding pre-albumin (TBPA) and albumin. TT4 has a higher binding affinity than T3, and this has been utilised in a test which assesses the available binding capacity for T3 in serum. The serum sample is incubated with radioactive T3 and a synthetic solid phase reagent which also binds T3. Equilibration is established between radioactive T3 binding to plasma proteins and to the solid phase and by determining the amount of radioactivity bound by the latter, the T3 uptake is calculated. Results are reported as a percentage of a standard serum sample.

Interpretation

In hypothyroidism, many binding sites on the serum proteins will not be occupied, so there will be an increased uptake of labelled T3 (>120%). In hyperthyroidism excess TT4 is in circulation, and there will be a reduction in the number of binding sites available for the labelled T3 and therefore the T3 uptake will be reduced (<90%).

Measuring T3 uptake can help with interpretation of inconclusive TT4 results. A serum sample from a hypothyroid dog will have a low TT4 and an increased T3 uptake. As mentioned above, reproductive hormones and certain drugs can alter the levels of the binding proteins and therefore affect the T3 uptake, so care must be taken if these factors are relevant.

FREE T4 (FT4)

Free T4 is that fraction of the total T4 not actually bound to protein and is the metabolically active form of the hormone. Measurement of FT4 concentration is therefore theoretically more relevant to function than the TT4. However, there is only a limited availability of this test at present for analysis of animal serum samples. Radioimmunoassay kits have been produced commercially for determination of FT4 and FT3 in man. Since the normal range for canine FT4 is comparable to the normal human range, these may be used for canine sera.

Interpretation

As with the total TT4 test, the FT4 assay suffers an area of overlap where serum from hypothyroid dogs may be within the lower limits of the normal range (7—33 pmol/l) and is also affected by the same non-thyroid disease conditions as TT4. FT4 should not be used as the sole method of diagnosis of hyperthyroidism in the dog. Recent investigation in Sweden (Larsson, 1987) recommends that the best diagnosis of hypothyroidism which can be performed on a single sample is to combine the results of FT4 and cholesterol assays.

FT4 concentration can be used to diagnose hyperthyroidism in cats, in which the normal range is similar to the canine normal range.

THYROID STIMULATING HORMONE (TSH) AND TSH STIMULATION

In humans the serum concentration of TSH is used as the routine screening test for hypothyroidism. Unfortunately, there is little immunoreactivity between antisera to human TSH and canine TSH and assays developed for human TSH are inappropriate for the canine hormone. A homologous radioimmunoassay has been described for canine TSH but it is not yet available in the United Kingdom.

Primary hypothyroidism due to thyroid gland malfunction can be most satisfactorily diagnosed by use of a thyroid stimulating hormone (TSH) stimulation test. (See also Chapter 2.)

A variety of protocols exist and the laboratory performing the assay should be consulted. The procedure used in Glasgow Veterinary School is:—
1. Take a resting blood sample.
2. Inject intravenously 1 I.U. of bovine TSH.
3. Collect a second blood sample 5 hours after the injection.
4. Allow to clot, centrifuge and remove serum.
5. Send both serum samples to the laboratory for TT4 assay.

Other centres use different doses, injection routes and collection times. For correct interpretation the procedure used must be the one recommended by the laboratory which will perform the TT4 assay.

Interpretation

As in all dynamic tests it is vital to interpret the result in respect of the protocol used and in relation to the expected values used by the laboratory undertaking the TT4 assays.

With the above protocol and in a normal dog, the stimulated TT4 level should be at least double the resting level and/or be greater than 30 nmol/l. The level in the hypothyroid animal will increase but it will not reach this level. For example, a hypothyroid dog with a resting TT4 in the region of 20 nmol/l will have a stimulated level of <30 nmol/l whereas a normal animal would exceed this limit. Hypothyroid dogs with a low resting TT4 may double their TT4 level on stimulation but it will not reach the 30 nmol/l threshold. The value of the threshold concentration of TT4 is that used in the author's laboratory and may vary between laboratories. In cases where there is still doubt after the TSH stimulation a therapeutic trial can be performed.

In cats the only use of a TSH stimulation test is for the diagnosis of hyperthyroidism in border-line cases.

The major problem with TSH stimulation is that the hormone is expensive and difficult to obtain though laboratories performing the TT4 assay may be able to provide the hormone. Currently, there are no British suppliers of pharmaceutical quality TSH.

TRH STIMULATION

A stimulation test based on thyrotrophin release hormone (TRH, Roche) has been described which can discriminate between secondary and tertiary hypothyroidism. TRH at a dose of 0.1mg/kg is injected intravenously. Ideally the *TSH* level should be monitored in serum before, and 6 hours after, injection, but as a canine TSH assay is not available in commercial laboratories, the change in TT4 level should be determined. In normal animals the TT4 should rise by 50% of the resting level in the 6 hour period, and a significant rise would be found in dogs with tertiary hypothyroidism due to a malfunction in the hypothalmus. Dogs with primary or secondary hypothyroidism show no rise in TT4 in response to TRH. At present, Roche will only supply TRH to hospital pharmacies in the UK.

ADRENOCORTICOID FUNCTION

Laboratory testing for adrenocorticoid function is concerned with the detection of hyperadrenocorticism (Cushing's syndrome) in the dog. Hypoadrenocorticism cannot be diagnosed on the basis of cortisol level as the normal range of cortisol (50–250 nmol/l) goes to the limit of sensitivity for most cortisol radioimmunoassays.

Cushing's syndrome is diagnosed by use of a dynamic test, as in a single resting sample from a dog with this disease the cortisol level is often in the normal range. The major screening tests available for Cushing's syndrome are the ACTH stimulation test and the low-dose dexamethasone suppression test. It is advisable to contact the laboratory to which the samples will be sent as interpretation of the result will depend on following their recommended procedure. The following protocol is based on procedures carried out at Glasgow Veterinary School.

ACTH STIMULATION

In the normal dog, ACTH stimulation causes the circulating cortisol level to — at the most — double. In pituitary-dependent hyperadrenocorticism, ACTH causes an exaggerated response, while with an adrenal tumour, a high cortisol will be found both before and after stimulation.

Procedure
1. Take a resting blood sample in a Li-heparin plasma tube (serum can also be used). As there is a diurnal variation in cortisol levels, it is recommended to perform the test in the morning.
2. Give an intramuscular injection of 0.25mg tetracosactrin (Synacthen, Ciba Labs.).
3. After 45 minutes take a second blood sample.
4. Centrifuge and remove plasma.
5. Send both plasma samples to the laboratory for cortisol analysis.

The protocol is different in the cat. For details see Chapter 4.

Interpretation

In the normal dog the resting plasma will have a cortisol level of <50–250 nmol/l and the stimulated cortisol level will not exceed 500 nmol/l being usually less than double the resting level.

In dogs with pituitary-dependent Cushing's syndrome the resting level may be within the normal range as above, but could be up to 300 nmol/l. On stimulation the cortisol level will give an exaggerated rise and is often >700 nmol/l. Cushing's syndrome would still be indicated when this level is not achieved if the resting level has more than tripled. A problem can occur in interpretation when a resting sample is at the high end of the normal range and the stimulated sample has a cortisol concentration in the range 500-700 nmol/l, but a three fold increase has not occurred. In these circumstances a dexamethasone suppression test would be advocated.

When Cushing's syndrome is produced by an adrenal tumour, the resting level of cortisol will be >200 nmol/l and the stimulated level will not be much higher.

In cases of primary hypoadrenocorticism in the dog, plasma cortisol levels are <50 nmol/l; no rise occurs after stimulation.

LOW DOSE DEXAMETHASONE SUPPRESSION

There are a variety of protocols for the dexamethasone suppression test and it is important to use the procedure recommended by the laboratory performing the analysis. For initial screening to detect hyperadrenocorticism, the low dose dexamethasone test is used, the procedure for which is as follows:-
1. Take a resting (i.e. baseline) sample of blood in a Li-heparin tube (serum can also be used).
2. Inject dexamethasone (intravenous or intra muscular) at a dose of 0.01mg/kg.
3. Take a second and third heparinised blood sample at 3 hours and 8 hours post injection.
4. If possible, centrifuge and remove plasma.
5. Send both plasma (or blood) samples to the laboratory for cortisol estimation.

Interpretation

With the low dose (0.01mg/kg) intravenous dose of dexamethasone, the plasma cortisol, in a normal dog, reaches less the half of the resting level at 3 hours and will still be <40 nmol/l at 8 hours. Dogs with Cushing's syndrome do not reach a level of <40 nmol/l at any time.

HIGH DOSE DEXAMETHASONE SUPPRESSION

While the low dose of dexamethasone will identify most dogs with hyperadrenocorticism, the high dose suppression test is designed to differentiate between dogs with pituitary dependent hyper-adrenocorticism and those with adrenal tumours. The test is performed as above for the low dose test except the dose of dexamethasone is 0.1mg/kg.

Interpretation

When the high dose (0.1mg/kg) intravenous protocol is used, the normal dog has a suppressed cortisol of less than half of the resting level at both 3 and 8 hours after injection, which is the same as for the low dose test. When an animal has pituitary-dependent Cushing's syndrome, the suppressed level will be less than half the resting level in either (or both) the 3 and 8 hour post-injection samples, while the cortisol concentration will not drop below half of the resting cortisol concentration in samples from dogs with adrenal tumours.

URINARY CORTICOID/CREATININE RATIO

A diagnostic test for hyperadrenocorticism based on the ratio of urinary cortisol to urinary creatinine has been reported (Rijnberk et al 1988) which was superior to the low dose dexamethasone test as a screen for hyperadrenocorticism. This test is not yet a routine analysis in veterinary laboratories in the United Kingdom and it should only be attempted if a laboratory has thoroughly validated a radioimmunoassay for use on canine urine samples. In the test, the concentrations of cortisol and creatinine are determined in two urine samples from consecutive mornings and the mean results used to calculate the ratio. The normal range for the canine urine corticoid/creatinine ratio is $1.2-6.9$ x 10^{-6} nmol/μmol.

ADRENOCORTICOTROPHIC HORMONE

Adrenocorticotrophic hormone (ACTH) is a highly conserved peptide, in that its aminoacid sequence is the same in most species. Therefore, radioimmunoassays for human ACTH can be used to measure canine or feline ACTH but only after thorough validation. However, the radioimmunoassay of ACTH is expensive, and is complicated by the instability of ACTH in plasma or serum. At present, the assay of ACTH is not available in the United Kingdom in veterinary diagnostic laboratories. Research or hospital laboratories could assay samples but, as mentioned previously, the assay should be validated for each species. Serum samples should be transported frozen in dry ice and in plastic vials as ACTH binds to glass. The normal plasma ACTH concentration in the dog is $20-100$ pg/ml. The use of corticotrophin release factor (CRF) in a dynamic test for ACTH and subsequent cortisol release has been proposed but, given the expense of CRF and the inherent problems of measuring the ACTH, there is little to be gained from this test of function of the pituitary-adrenal axis.

STEROID INDUCED ALKALINE PHOSPHATASE (SIAP)

Routine biochemistry and haematology can be of some benefit in the diagnosis of Cushing's syndrome, but the only test which is specific for the disease is steroid induced alkaline phosphatase. This alkaline phosphatase isoenzyme is produced by the liver in response to raised levels of cortisol. It can be induced experimentally by prednisolone administration and is a frequent finding in cases of iatrogenic Cushing's syndrome as well as the naturally occurring disease.

SIAP has a number of properties which distinguish it from liver or bone alkaline phosphatase and these have been used as the basis of alternative biochemical tests. SIAP has a greater electrophoretic mobility, a higher resistance to inactivation by heat, has a different immunoreactivity and exhibits greater inhibition of its activity by L-phenylalanine (L-phe). The latter phenomenon is utilised in the biochemical test employed at Glasgow Veterinary School.

The test for SIAP can be performed on serum or plasma (heparinised) as an initial check and a dynamic test then used to confirm the result. Alternatively, it can be performed on the resting sample of an ACTH stimulation or dexamethasone suppression test to help clarify equivocal results. Although relatively easy to perform compared to the immunoassays required for cortisol, the assay for SIAP should be carried out by laboratories familiar with the technique.

Interpretation

Usually, over 90% of the alkaline phosphatase present in the circulation of dogs with Cushings syndrome is SIAP. SIAP can be found in a number of other conditions, but the finding that SIAP is present in an animal suspected of Cushing's syndrome implies that excessive corticosteroids have been present in the circulation. A dynamic test should be undertaken for further confirmation.

ADRENAL MEDULLARY FUNCTION

Although in humans the estimation of catecholamine metabolites in urine is a routine screening test for pheochromocytomas, this is not a test available in veterinary diagnostic laboratories. However, the urine concentration of one of the major metabolites, vanillylmandelic acid (VMA), in the dog is 0.6—15mg/24 hour. For this test, urine has to be collected over 24 hours in a beaker of 15ml of 6mol/l HC1. A hospital or research laboratory may then be able to determine the urine VMA content.

PANCREATIC ENDOCRINE FUNCTION

Although the pancreas secretes both glucagon and insulin, it is measurement of the latter which has diagnostic value. Insulin assay has only a limited availability but is performed by Serono Labs. The utility of a serum insulin assay is in diagnosis of islet cell tumours (insulinoma) and possibly in differentiation of different types of diabetes mellitus.

INSULINOMA (ISLET CELL TUMOUR)

Approximately 60% of islet cell tumours are functionally active in that they secrete insulin to produce hyperinsulinaemia, which in turn leads to hypoglycaemia.

The normal range of insulin level in the dog is 5—40 μIU/l and in cases of insulinoma, this will rise to >85 μIU/l. Results which can occur in the intermediate area of 40—80 μIU/l would be indicative of insulinoma if the blood glucose was at a hypoglycaemic level.

DIABETES MELLITUS

The diagnosis of diabetes mellitus does not require an insulin assay to be performed as the classic signs of raised blood and urine glucose, ketotic urine and acetone on the breath are much easier and cheaper to perform. In those cases where there is any doubt, a glucose tolerance test can be performed. Glucose at a dose of 1g/kg body weight is given orally and blood samples taken at 15—30 minute intervals over the next two hours.

However, diabetic dogs can be classified into two types and identification of the type of disease is relevant to treatment. There are dogs in which the diabetic condition is a direct result of low blood insulin (hypoinsulinaemic) but there is another group in which insulin levels are actually higher than normal (hyperinsulinaemic). In this latter group tissues which are usually stimulated by insulin to absorb glucose from the blood, no longer respond. The reason for the development of a reduced response to insulin is not clear but these animals often have associated hypercortisolaemia, hyperlipaemia or hyperprogestaemia.

As dogs with hyperinsulinaemia already have an excess of endogenous hormone, treatment with injected insulin will be ineffective and these dogs are 'insulin resistant'. Use of an insulin assay will identify dogs with this condition and treatment can be adjusted at an early stage.

Intrepretation

Diabetes mellitus is diagnosed by a dog having a fasting blood glucose level of >7 mmol/l, but the level is often >15 mmol/l when first presented. The result of a glucose tolerance test in a normal dog is that the blood glucose will be back within the normal range of 2.5—5 mmol/l within 2 hours of the glucose load. In a diabetic the return to normal is much extended.

The majority of diabetics will have a serum insulin below the normal range (5—40 μIU/l) while those with hyperinsulinaemia and therefore likely to be insulin resistant, will be above the normal range.

PARATHYROID FUNCTION

In humans, the estimation of serum parathyroid hormone (PTH) concentration is a valuable procedure in the diagnosis of both hyper- and hypo-parathyroidism. Although there is considerable sequence homology between PTH of different species and assays for human PTH have been validated for use with canine serum, there are no veterinary diagnostic laboratories in which this test is available. If a research or hospital laboratory can be persuaded to assay canine PTH, their method must be validated and a normal range established for the particular assay.

REPRODUCTIVE HORMONES

The analysis of reproductive hormones in small animals is not as prevalent as in larger species where pregnancy diagnosis is possible by immunoassay of hormones. In the bitch, it is difficult to differentiate between the pregnant and non-pregnant female on the basis of steroid hormone level.

In small animals, reproductive hormone analysis is performed (1) to confirm that castration or spaying has been carried out successfully, (2) in detection of hormone-secreting tumours and (3) in the determination of oestrus so that artificial insemination can be performed at the optimum time.

PROGESTERONE

The analysis of plasma progesterone is performed on daily samples for the determination of oestrus in the bitch for coordination of artificial insemination. Serum progesterone rises from a negligible level during anoestrus to a level of 0.1—1 nmol/l in proestrus. An oestrus occurs, the progesterone rises more rapidly to reach 50 nmol/l by the start of metoestrus. If daily serum samples are assayed for progesterone, insemination should take place when the level reaches 30 nmol/l, as ovulation has taken place. The advent of commercial kits for the rapid detection of serum progesterone by enzyme-linked immunosorbent assay (Ovucheck, Cambridge Life Sciences) means that this approach could be carried out by a practice laboratory. This may be necessary as rapid results are required so that the optimal time for insemination is detected. Kits for sale to veterinary practitioners are designed for pregnancy diagnosis in cattle but one of the kits at least has been validated for use with canine plasma (Ovuchek, Cambridge Veterinary Sciences).

OESTRADIOL

Detection of greater than basal levels of oestradiol (ie >50 pmol/l) in a spayed bitch or queen indicates that there is residual active ovarian tissue present.

Sertoli cell tumours in the dog may secrete significant amounts of oestradiol and therefore, when this is suspected, the analysis of serum oestradiol will help to confirm the diagnosis.

TESTOSTERONE

Testosterone has a normal range in the adult dog of 3—30 nmol/l. In the castrated animal the level of testosterone falls to <0.5 nmol/l. In the cat, the normal range is similar, as is the response to castration.

REFERENCES

GERSHENGORN, M. C., GLINOER, D. and ROBBINS, J. (1980). Transport and metabolism of thyroid hormones. In: *The Thyroid Gland.* (ed. M. De Visscher) p 81. Raven Press, New York.

LARSSON, M. (1987). *Diagnostic methods in canine hypothyroidism and the influence of nonthyroidal illness on thyroid hormones and thyroxine-binding proteins.* Swedish University of Agricultural Sciences, Uppsala.

RIJNBERK, A., VAN WEES, A. and MOL, J. A. (1988). Assessment of two tests for the diagnosis of canine hyperadrenocorticism. *Vet. Rec.* **122** 178.

FURTHER READING

BURKE, T. J. (1986). (ed.) *Small Animal Reproduction and Infertility.* Lea and Febiger, Philadelphia.

CHASTAIN, C. B. (1982). Canine hypothyroidism. *J. Am. vet. med. Ass.* **181**, 349.

KANEKO, J. J. (1980). *Clinical Biochemistry of Domestic Animals,* 3rd ed., Academic Press, New York.

CHASTAIN, C. B. and GANJAM, V. K. (1986). *Clinical Endocrinology of Companion Animals.* Lea and Febiger, Philadelphia.

REFERENCE RANGES FOR HORMONES OF DOGS AND CATS

These reference ranges are given as a guide and should not be used for comparison to results from clinical samples. The reference range from the laboratory analysing the sample should be used for the interpretation of results.

Hormone	Dog	Cat	Units
Thyroxine	13—50	19—65*	nmol/l
Triiodothronine	0.2—1.6*	0.6—2.0*	ng/ml
T3 Uptake	90—120*	90—120*	%
Free TT4	7.5—50	—	pmol/l
Cortisol	50—250	—	nmol/l
Insulin	5—40*	—	uIU/l
Progesterone			
Anoestrus	<2	<2	nmol/l
Luteal phase	60—90	—	nmol/l
Follicular phase	2—6	<10*	nmol/l
Mid-pregnancy	60—90	60—120	nmol/l
Late-pregnancy	15—30	25—60	nmol/l
Oestradiol			
Anoestrus	<30	<30	pmol/l
Oestrus	45—90	30—150	pmol/l
Metestrus	60—90	<30	pmol/l
Male	40—190*	—	pmol/l
Testosterone (Male)	1.5—26*	>1*	nmol/l

Quoted with the permission of Serono Laboratories (U.K.) Ltd.

LH 12
    in the bitch 127
    at ovulation 141
    deficiency 13, 23
    in the dog 121
    in the queen, at ovulation 144-5
    'surge' 127, 128
    in the tom 145
liothyronine sodium 53
liver, effect of glucocorticoids on 75, 76
Losec 198
low-dose dexamethasone suppression test
    90-1, 92, 211-12
low T3 syndrome 27
low T4 state of medical illness 27
luteinising hormone see LH
lymphocytic thyroiditis 38, 48
lymphoma 202
lymphopenia 83

mammary hypertrophy, feline 151
mammary nodules, canine 130
mammary tumours, oestrogen-dependent 140
mast cell degranulation 197, 198
matings, multiple, feline 145
medullary carcinoma of the thyroid 40-1
medullary washout 161-2
melanocyte stimulating hormone
    (melanotrophin) 12
MEN syndromes 38
mesorchium 121
mesosalpinx 127
mesovarium 127
metformin 111
methimazole see MMI
metoestrus
    canine 129
        acromegaly during 138
        diabetes mellitus during 138
    feline 144
metyrapone 95-6
miliary eczema 151
mineralocorticoids 73
    deficiency 97
    functions 77
    regulation of release 76-7
misalliance
    canine 137
    feline 150
mithramycin (Mithracin) 64, 204
mitotane therapy 87-8, 93-4, 95
    hypoadrenocorticism following 96
MMI
    long-term therapy 47
    pre-thyroidectomy 44
monoclonal gammopathy,
    tumour-associated 199
MSH 12
multiple endocrine neoplasia syndromes 38
multiple myeloma 202
muscle
    adrenergic effects on 78
    effect of glucocorticoids on 76
    wasting 81-2, 171
        see also weakness
myasthenia gravis
    tumour-associated 198, 205
myotonia 82

nafarelin 136
natriuretic factors 158
nephrocalcinosis
    in hyperparathyroidism 62

after vitamin D therapy 71
nephrotic syndrome 164
neurogenic diabetes insipidus 14-15, 165
    secondary 160
neurohypophysis 9, 10
neuromuscular dysfunction
    in canine hypothyroidism 51
    in hypoparathyroidism 68
nidation, prevention of
    canine 137
    feline 150
Nizoral 94
nocturia 155, 159
noradrenaline
    oversecretion 101-2
    release and effects 77-8

obesity
    definition 181
    in diabetes mellitus 107, 182, 185
    diagnosis of cause 181-3
    in hypothyroidism 34, 50, 182, 185-6
    in insulinoma 182, 187
    in pituitary dwarfism 186
oestrogens
    assay 146, 214
    in the bitch 127, 128
        at ovulation 141
        in pregnancy diagnosis 141
    in the queen
        in the oestrous cycle 144
        at ovulation 145
        in pregnancy 145
oestrogens, therapeutic
    adverse effects 122, 131
    in the bitch 130-1
        in misalliance 137
        in pseudopregnancy 137
    in the dog 122
        in aggressive behaviour 123
        in prostatic hyperplasia 124
    in the queen 150
oestrous cycle
    canine 128-9
        control of 134-6
        irregular 137
    feline 143, 144
oestrual display, feline 144, 149
oestrus
    canine 128
        first 136
        induction 136
        post-ovariectomy 140
        prevention 134, 135
        silent 136
        suppression 134, 135
    feline 144
        failure of 146-7
        induction 147-8
        suppression 148-50
omeprazole 198
Oncovin 39
optic disc oedema 13
oral hypoglycaemic therapy 111
osteitis fibrosa cystica 62
osteoporosis 89
ovarian cysts, feline 146
ovarian follicles
    canine 127
    feline 144
ovarian imbalance
    type 1 174
    type 2 141, 174
oviarectomy, sequelae 140

ovaries 127
ovariohysterectomy
    in acromegaly 17
    in pregnancy termination 138-9
overeating 182
overhydration 155
ovulation
    canine
        confirmation of 141
        prediction of 128, 140-1
    feline 144-5
        confirmation of 146
        failure of 147
        induction 148
oxyphil cells 59
oxytocin 10, 12,
    therapeutic 132-3, 139

pancreas
    anatomy 105
    disorders of function 106-19
    function tests 213
    histology 105
    hormone secretion 105-6
    tumours 116-19
pancreatitis, post-operative 118
pancytopenia, tumour-associated 199, 205
panhypopituitarism 13
papillary adenocarcinoma, feline 33, 40
parafollicular cells 25
    carcinoma of 40-1
paraneoplastic syndromes
    ectopic 200, 201-5
    topic 197-200
parathyroid glands 25
    accessory tissue 25, 59
    anatomy and histology 59
    disorders function 60-71
    function tests 62, 214
    hormone secretion 59-60
    hyperplasia 60
    tumours 202
parathyroid hormone see PTH
Parlodel 95, 133, 137
parturition, canine, hormonal control 129
Periactin 94
peripheral neuropathy, diabetic 114
peritoneal dialysis 66
peritonitis 183
phaeochromocytoma 101-2, 182, 213
phentolamine 102
phosphate binders 66
pituitary gland
    anatomy and histology 9
    disorders related 12-23
    effect of glucocorticoids on 76
    function tests 208
    hormone secretion 10-12
    irradiation 95
    tumours 12-13, 79-80, 85, 159
placenta
    retention 139
    sub-involution of sites 139
pneumoperitoneum 183
pollakiuria 155
polydipsia 14, 61, 81, 107, 171, 182
    causes 164-5
    clinical examination 157, 160
    definition 155
    history-taking 157, 158-60
    investigations 160-2
    pathophysiological classification 161-2